Anaesthesia: Review 8

Contents and contributors to *Anaesthesia Review* 7

ISBN 0 443 04216 0

You can place your order by contacting your local medical bookseller or the Sales Promotion Department, Robert Stevenson House, 1–3 Baxter's Place, Leith Walk, Edinburgh EH1 3AF, UK

Tel: (031) 556 2424; Telex: 727511 LONGMN G; Fax: (031) 558 1278

Look out for *Anaesthesia Review* 9 in May 1992

Anaesthesia:
Review 8

Edited by

Leon Kaufman MD, FFARCS

Consulting Anaesthetist, University College Hospital, London, and St Mark's Hospital, London; Honorary Senior Lecturer, Faculty of Clinical Sciences, University College, London, UK

CHURCHILL LIVINGSTONE
EDINBURGH LONDON MELBOURNE NEW YORK AND TOKYO 1991

CHURCHILL LIVINGSTONE
Medical Division of Longman Group UK Limited

Distributed in the United States of America by
Churchill Livingstone Inc., 1560 Broadway, New York,
N.Y. 10036, and by associated companies, branches
and representatives throughout the world.

First published 1991

ISBN 0-443-04384-1
ISSN 0263-1512

British Library Cataloguing in Publication Data
Anaesthesia—Review 8
  1. Anaesthesia—Periodicals
  617′.96′05   RD78.3

Library of Congress Cataloging/Card Number 88-656263

Printed in Great Britain at The Bath Press, Avon

Preface

It is gratifying to note the welcome response of readers to *Anaesthesia Review* which also appears to have achieved a high rating in the list of reading material chosen by examination candidates. On the other hand, critics of the series have varied in their comments—a chapter may gain praise from some and adverse comment from others.

The pattern of presentation remains unchanged. Some chapters are presented in a formal essay on subjects that required re-appraisal, including the problem of halothane hepatitis and the hazards of central venous catheterization. The section on medical gases has been completed, while a study by those actively engaged in obstetrics considers in detail the effects of anaesthesia on the fetus. The role of hypoxia and control of breathing is discussed by trans-Atlantic colleagues, while the management of acute asthma serves as a reminder of the potential lethal complications. The mechanisms of sweating are also reviewed. Audit of medical activities is very fashionable and rapid progress has been made in the field of anaesthesia.

Recent papers on medicine relevant to anaesthesia, endocrinology and pain are collated, and may also be of interest to those engaged in further education and research. Readers are encouraged to read the original papers which are often controversial and appear to contradict established values. The mechanisms of the sleep apnoea syndrome have become more apparent as can be seen from the number of papers on this subject.

Contributors are thanked for the prompt presentation of their chapters while the publishers are congratulated on the rapid publication of this issue. Mrs M. Pitts and Word Perfect 5.1 are praised for the arduous task of preparing *Review 8*.

London 1991   L.K.

Contributors

A John Asbury MB ChB FFARCS PhD
Senior Lecturer in Anaesthesia, and Honorary Consultant Anaesthetist, Western Infirmary, Glasgow, UK

Simon Cottam MB ChB FFARCS
Lecturer in Anaesthetics, King's College Hospital, London, UK

John Eason FFARCS MRCP
Senior Lecturer in Anaesthetics and Intensive Care, and Honorary Consultant, St Mary's Hospital, London, UK

R S C Howell MB BS D ObstRCOG FFARCS
Consultant Anaesthetist, Walsgrave Hospital, Coventry, UK

Leon Kaufman MD FFARCS
Consulting Anaesthetist, University College Hospital, and St Mark's Hospital, London; Honorary Senior Lecturer, Faculty of Clinical Sciences, University College, London, UK

C S Martin FFARCSI
Registrar in Anaesthetics, Western Infirmary, Glasgow, UK

B M Morgan MB ChB FFARCS
Senior Lecturer in Obstetric Anaesthesia, Royal Postgraduate Medical School Institute of Obstetrics and Gynaecology, Queen Charlotte's Hospital, London, UK

Paul Morrison BM BS FFARCS
Senior Registrar, Department of Anaesthetics, The Queen Elizabeth Hospital, Birmingham, UK

P Nandi MB BS MRCP FFARCS
Senior Registrar, Department of Anaesthetics, University College Hospital, London, UK

James M Neuberger DM MRCP
Consultant Physician, and Honorary Senior Clinical Lecturer, The Queen Elizabeth Hospital, Birmingham, UK

Saxon A Ridley MB BS FFARCS
Senior Registrar, Department of Anaesthetics, Western Infirmary,
Glasgow, UK

J Secker-Walker BSc MB BS FFARCS
Senior Lecturer, University College, London; Consultant Anaesthetist,
Bloomsbury and Islington Health Authority, London, UK

John A Temp MD
Resident, Department of Anesthesiology, UCLA School of Medicine,
Los Angeles, USA

Denham S Ward MD PhD
Associate Professor, Department of Anesthesiology, UCLA School of
Medicine, Los Angeles, USA

Contents

1. Medicine relevant to anaesthesia (1)

L. Kaufman

CARDIOVASCULAR SYSTEM

HYPERTENSION

The precise etiology of hypertension is still unknown and various theories are still being propounded. Julius & Weder (1989) expressed the view that in hypertension, blood pressure is set at a higher level, but the regulation of the pressure is normal. There is a relationship between blood pressure and the hyper-response to mental stress. The regulation of blood pressure and blood pressure variability are two independent factors. The haemo-dynamics of hypertension is still subject to debate, and recent studies have shown that there is no increase in oxygen delivery to tissues, which had been thought to be the reason for the increased peripheral vascular resistance (Leading article, Lancet 1990a).

Excess secretion of hormones leads to hypertension; hypertension due to excess mineralocorticoids is rare, the commonest agent being excess of aldosterone. Excessive administration of steroids and glucocorticoids also lead to hypertension such as is seen in Cushing's syndrome. Studies following short term administration of cortisol or ACTH revealed a rise in blood pressure within 3–5 days, accompanied by a loss of potassium and retention of sodium while blood volume and extracellular fluid volume increased. Cortisol acts through type I receptors (mineralocorticoids) or type II receptors (glucocorticoids) and modifies the mechanisms which regulate blood pressure. It is possible that glucocorticoids act centrally, affecting the sympathetic activity or the increased peripheral resistance directly, and they may increase the vascular responsiveness of vasopressors.

Tumours of the adrenal medulla give rise to hypertension, notedly that of phaeochromocytoma. Growth hormone is a further cause of hypertension, but the causes are still not clear. There is sodium retention and myocardial hypertrophy. Hyperthyroidism is associated with hypertension, with increased cardiac output, heart rate and stroke volume while peripheral resistance is reduced. Other hormones known to affect blood pressure are AVP, increased plasma renin activity, while diabetes (type I) is also impli-cated. Androgens also increase blood pressure. The role of hormones and hypertension is further discussed by Fraser et al (1989). Hypertension complicates at least 10% of all pregnancies; hypertension occurred alone or with proteinuria, and was associated with an increase of sodium and water retention due to impaired renal function (Marlettini et al 1989).

A further possible cause of hypertension has been postulated, in that there might be an increase in the density of alpha-2 and beta-2 receptors, but this has been disproven by Graafsma et al (1989). They found that there is no difference in the adrenaline receptor density under baseline conditions or following mental stress.

Elderly patients with hypertension are more likely to develop hypotensive episodes and the commonest causes are orthostatic, postprandial, nitrate intolerance and atrial fibrillation (Lipsitz 1989a). The incidence of orthostatic hypotension is 20% in patients over 65, and 30% in those over 75 years of age. Causes may be associated with age, reduction of blood volume, medication, autonomic insufficiency, drug therapy including fludrocortisone, indomethacin and the recently introduced alpha-adrenergic agonists such as phenylpropranolamine and midodrine (Lipsitz 1989b).

Treatment

The treatment of mild to moderate hypertension has been reviewed by Lewis & Maclean (1990) and although hypertension is a major cause of stroke and myocardial infarction, there is still debate regarding the indications for therapy. Although it appears to be accepted that mild hypertension results in complications, consensus seems to emerge that treatment should be directed to those with diastolic pressure exceeding 100 mmHg, especially if there are signs of other risk factors such as left ventricular hypertrophy (see Lewis & Maclean 1990).

Diuretics such as thiazides are considered to be the first choice of treatment of hypertension in the elderly, whereas beta-blockers such as atenolol have been advocated in younger patients (Schnaper 1989). If this therapy is unsuccessful, calcium antagonists such as nifedipine or verapamil have been recommended while the third line of treatment involves the use of angiotensin-converting enzyme (ACE) inhibitors, especially in hypertensive diabetics.

Captopril results in venous and arterial dilatation in patients with congestive cardiac failure (Capewell et al 1989). ACE inhibitors can be safely given to patients with asthma, in contrast to beta-adrenergic blocking agents (Riska et al 1990). Cerebral blood flow is maintained, possibly due to an action on locally produced angiotensin II (Waldemar & Paulson 1989, see also McInnes & Sever 1989). ACE inhibitors may have a place in the acute phase of myocardial infarction (Leading article, Lancet 1989a). Indomethacin attenuates the antihypertensive effect of captopril, but there is little interaction between enalapril, another ACE inhibitor (Koopmans et al 1989).

ACE inhibitors have unusual respiratory complications including persistent non-productive cough. It has been suggested that this may be due to bradykinin which may accumulate in the presence of ACE inhibitors while prostaglandins may also be implicated (Berkin 1989).

As hypertension and diabetes often co-exist, there is a possibility that treatment may affect the sympathetic response to hypoglycaemia. Although clonidine inhibits ACTH and catecholamine release, Guthrie et al (1989) found that clonidine did not impair the sensitivity of insulin or recovery from hypoglycaemia.

The renal effects of antihypertensive drugs have been discussed by Schlueter & Batlle (1989), showing that calcium entry blockers and ACE inhibitors increase glomerular filtration rate and renal blood flow in patients with hypertension, and prevent tubular reabsorption of sodium. They may limit the progression of renal disorders. In contrast, beta-blockers cause a small decrease in renal blood flow and glomerular filtration rate. Alpha-blockers such as prazosin do not appear to affect renal function. However, care must be taken with the use of ACE inhibitors in patients who are developing renal artery stenosis.

Nitric oxide

The vascular endothelium produces a labile relaxing factor which is synthesized from L-arginine (Vallance et al 1989), but it also releases vasoconstrictors such as endothelin-1 which is more potent than angiotensin II. Plasma levels are elevated in myocardial infarction, pulmonary or essential hypertension (see Vane et al 1990). Nitric oxide (NO) not only promotes vasorelaxation but also inhibits platelet adhesion and aggregation (Griffith & Randall 1989). This affects the blood viscosity and flow-induced dilatation (Melkumyants & Balashov 1990). It has however been suggested that the endothelium derived relaxant factor is not identical to that of NO (Long & Berkowitz 1989). However, the endothelium mediated vasodilatation is impaired in essential hypertension (Panza et al 1990). It has been postulated that there is impairment of the endothelium derived relaxant factor in patients with Eisenmenger's syndrome (Dinh Xuan et al 1989). This finding would possibly affect the treatment of pulmonary hypertension which has been known to be divided into three subtypes— plexogenic pulmonary arteriopathy due to abnormalities of endothelial structure; thromboembolic pulmonary arteriopathy due to endothelial cell injury and veno-occlusive disease. The division of these subtypes might explain the failure of therapy. Secondary pulmonary hypertension without endothelial damage readily responds to therapy when the primary cause such as mitral stenosis or hypoxic lung disease is reversed (Rich & Brundage 1989).

MYOCARDIAL INFARCTION

Myocardial infarction is associated with pre-existing coronary atherosclerosis, alterations of coronary artery flow and damage to the intima of the coronary artery. The damaged endothelium releases factors which cause platelet aggregation, with alterations in electrolytes such as calcium, sodium and potassium. This phase occupies approximately 6 h during which time treatment set on restoring the myocardial oxygen supply is more likely to be effective; then there is stretching and dilatation of the injured myocardium with a possibility of aneurysm developing, septal wall rupture, and extension of the area of infarction with an increase in MB isoenzyme (Pepine 1989). Non-Q-wave myocardial infarction indicates a smaller infarct and the short term prognosis is better than those with Q-waves; however, they are more likely to have reinfarction (Leading article, Lancet 1989b). Serum cortisol levels are raised in patients with ischaemic chest pain due to myocardial infarction, but remain within the normal range for those with angina (Bain et al 1989).

Circadian rhythm influences the possibility of myocardial infarction with an increase between 06:00 and 12:00 (Muller et al 1989). The cause of sudden death is often multifactorial in patients with advanced heart disease. Thirty-eight percent were due to ventricular tachycardia or fibrillation while others had acute or recent infarction, hyperkalaemia, bradycardia or electromechanical dissociation (Luu et al 1989).

Survival rate following the first myocardial infarction is unpredictable; patients with a normal response to exercise testing have a good prognosis and require little further investigations. Patients under 50 years of age, without primary hyperlipidaemia usually have single vessel disease whereas older patients are more likely to have multivessel disease (Moss & Benhorin 1990). Patients who have had a cardiac transplant seldom have chest pain or characteristic ECG changes following an infarct, and the mortality is high (Gao et al 1989). In patients whose ECG is normal or non-specific, there is a long delay between the onset time and the confirmatory diagnosis by creatine kinase levels which are lower than those whose ECG is abnormal. The mortality rate is also less (Rouan et al 1989). Oxygen consumption is significantly higher in those who fail to survive from myocardial infarction. An increase in P-50 is also higher in non-survivors implying that there is precarious oxygen transport and consumption balance in peripheral tissue (Sumimoto et al 1989).

The concept of reperfusion injury is still controversial and can be minimized by the use of beta-adrenergic blocking agents (Opie 1989). Oxygen radicals are generated during periods of ischaemia followed by reperfusion, but there is no evidence that oxygen radicals-scavenging agents are beneficial (Kloner et al 1989). The role of oxygen free radicals in ischaemic/reperfusion myocardial injury have also been discussed by Barta (1989), while Prasad et al (1989) felt that scavenging of oxygen free radicals would be beneficial.

ELECTROMECHANICAL DISSOCIATION

This condition results in cardiac arrest in which there is inadequate cardiac output despite apparent normal ECG complexes. It has been suggested that the condition occurs when a large area of the myocardium is ischaemic. Calcium ions appear to be involved as the condition can be simulated by contrast material containing EDTA and sodium citrate. Beta-adrenergic agents appear to be ineffectual but alpha-agonists such as adrenaline are satisfactory. The role of bicarbonate and calcium ions is not proven, although calcium channel blockers increase the success rate of resuscitation. Atropine has not been found to be of particular value. Secondary electromechanical dissociation may occur in massive pulmonary embolism, acute cardiac tamponade, tension pneumothorax, haemorrhage and myocardial ischaemia; treatment involves that of the primary condition (Charlap et al 1989).

ANGINA

The role of adenosine in the pathogenesis of anginal pain is discussed by Crea et al (1990) who found that adenosine is partially responsible for the anginal pain during myocardial ischaemia and this is antagonized by aminophylline. However, it does have a specific action on the AV node and is effective in the termination of supraventricular tachycardia (Belardinelli & Lerman 1990). Decreased coronary blood flow or increased myocardial oxygen demand are not the only criteria for angina as there are also metabolic, hormonal and haemodynamic factors (Collins & Fox 1990).

Unstable angina which is characterized by severe transient myocardial ischaemia has been classified by Braunwald (1989). Unstable angina may be rated according to severity (1 to 3) or according to circumstances when the angina occurs, e.g. secondary unstable angina, primary unstable angina and post-infarction unstable angina.

SUDDEN CARDIAC DEATH

Ventricular fibrillation is the first arrhythmia to be detected in 75% of patients suffering from acute cardiovascular collapse and only occasionally is ventricular tachycardia recorded. Thus early defibrillation is essential to ensure a satisfactory recovery with little neurological damage. Unfortunately there is a high recurrent rate of ventricular fibrillation in survivors (Greene 1990).

Topaz et al (1989) identified two groups of patients who have survived sudden cardiac arrest: one group had definite cardiac or respiratory pathology such as cardiomyopathy, mitral valve prolapse and tetralogy of Fallot. Another group had an apparent normal heart but some were found to have Wolff–Parkinson–White syndrome. In patients who were over 70 years there was usually a history of heart failure, dyspnoea and medication with digoxin and diuretics. Younger patients complained of chest pain and in 42% of this group, ventricular fibrillation was the initial arrhythmia whereas in the elderly it was only 22%. Resuscitation of elderly patients was just as successful as that of younger patients, but the long term survival rate was twice as great in the younger age group (Tresch et al 1990). Automatic defibrillators have been suggested for long term survival (Leading article, Lancet 1988), but Walls et al (1989) advised against the implanting of permanent internal cardiac defibrillators as it might impede successful defibrillation externally should it become necessary.

Cardiac arrest

Studies in animals have shown the value of coronary perfusion pressure in predicting the outcome of resuscitation following cardiac arrest. Paradis et al (1990) have confirmed these studies in man as placement of catheter in the right atrium and the aorta arch via the femoral artery is routine practice in their department; their results indicate that only patients whose coronary perfusion pressures reached 15 mmHg or more had a spontaneous return of circulation.

HYPOXIA AND MYOCARDIAL FUNCTION

Transient myocardial dysfunction occurred following severe hypoxia associated with drug overdosage, and there was pulmonary oedema which was believed to be of cardiac origin (Smith et al 1989). There is a significant increase in heart rate in response to isocapnic hypoxia but in the condition of hyperoxia, the increase in heart rate is insignificant (Sanders & Keller, 1989).

Opioids

Saini et al (1989) have demonstrated the effects of opioids on the incidence of ventricular fibrillation following acute myocardial ischaemia. Fentanyl which has mu-agonist activity increases the fibrillation rate whereas buprenorphine, a partial mu-agonist has little effect, although it does reduce heart rate and arterial pressure.

Bicarbonate

Although sodium bicarbonate may be administered following cardiac arrest to correct the resulting acidosis, its use in the management of cardiac disease has not been questioned until recently. Bersin et al (1989) noted that an infusion of bicarbonate impaired arterial oxygenation and reduced the myocardial oxygen consumption. Blood lactic levels increased which might lead in some cases to myocardial ischaemia. However, in patients who are on dialysis, bicarbonate may improve the cardiovascular function (Ayus & Krothapali 1989). In critically ill patients who have lactic acidosis, bicarbonate had no significant effect in improving the myocardial contractility and cardiac output. The $Paco_2$ rose while plasma ionized calcium fell (Cooper et al 1990) (see also Fernandez et al 1989 for discussion on bicarbonate distribution space).

CONGESTIVE CARDIAC FAILURE

The pharmacology of positive inotropic agents including the use of dopamine, dobutamine and dopexamine in the management of acute heart failure have been outlined by Parratt (1989). The treatment of congestive cardiac failure involves the reduction of cardiac work load by vasodilatation, reduction of blood volume by diuretics and an increase in myocardial contractility by positive inotropic agents. The use of digoxin is criticized for its low therapeutic index and this has led to the search for agents with inotropic activity. These include selective cardiac phosphodiesterase inhibitors (PDE) and alpha-1 adrenoceptor stimulants of the phosphoinositide pathway (v. der Leyen et al 1989). The phosphodiesterase inhibitors such as enoximone and imazodan inhibit the phosphodiesterase in myocardial cells, leading to increased cAMP levels. Severe cardiac congestive failure has been treated by the use of metolazone which is a potent sulphonamide diuretic with good overall results. Side effects include hypokalaemia, hyponatraemia and possible renal impairment (Kiyingi et al 1990).

Assessment of response to cardiac failure is always subjective and Feinstein et al (1989) have proposed an index based on dyspnoea and fatigue. Cardiomyopathy of overload is discussed by Katz (1990, see also Shub 1989). Cardiac hypertrophy is an effective response in the short term but when the clinical condition becomes chronic, the changes in the heart muscles lead to cell death. Echocardiography can identify left ventricular hypertrophy and an increase in left ventricular mass indicating a higher incidence of mortality (Levy et al 1990).

Midazolam, a short acting benzodiazepine may be used to produce sedation in patients undergoing diagnostic and endoscopic procedures, even in patients with cardiovascular disorders. Congestive cardiac failure reduces the clearance of midazolam by 30%, but the drug appears to be well tolerated with little adverse effects (Patel et al 1990).

Cardiovascular reflexes

Simple non-invasive tests of cardiovascular reflex function reveal that there are two groups of patients: those with a small reflex response associated with a fall in cardiac output during tilting; and those who have a hyperactive reflex associated with a tendency to develop vasovagal attack

(Wahbha et al 1989). Transient bradycardia may be a cause of syncope (Fujimura et al 1989), and the reversal of bradycardia with atropine may not necessarily restore the blood pressure (Scherrer et al 1990).

In obese patients there is a high frequency of cardiac autonomic dysfunction which may account for the increased incidence of sudden death (Rossi et al 1989).

CARDIAC SURGERY

Coronary bypass surgery is still associated with neurological complications including cerebrovascular accidents, retinal damage and even psychosis. The mechanisms of cerebral damage are thought to be macroembolism, microembolism and inadequate cerebral perfusion. Shaw et al (1989) have discussed factors that are likely to be associated with neurological complications including the duration and severity of the vascular disease prior to surgery, peripheral vascular disease, history of heart failure, diabetes, difficulty in terminating bypass, mean arterial pressure levels of less than 40 mmHg at operation, a fall of haemoglobin during surgery, prolonged stay in the intensive care unit and difficulty in controlling blood pressure in the post-operative period. Bypass involving hypothermia may lead to phrenic nerve damage during the application of cold solutions to the heart. Hypothermia leads to demyelination and degeneration of the axon (see Leading article, Lancet 1990b).

Lowering the flow rates may decrease non-coronary collateral blood flow, thus improving myocardial perfusion but with a flow rate of less than $1.5 \, l \, min^{-1}/m^2$, oxygen uptake is reduced (Alston et al 1989). Blood volume is reduced in patients with stable angina pectoris, but this does not improve after coronary artery bypass grafting (Ivert et al 1989). Enolase, an iso-enzyme, may be a sensitive marker of heart damage during coronary bypass surgery (Usui et al 1989). There is delayed myocardial recovery following cardioplegic arrest, and this is due to the low post-operative concentrations of ATP (Weisel et al 1989). Van Lente et al (1989) found that creatine kinase MB activity is reasonably accurate in detecting peri-operative myocardial infarction.

The administration of alfentanil during cardiac surgery does not abolish the adrenergic response to intubation and cardiac surgery. The elimination half-life was prolonged after cardiopulmonary bypass and did not allow for an early removal of the endotracheal tube (Robbins et al 1990).

CARDIOVASCULAR DISEASE AND SURGERY

Predicting the outcome of non-cardiac surgery in patients with cardiovascular disease is still subject to debate. There have been many indices of outcome, the most popular has been that reported by Goldman et al (1977). Improvement in monitoring and post-operative care plays a significant part in determining the outcome, while it is essential to have a close liaison between cardiologists and anaesthetists. Many of the problems have been reviewed by Mangano (1990) who found that peri-operative cardiac morbidity appears to be one of the biggest causes of death following operation. These include peri-operative myocardial infarct, unstable angina, congestive cardiac failure, dysrhythmias or cardiac arrest. Other reasons for poor outcome are a recent myocardial infarction or the presence of congestive cardiac failure. Changes in pulse rate at operation did not appear to be helpful in predicting potential problems, but prolonged increases or decreases of 20 mmHg or more in mean arterial pressure caused a significant rise in post-operative cardiac arrest, ischaemia or myocardial infarction (Charlson et al 1989).

For patients undergoing peripheral vascular surgery, Raby et al (1989) found that pre-operative ECG monitoring was of value in assessing cardiac risk, in that the absence of ischaemia suggested a good prognosis. However, Ouyang et al (1989) in a similar study found a very high incidence of silent post-operative myocardial ischaemia. Mullins & Garrison (1989) studied the effect of infusion of normal saline in high-risk surgical patients, and found that the fractional change in blood volume was of value in predicting the outcome of non-cardiac surgery. In the elderly, Gerson et al (1990) advocated that exercise tolerance was of value in predicting the outcome of non-cardiac thoracic surgery in relation to the incidence of cardio-pulmonary complications. Freeman et al (1989) felt that clinical history and examination were the most important components of pre-operative assessment to monitor the risk of invasive cardiac investigations.

Eagle & Boucher (1989) also expressed concern that cardiac risk may be increased in response to surgical stimulation in patients at a high risk. On the other hand, non-invasive tests may be expensive and therefore a re-evaluation of the clinical assessment of patients with previous cardiac disease should be taken into consideration. This involves consideration of the type of surgery, e.g. emergency, aortic, vascular, intrathoracic or abdominal, which appears to have a high risk of post-operative coronary complications. Young women and those patients without a cardiac history had the least risk at operation, whereas the risk increased in older patients with chest pain or in patients with coronary disease such as angina or previous myocardial infarction.

Pre-operative assessment could differentiate patients into medium or high risk. The incidence of myocardial insufficiency at operation in moderate or high risk patients was only of the order of 5 to 10%, and the death rate was only 0 to 2%. Eagle & Boucher (1989) noted that invasive tests are not without risk and that non-invasive investigations appear to identify many of the patients likely to have post-operative cardiac problems. Continuous ECG monitoring may uncover other abnormalities, but patients with cardiac hypertrophy may have ST depression which is not due to coronary disease.

Dipyridamole–thallium imaging appears to be a more successful index of identifying patients likely to have post-operative cardiac complications (Lette et al 1990), especially in patients unable to undergo exercise testing. The problem of exercise testing is often non-specific and may also be modified by advanced age, peripheral vascular disease, neurological disorders or even by beta-blockers. Dipyridamole causes a marked vaso-dilatation of coronary vessels with an increase in coronary blood flow. If there is damage to the heart due to reduced blood flow in coronary vessels, less thallium is taken up by the myocardium during scanning than the rest of the heart which is supplied by normal blood vessels. After the period of vasodilatation, the thallium redistributes in the damaged areas supplied by stenotic coronary arteries.

Myotonic dystrophy

Patients with congenital myotonic dystrophy have no symptoms, but their echocardiograms are abnormal and conduction defects are the main ECG changes (Forsberg et al 1990).

Catecholamines

Venter et al (1989) put in perspective the relationship between adrenergic and muscarinic cholinergic receptors and how they evolved from a common ancestor. This may explain the anomaly of sweating, in that the innervation is sympathetic but the mechanism is cholinergic. Benfey (1990) has drawn attention to the fact that the myocardium contains not only beta-adreno-receptors but also alpha-1 receptors for which adrenaline and noradrenaline have a higher affinity. Hypoxia increases the density of alpha-1 receptors. Cardiac arrhythmias during coronary artery occlusion and reperfusion have a potential significance in man, in that sudden cardiac death may occur without the presence of intraluminal thrombi.

The effects of intravenous catecholamines and insulin on plasma volume have been investigated by Hilsted et al (1989). Infusions of adrenaline increased peripheral venous packed cell volume, although noradrenaline was without effect at low concentrations. At high concentrations of adrenaline, packed cell volume increased, plasma volume decreased and intravascular mass of albumin decreased. Infusions of insulin led to an increase in transcapillary escape rate of albumin and a decrease in intra-vascular albumin. The changes in packed cell volume, plasma volume and albumin during hypoglycaemia are therefore due to the combined effects of adrenaline and insulin.

Small doses of L-tyrosine lead to hypertension and tachycardia while high doses produce hypotension and bradycardia. The inhibitory effects of L-tyrosine appear to be peripheral rather than central (Ekholm &

2

Karppanen 1989). Infusions of isoprenaline result in an increase in cardiac output with a rise in total body clearance, whereas the haemodynamic effects of isoprenaline affect its own pharmacokinetics (Ludwig et al 1989).

Although it is widely believed that alpha-1 receptors are located at post-synaptic sites and alpha-2 receptors at pre-synaptic sites, there is evidence that there are also alpha-2 receptors at post-synaptic sites. Stimulation of alpha-1 and alpha-2 receptors post-synaptically causes an influx of extra-cellular calcium ions, and it may be the mechanism of the effect of calcium blockade (Van Zwieten 1989).

Antiarrhythmic agents

Antiarrhythmic agents are classified in four categories according to that proposed by Vaughan Williams (1970) and updated by Harrison et al (1981).

Class I agents are essentially drugs which block the sodium channels, *Class II* are beta-adrenergic blocking agents, *Class III* are drugs which prolong the cardiac action potential and *Class IV* are calcium channel blockers. Frumin et al (1989) have emphasized the fact that not only are the mechanisms of arrhythmia complex, the drugs themselves have 'mixed' actions and that the classification was probably based on the actions of drugs on normal cardiac muscle fibres.

Class I agents (sodium channel blockers)

Class I agents are divided in three groups: 1A, 1B and 1C and the actions of drugs within the subgroups may not necessarily be predictable or effi-cacious. This is not surprising in view of the fact that sodium channels can exist in three states; resting, activated, and inactivated (see Davies & Camm 1987). Class I agents include intravenous local anaesthetic agents, e.g. lignocaine. If protein binding is reduced, plasma lignocaine may reach toxic levels. Routledge et al (1989) assessed the factors affecting free plasma lignocaine concentrations and found that loading and maintenance doses can be given according to body weight, but in the presence of Killip Class II heart failure the dose should be reduced by 20%.

Beta-adrenergic blocking agents

Beta-adrenergic blocking agents may have a central side effect in that patients complain of feeling sleepy. Pearson et al (1989) have demonstrated a central hypotensive action of the drug atenolol, and this is selective for the (−)enantiomer.

Propranolol has also been used for the treatment of portal hypertension, reducing heart rate and cardiac output with a reduction in portal pressure. However, Mastai et al (1989) have demonstrated that propranolol causes a significant reduction of hepatic artery flow in patients with cirrhosis. There is a potential possible role for propranolol in the acute phase of sepsis as it reduces negative nitrogen balance and decreases 3-methylhistidine excretion (Dickerson et al 1990).

Labetalol. Labetalol is an alpha-1 and beta-adrenergic antagonist which is used as an antihypertensive agent. Age is always considered as a factor to affect the metabolism of drugs, but Rocci et al (1989) were unable to demonstrate that age affected the oral clearance of labetalol, especially in those undergoing prolonged therapy with the agent.

Epanolol. Epanolol is a beta-1 partial agonist with agonist activity of approximately 20% of that of isoprenaline. It has little effect on the cardiac haemodynamic parameters at rest but during exercise it reduces heart rate and blood pressure, an effect lasting for more than 24 h. It thus may have a place in the management of patients with angina as it is likely to produce less side effects (Harry 1989).

Pindolol. The mode of action of pindolol is not only its non-selective beta-antagonist activity but it also acts by affecting the opioid receptors centrally (Jones & Tackett 1989).

Xamoterol. Xamoterol is a selective beta-1 adrenergic partial agonist; in low concentration it stimulates beta-1 receptors while in high concentrations it blocks both beta-1 and beta-2 receptors. The use of xamoterol has been advocated in mild cardiac failure, but in patients with severe cardiac failure it is contraindicated. Also, it should not be used in patients with airway obstruction or in those treated with ACE inhibitors (The Xamoterol in Severe Heart Failure Study Group 1990, Leading article, Lancet 1990c, Drug and Therapeutics Bulletin 1990).

Miscellaneous effects. Beta-adrenoceptor antagonists have been developed which are said to be selective with little effect on the airway, but this is not necessarily so in patients with asthma. Dilevalol and atenolol have no significant effect on pulmonary function and airway responsiveness in most subjects without asthma, although with prolonged use dilevalol may cause significant airway obstruction (Boulet et al 1990).

Response to moderate hypoglycaemia is affected by beta-antagonists such as propranolol, atenolol and metoprolol which prevent the rise in systolic and the fall in diastolic pressures associated with hypoglycaemia. All drugs augmented sweating but had little effect on awareness. Beta-adrenergic blockade enhanced the rise in plasma adrenaline seen during hypoglycaemia (Kerr et al 1990).

Calcium blockers have been used increasingly with beta-adrenergic blockers in the management of hypertension, but there might possibly be drugs interactions. Schoors et al (1990) found that nicardipine decreased the clearance of propranolol but did not augment its action and there was no serologistic action between the drugs.

Calcium channel blockers

The mechanisms of calcium channel blocking agents are discussed by Schwartz (1989); there are three subtypes of calcium channels designated as L, T and N, and it is the L subtype that is sensitive to calcium antagonists. The L channel has five subunits designated as alpha-1, alpha-2, beta, gamma and delta. Alpha-1 contains the receptors with three classes of calcium antagonists. Felodipine, a calcium antagonist with diuretic activity also was a preferred treatment of hypertension by Sudhir et al (1989), as it had fewer metabolic side effects. Nifedipine has also been used successfully in the acute management of high altitude pulmonary oedema (Oelz et al 1989). An attempt to use nifedipine to promote peripheral blood flow, to protect a skin-flap survival in plastic surgery was unsuccessful (Emery et al 1990).

Other possible uses of calcium entry blockers include the attempt to influence gastrointestinal disorders by inhibiting gastric activity, but drugs such as nifedipine, verapamil and diltiazem have profound cardiovascular effects (De Ponti et al 1989).

Although calcium channel blockers are effective in the treatment of hypertension and cardiac arrhythmias, developments have taken place to produce agents which open potassium channels. Cromakalim acts in this manner and appears to improve cardiac performance by arteriolar vaso-dilation (Thomas et al 1990).

Antibiotics

Recommendations for antibiotic prophylaxis of infective endocarditis have been outlined by the Endocarditis Working Party of the British Society for Antimicrobial Chemotherapy (1990). For dental treatment under local or no anaesthesia, amoxycillin 3 g one hour prior to dental surgery is advised, and for those allergic to penicillin the drugs recommended are erythromycin 1.5 g or clindamycin 600 mg. For dental procedures under general anaesthesia, amoxycillin 1 g intramuscularly before induction with 0.5 mg given 6 h later is recommended. It is advised that patients who have prosthetic heart valves, those who are allergic to penicillin or had a previous attack of endocarditis should be referred to hospital. Vancomycin 1 g is recommended in those patients who are allergic to penicillin. It is also advised that antibiotic cover is provided for patients having surgery or instrumentation of the upper respiratory tract, genitourinary instru-mentation, obstetrics and gynaecological procedures as well as gastro-intestinal procedures. Regarding patients who have mitral valve prolapse, antibiotics are only advised when there is an associated systolic murmur. It is worth noting that there are 4000 deaths per annum in the United States from mitral valve prolapse (Devereux et al 1989).

Coagulation and anticoagulants

Malignancy

There is an increase in venous thrombosis in patients with malignancy. There is a hypercoagulable state due to thrombin generation, fibrinogen to fibrin conversion and the impairment of fibrinolysis (Rocha et al 1989). A single injection of tumour necrosis factor led to the formation of activated factor X and prothrombin, probably through the extrinsic mechanism (Van Der Poll et al 1990).

Stress

Adrenaline and AVP released in high concentrations in response to stress increase levels of factor XIII, whereas insulin, cortisol and sex steroids result in a smaller and long term response. There is an increase of inhibitor of plasminogen activators with the suppression of fibrinolysis (Grant & Medcalf 1990).

Treatment

Streptokinase has been advocated to recanalize occluded coronary arteries, but recent studies indicated that recombinant tissue-type plasminogen activator is more successful. It is similar to that of physiological plasminogen activator and does not give antibody responses (Collen et al 1989).

The value of thrombolytic therapy in intensive care situations has been reviewed by De Bono (1990), with suggestions that they may also have a place in reducing the incidence of stroke and possibly in the treatment of mesenteric ischaemia.

Replacement of heart valves with mechanical prosthesis may result in thrombosis and arterial thromboembolism. Saour et al (1990) advocated that a moderate anticoagulation (prothrombin time ratio about 1.5) offered protection with reduced complications, compared to that with intensive regimes with warfarin. Travis et al (1989) have issued guidelines on perioperative anticoagulant control and it seems that it is safe to omit anticoagulants six days before patients undergo non-cardiac surgery, and then administer heparin before operation and 36 h later. They suggested that it is safe to operate on patients on warfarin undergoing dental or cataract surgery, but there were reservations regarding intramuscular analgesia and central venous cannulation. The guidelines suggested maintaining the international normalized ratio (INR) of < 1.5 at operation, and returning to full anticoagulation in the post-operative period. In patients with prosthetic valves, they recommend intravenous heparin of 15 000 units for 12 h started 24 h after the last dose of warfarin, aiming to have the activated partial thromboplastin time at 70–100 s. Heparin should be discontinued 6 h before surgery and both the INR and activated partial thromboplastin time should be checked 1 h before surgery. In patients with mitral valve replacement, the risk of emboli is higher than with aortic prostheses and in these circumstances, when warfarin is discontinued aspirin and dipyridamole is given. Patients on anticoagulants for other reasons other than for mechanical cardiac valves, surgery is safe after omitting three doses of warfarin. INR should be checked on admission and after operation. If the risk of thromboembolism is high, post-operative heparin infusion can be commenced.

For patients on heparin, the use of protamine sulfate is the recommended antidote but it does impair oxygen consumption which may account for the toxic effects (Wakefield et al 1989).

Miscellaneous agents

Atropine

Atropine blocks the parasympathetic activity on the heart, improving AV conduction and increasing the heart rate. In low doses, atropine stimulates parasympathetic activity. Das (1989) emphasized the use of constant ECG monitoring during the administration of atropine in patients with myocardial infarction, in that small doses may increase bradycardia while large doses may give rise to tachyarrhythmias.

Contrast media

Cardiovascular effects of contrast media result in an initial increase in myocardial contractility by depression of ventricular function. Vasodilatation and hypotension are succeeded by rebound phenomena involving reflex sympathetic stimulation. In addition, there are increased levels of vasopressin and atrial natriuretic hormone. Radiopaque media which are non-ionic and of low osmolality often reduce side effects, especially if there is little action on calcium ions (Dawson 1989).

Lithotripsy

Blood pressure changes occur following extracorporeal shock wave lithotripsy. Side effects of the technique include a decrease in renal function, liability to new stone formation and an increase in blood pressure. There was a marked rise in diastolic pressure after treatment and long term significance of this is unknown (Lingeman et al 1990).

Erythropoietin

There are at least five haemopoietic growth factors of which erythropoietin is one (Groopman et al 1989). Hypoxia increases erythropoietin production

(Ueno et al 1989) which improves the haemopoietic response in patients on dialysis for renal failure. It also leads to an improvement of cardio-respiratory function with a decrease in left ventricular mass (MacDougall et al 1990). In ischaemic acute renal failure, there is red cell trapping as there is an increase in the permeability of the renal capillaries with loss of plasma and haemoconcentration, obstructing further the renal blood flow (Bayati et al 1990). Attempts to demonstrate the high affinity of erythropoietin receptors have proved inconclusive (Means et al 1989). In conditions where there are myeloproliferative disorders such as primary thrombocythaemia, anagrelide produces thrombocytopenia and it may have a place in therapy (Silverstein et al 1988).

CARCINOID SYNDROME

Coupe et al (1989) reported on the clinical course and treatment of 63 patients with carcinoid syndrome. Poor prognosis was associated with marked weight loss and high secretion of 5-hydroxyindole acetic acid (5-HIAA). Treatment involved the use of hepatic artery embolization or hepatic resection. Drug therapy with parachlorophenylalanine decreased 5-HIAA excretion and reduced symptoms, but toxic effects such as depression and psychiatric disturbances were recorded. Other drugs included cyproheptadine which antagonized the action of 5-HT on smooth muscle. Ketanserin produced profound postural hypotension. Methysergide, although of value, caused retroperitoneal fibrosis while a 5-HT_3 receptor blocker improved diarrhoea but not flushing. Somatostatin analogue, Sandostatin, led to a reduction in the frequency of flushing and diarrhoea and in some patients a reduction of 5-HIAA. Vinik & Moattari (1989) reported that somatostatin analogue abolished diarrhoea in 80% of patients, flushing and wheezing in 100% of patients and even myopathy in one patient. Blood serotonin levels were unchanged but the urine 5-HIAA fell in 75% of patients. Kvols (1989) reported that somatostatin analogue is effective in preventing life-threatening carcinoid crisis.

KIDNEY

Renal function

DiBona (1989) has reviewed the neural control of renal function, emphasizing the effect of efferent renal sympathetic activity which affects blood flow, glomerular filtration rate, the reabsorption of water, sodium and other ions as well as controlling the release of renin, prostaglandins and other vasoactive agents. The efferent nerves are also involved in excessive retention of sodium which leads to the oedema seen in congestive cardiac failure. Post-efferent and afferent nerves are involved in the development of hypertension. In addition, angiotensin II also affects renal haemodynamic activity and tubular function, but the relationship between the sympathetic nerves and angiotensin II is still unclear (Johns 1989).

Cytochrome P450-dependent arachidonic acid metabolism may stimulate peptide release and may be involved in the pathogenesis of essential hypertension (Schwartzman et al 1990). On the other hand, the kidney appears to have an antihypertensive function releasing the hormone medullipin I, which is converted to medullipin II in the liver and requires the presence of cytochrome P-450 (Muirhead et al 1989).

There are many other hormones acting in the kidney, the clinical importance of which is still not understood. For example, adenosine receptors have been demonstrated in the cortical collecting tubules and this is involved in the mobilization of intracellular calcium (Arend et al 1988). Calcium channel blockers also act in the kidney by improving the glomerular filtration rate, renal blood flow and excretion of electrolytes (Chan & Schrier 1990). Intravenous clonidine promotes natriuresis, possibly by an extrarenal action (Blandford & Smyth 1989). Finkel et al (1989) have studied the distribution of renal vasopressin receptors (V_1); high levels of circulating AVP decrease the number of AVP receptors. In critically ill patients, oliguria is not uncommon and is associated with hypoperfusion of the kidney and an excess of AVP. Hypovolaemic patients could increase the urine output in response to 500 ml of normal saline (Zaloga & Hughes 1990). Low dose dopamine increases renal blood flow without causing a significant increase in urine output (Schwartz et al 1988); however Kaufman & Bailey (1987) have demonstrated that low dose bumetanide not only promoted diuresis during operation, but also attenuated the increased levels of AVP seen following surgical stimulation.

Diuretics

Thiazide diuretics lead to hypokalaemia and this is augmented in the presence of adrenaline given in association with local analgesia. Lipworth et al (1989) reported a similar interaction with diuretics in patients given high doses of inhaled albuterol for the treatment of asthma. Beneficial effects of thiazide diuretics include a reduction in the risk of hip fracture. This effect is restricted to thiazides and may be due to their action on reducing urine excretion of calcium and thus improving calcium balance (LaCroix et al 1990).

ACE inhibitors increase the diuresis of frusemide, promoting the excretion of sodium, potassium and dopamine but the mechanism for this is still unclear (MacDonald et al 1989). It has little effect on acid balance or ions in the CSF during acute respiratory acidosis (Javaheri et al 1989). However it reduces the intrapulmonary shunt in patients while being ventilated with gaseous exchange problems. As the cardiac output was unchanged it was assumed that the drug had a direct action on the pulmonary vasculature (Baltopoulos et al 1989). Frusemide is least effective when given in a bolus intravenous dose (Alvan et al 1990). In obese animals, frusemide causes liver and renal damage as it has a low lipid solubility and it may well be the result from increased concentrations in the lean body mass (Corcoran et al 1989). The pharmacokinetics of bumetanide in healthy patients and those with congestive cardiac failure is similar, irrespective of whether the drug is given orally or intravenously (Cook et al 1988).

For a detailed discussion of molecular mechanisms of diuretic agents see Breyer & Jacobson (1990).

Alfentanil

It might be expected that in patients with chronic renal failure, with decreased protein binding, that the metabolism of alfentanil might be affected. Bower & Sear (1989) failed to demonstrate any difference in the elimination half-life and volume of distribution in patients with chronic renal disease or in normal patients. It is possible that the increase in the unbound state of the drug may affect its potency. The main alfentanil binding is not with albumin but alpha-1-acid glycoprotein.

REFERENCES

Alston R P, Singh M, McLaren A D 1989 Systemic oxygen uptake during hypothermic cardiopulmonary bypass. Effects of flow rate, flow character, and arterial pH. J Thorac Cardiovasc Sur 98: 757–768
Alvan G, Helleday L, Lindholm A, Sanz E, Villen T 1990 Diuretic effect and diuretic efficiency after intravenous dosage of frusemide. Br J Clin Pharmacol 29: 215–219
Arend L J, Burnatowska-Hledin M A, Spielman W S 1988 Adenosine receptor-mediated calcium mobilization in cortical collecting tubule cells. Am J Physiol 255: C581–588
Ayus J C, Krothapalli R K 1989 Effect of bicarbonate administration on cardiac function. Am J Med 87: 5–6
Bain R J I, Poeppinghaus V J I, Jones G M, Peaston M J T 1989 Cortisol level predicts myocardial infarction in patients with ischaemic chest pain. Int J Cardiol 25: 69–72
Baltopoulos G, Zakynthinos S, Dimopoulos A, Roussos C 1989 Effects of furosemide on pulmonary shunts. Chest 96: 494–498
Barta E 1989 The role of free oxygen radicals in the mechanism of ischaemic-reperfusion myocardial injury. Physiol Bohemoslov 38: 385–388
Bayati A, Christofferson R, Kallskog O, Wolgast M 1990 Mechanism of erythrocyte trapping in ischaemic acute renal failure. Acta Physiol Scand 138: 13–23
Belardinelli L, Lerman B B 1990 Electrophysiological basis for the use of adenosine in the diagnosis and treatment of cardiac arrhythmias. Br Heart J 63: 3–4
Benfey B G 1990 Minireview: Function of myocardial α-adrenoceptors. Life Sci 46: 743–757
Berkin K E 1989 Respiratory effects of angiotensin converting enzyme inhibition. Eur Respir J 2: 198–201
Bersin R M, Chatterjee K, Arieff A I 1989 Metabolic and hemodynamic consequences of sodium bicarbonate administration in patients with heart disease. Am J Med 87: 7–14
Blandford D E, Smyth D D 1989 Enhanced natriuretic potency of intravenous clonidine: extrarenal site of action? Eur J Pharmacol 174: 181–188
Boulet L P, Lacourciere Y, Milot J, Lampron N 1990 Comparative effects of dilevalol and atenolol on lung function and airway response to methacholine in hypertensive subjects. Br J Clin Pharmacol 29: 725–731
Bower S, Sear J W 1989 Disposition of alfentanil in patients receiving a renal transplant. J Pharm Pharmacol 41: 654–657

Braunwald E 1989 Unstable angina. A classification. Circulation 80: 410–414
Breyer J, Jacobson H R 1990 Molecular mechanisms of diuretic agents. Ann Rev Med 41: 265–275
Capewell S, Taverner D, Hannan W J, Muir A L 1989 Acute and chronic arterial and venous effects of captopril in congestive cardiac failure. Br Med J 299: 942–945
Chan L, Schrier R W 1990 Effects of calcium channel blockers on renal function. Ann Rev Med 1990: 289–302
Charlap S, Kahlam S, Lichstein E, Frishman W 1989 Electromechanical dissociation: diagnosis, pathophysiology, and management. Am Heart J 118: 355–360
Charlson M E, MacKenzie R, Gold J P et al 1989 The preoperative and intraoperative hemodynamic predictors of postoperative myocardial infarction or ischemia in patients undergoing noncardiac surgery. Ann Surg 210: 637–648
Collen D, Lijnen H R, Todd P A, Goa K L 1989 Tissue-type plasminogen activator. A review of its pharmacology and therapeutic use as a thrombolytic agent. Drugs 38: 346–388
Collins P, Fox K M 1990 Pathophysiology of angina. Lancet 335: 94–96
Cook J A, Smith D E, Cornish L A, Tankanow R M, Nicklas J M, Hyneck M 1988 Kinetics, dynamics, and bioavailability of bumetanide in healthy subjects and patients with congestive heart failure. Clin Pharmacol Ther 44: 487–500
Cooper D J, Walley K R, Wiggs B R, Russell J A 1990 Bicarbonate does not improve hemodynamics in critically ill patients who have lactic acidosis. A prospective, controlled clinical study. Ann Intern Med 112: 2–498
Corcoran G B, Salazar D E, Chan H H 1989 Obesity as a risk factor in drug-induced organ injury. III. Increased liver and kidney injury by furosemide in the obese overfed rat. Toxicol Appl Pharmacol 98: 12–24
Coupe M, Levi S, Ellis M, Clarke B, Morris J A, Alstead E A, Allison D J, Hodgson H J F 1989 Therapy for symptoms in the carcinoid syndrome. Q J Med 73: 1021–1036
Crea F, Pupita G, Galassi A R, El-Tamimi H, Kaski J C, Davies G, Maseri A 1990 Role of adenosine in pathogenesis of anginal pain. Circulation 81: 164–172
Das G 1989 Cardiac effects of atropine in man: an update. Int J Clin Pharmacol Ther Toxicol 27: 473–477
Davies D W, Camm A J 1987 A classification of antiarrhythmic drugs and common cardiac arrhythmias. In: Kaufman L (ed) Anaesthesia Review 4. Churchill Livingstone, London, pp 73–79
Dawson P 1989 Cardiovascular effects of contrast agents. Am J Cardiol 64: 2E–9E
De Bono D P 1990 Thrombolysis in the intensive therapy unit. Intensive Ther Clin Monit 11: 25–28
De Ponti F, D'Angelo L, Frigo G M, Crema A 1989 Inhibitory effects of calcium channel blockers on intestinal motility in the dog. Eur J Pharmacol 168: 133–144
Devereux R B, Kramer-Fox R, Kligfield P 1989 Mitral valve prolapse: causes, clinical manifestations, and management. Ann Intern Med 111: 305–317
DiBona G F 1989 Neural control of renal function: cardiovascular implications. Hypertension 13: 539–548
Dickerson R N, Fried R C, Bailey P M, Stein T P, Mullen J L, Buzby G P 1990 Effect of propranolol on nitrogen and energy metabolism in sepsis. J Surg Res 48: 38–41
Dinh Xuan A T, Higenbottam T W, Clelland C, Pepke-Zaba J, Cremona G, Wallwork J 1989 Impairment of pulmonary endothelium-dependent relaxation in patients with Eisenmenger's syndrome. Br J Pharmacol 99: 9–10
Drug and Therapeutics Bulletin 1990 Xamoterol—more trouble than it's worth? 28: 53–54
Eagle K A, Boucher C A 1989 Cardiac risk of noncardiac surgery. N Engl J Surg 321: 1330–1332
Ekholm S, Karppanen H 1989 Cardiovascular effects of L-tyrosine: influence of blockade of tyrosine metabolism. Eur J Pharmacol 163: 209–217
Emery F M, Kodey T R, Bomberger R A, McGregor D B 1990 The effect of nifedipine on skin-flap survival. Plast Reconstr Surg 85: 61–63
Endocarditis Working Party of the British Society for Antimicrobial Chemotherapy 1990 Antibiotic prophylaxis of infective endocarditis. Lancet 335: 88–89
Feinstein A R, Fisher M B, Pigeon J G 1989 Changes in dyspnea–fatigue ratings as indicators of quality of life in the treatment of congestive heart failure. Am J Cardiol 64: 50–55
Fernandez P C, Cohen R M, Feldman G M 1989 The concept of bicarbonate distribution space: the crucial role of body buffers. Kidney Int 36: 747–752

Finkel M S, Mendelsohn F A O, Quirion R, Zamir N, Keiser H R 1989 Physiologic regulation and distribution of the renal vasopressin receptor. Pharmacology 39: 165–175

Forsberg H, Olofsson B-O, Eriksson A, Andersson S 1990 Cardiac involvement in congenital myotonic dystrophy. Br Heart J 63: 119–121

Fraser R, Davies D L, Connell J M C 1989 Hormones and hypertension. Clin Endocrinol 31: 701–746

Freeman W K, Gibbons R J, Shub C 1989 Preoperative assessment of cardiac patients undergoing noncardiac surgical procedures. Mayo Clin Proc 64: 1105–1117

Frumin H, Kerin N Z, Rubenfire M 1989 Classification of antiarrhythmic drugs. J Clin Pharmacol 29: 387–394

Fujimura O, Yee R, Klein G J, Sharma A D, Boahene K A 1989 The diagnostic sensitivity of electrophysiologic testing in patients with syncope caused by transient bradycardia. N Engl J Med 321: 1703–1707

Gao S Z, Schroeder J S, Hunt S A, Billingham M E, Valantine H A, Stinson E B 1989 Acute myocardial infarction in cardiac transplant recipients. Am J Card 64: 1093–1097

Gerson M C, Hurst J M, Hertzberg V S et al 1990 Prediction of cardiac and pulmonary complications related to elective abdominal and noncardiac thoracic surgery in geriatric patients. Am J Med 88: 101–107

Goldman L, Caldera D L, Nussbaum S R et al 1977 Multifactorial index of cardiac risk in noncardiac surgical procedures. N Engl J Med 297: 845–850

Graafsma S J, van Tits L J, van Heijst P et al 1989 Adrenoceptors on blood cells in patients with essential hypertension before and after mental stress. J Hypertens 7: 519–524

Grant P J, Medcalf R L 1990 Hormonal regulation of haemostasis and the molecular biology of the fibrinolytic system. Clin Sci 78: 3–11

Greene H L 1990 Sudden arrhythmic cardiac death—mechanisms, resuscitation and classification: the Seattle perspective. Am J Cardiol 65: 4B–12B

Griffith T, Randall M 1989 Nitric oxide comes of age. Lancet II: 875–876

Groopman J E, Molina J-M, Scadden D T 1989 Hematopoietic growth factors—biology and clinical applications. N Engl J Med 321: 1449–1459

Guthrie G P Jr, Kotchen T A, Van Loon G R 1989 Effect of transdermal clonidine on the endocrine responses to insulin-induced hypoglycemia in essential hypertension. Clin Pharmacol Ther 45: 417–423

Harrison D C, Winkle R A, Sami M, Mason J W 1981 Encainide: A new and potent antiarrhythmic agent. In: Harrison D C (ed) Cardiac Arrhythmias: a Decade of Progress. G K Hall, Boston, pp 315–330

Harry J D 1989 Clinical pharmacology of epanolol—pharmacodynamic aspects. Drugs 38 (suppl 2): 18–27

Hilsted J, Christensen N J, Larsen S 1989 Effect of catecholamines and insulin on plasma volume and intravascular mass of albumin in man. Clin Sci 77: 149–155

Ivert T, Pehrsson S K, Landou C, Magder S, Holmgren A 1989 Blood volume after coronary artery bypass grafting. Clin Physiol 9: 547–554

Javaheri S, Freidel J F, Davis P J 1989 Furosemide and cerebrospinal fluid ions during acute respiratory acidosis. J Appl Physiol 67: 563–569

Johns E J 1989 Role of angiotensin II and the sympathetic nervous system in the control of renal function. J Hypertens 7: 695–701

Jones L F, Tackett R L 1989 Catecholaminergic and opioidergic mechanisms involved in the hypotensive response of pindolol. Eur J Pharmacol 165: 123–128

Julius S, Weder A B 1989 Brain and the regulation of blood pressure: a hemodynamic perspective. Clin Exp Hypertens 11 (suppl 1): 1–19

Katz A M 1990 Cardiomyopathy of overload. A major determinant of prognosis in congestive heart failure. N Engl J Med 322: 100–116

Kaufman L, Bailey P M 1987 Intravenous bumetanide attenuates the rise in plasma vasopressin concentrations during major surgical operations. Br J Clin Pharmacol 23: 237–240

Kerr D, MacDonald I A, Heller S R, Tattersall R B 1990 β-adrenoceptor blockade and hypoglycaemia. A randomised, double-blind, placebo controlled comparison of metoprolol CR, atenolol and propranolol LA in normal subjects. Br J Clin Pharmacol 29: 685–693

Kiyingi A, Field M J, Pawsey C C, Yiannikas J, Lawrence J R, Arter W J 1990 Metolazone in treatment of severe refractory congestive cardiac failure. Lancet 335: 29–37

Kloner R A, Przyklenk K, Whittaker P 1989 Deleterious effects of oxygen radicals in ischemia/reperfusion. Resolved and unresolved issues. Circulation 80: 1115–1127

Koopmans P P, Van Megen T, Thien T, Gribnau W J 1989 The interaction between indomethacin and captopril or enalapril in healthy volunteers. J Intern Med 226: 139–142

Kvols L K 1989 Therapy of the malignant carcinoid syndrome. Endocrinology and metabolism—Clinics of North America 18: 557–568

LaCroix A Z, Wienpahl J, White L R et al 1990 Thiazide diuretic agents and the incidence of hip fracture. N Engl J Med 322: 286–290

Leading article 1988 Automatic defibrillators. Lancet 1: 1199–1201

Leading article 1989a ACE inhibitors after myocardial infarction. Lancet II: 1133–1134

Leading article 1989b Non-Q-wave myocardial infarction. Lancet II: 899–900

Leading article 1990a Haemodynamics of hypertension. Lancet 335: 83–84

Leading article 1990b Phrenic nerve trauma and cardiac surgery. Lancet 335: 1373

Leading article 1990c New evidence on xamoterol. Lancet 336: 23–24

Lette J, Waters D, Lassonde J et al 1990 Postoperative myocardial infarction and cardiac death. Ann Surg 211: 84–90

Levy D, Garrison R J, Savage D D, Kannel W B, Castelli W P 1990 Prognostic implications of echocardiographically determined left ventricular mass in the Framingham Heart study. N Engl J Med 322: 1561–1566

Lewis R V, Maclean D 1990 Treatment of mild–moderate hypertension. Hosp Update April: 331–334

Lingeman J E, Woods J R, Toth P D 1990 Blood pressure changes following extracorporeal shock wave lithotripsy and other forms of treatment of nephrolithiasis. JAMA 263: 1789–1794

Lipsitz L A 1989a Altered blood pressure homeostasis in advanced age: clinical and research implications. J Gerontol 44: M179–M183

Lipsitz L A 1989b Orthostatic hypotension in the elderly. N Engl J Med 321: 952–957

Lipworth B J, McDevitt D G, Struthers A D 1989 Prior treatment with diuretic augments the hypokalemic and electrocardiographic effects of inhaled albuterol. Am J Med 86: 653–657

Long C J, Berkowitz B A 1989 What is the relationship between the endothelium derived relaxant factor and nitric oxide? Life Sci 45: 1–14

Ludwig J, Halbrugge T, Vey G, Walter J, Graefe K-H 1989 Haemodynamics as a determinant of the pharmacokinetics of and the plasma catecholamine responses to isoprenaline. Eur J Clin Pharmacol 37: 493–500

Luu M, Stevenson W G, Stevenson L W, Baron K, Walden J 1989 Diverse mechanisms of unexpected cardiac arrest in advanced heart failure. Circulation 80: 1675–1680

MacDonald T M, Craig K, Watson M L 1989 Frusemide, ACE inhibition, renal dopamine and prostaglandins: acute interactions in normal man. Br J Clin Pharmacol 28: 683–694

MacDougall I C, Lewis N P, Saunders M J et al 1990 Long-term cardiorespiratory effects of amelioration of renal anaemia by erythropoietin. Lancet 335: 489–493

McInnes G T, Sever P S (eds) 1989 The relationships between structure and effects of ACE inhibitors. Br J Clin Pharmacol 28 (suppl 2): 93S–189S

Mangano D T 1990 Perioperative cardiac morbidity. Anesthesiology 72: 153–184

Marlettini M G, Cassani A, Morselli Labate A M, Crippa S, Contarini A, Orlandi C 1989 Clinical and biochemical aspects of pregnancy-induced hypertension. Clin Exp Hypertens 11: 1565–1584

Mastai R, Bosch J, Bruix J, Navasa M, Kravetz D, Rodes J 1989 β-blockade with propranolol and hepatic artery blood flow in patients with cirrhosis. Hepatology 10: 269–272

Means R T Jr, Krantz S B, Sawyer S T, Gilbert H S 1989 Erythropoietin receptors in polycythemia vera. J Clin Invest 84: 1340–1344

Melkumyants A M, Balashov S A 1990 Effect of blood viscosity on arterial flow induced dilator response. Cardiovasc Res 24: 165–168

Moss A J, Benhorin J 1990 Prognosis and management after a first myocardial infarction. N Engl J Med 322: 743–753

Muirhead E E, Byers L W, Capdevila J, Brooks B, Pitcock J A, Brown P S 1989 The renal antihypertensive endocrine function: its relations to cytochrome P-450. J Hypertens 7: 361–369

Muller J E, Tofler G H, Stone P H 1989 Circadian variation and triggers of onset of acute cardiovascular disease. Circulation 79: 733–743

Mullins R J, Garrison R N 1989 Fractional change in blood volume following normal saline infusion in high-risk patients before noncardiac surgery. Ann Surg 209: 651–661

Oelz O, Maggiorini M, Ritter M et al 1989 Nifedipine for high altitude pulmonary oedema. Lancet II: 1241–1244

Opie L H 1989 Reperfusion injury and its pharmacologic modification. Circulation 80: 1049–1062

Ouyang P, Gerstenblith G, Furman W R, Golueke P J, Gottlieb S O 1989 Frequency and significance of early postoperative silent myocardial ischemia in patients having peripheral vascular surgery. Am J Cardiol 64: 1113–1116

Panza J A, Quyyumi A A, Brush J E Jr, Epstein S E 1990 Abnormal endothelium-dependent vascular relaxation in patients with essential hypertension. N Engl J Med 323: 22–27

Paradis N A, Martin G B, Rivers E P et al 1990 Coronary perfusion pressure and the return of spontaneous circulation in human cardiopulmonary resuscitation. JAMA 263: 1106–1113

Parratt J R 1989 The pharmacology of positive inotropic agents in acute heart failure. Appl Cardiopulmonary Pathophysiol 3: 85–93

Patel I H, Soni P P, Fukuda E K, Smith D F, Leier C V, Boudoulas H 1990 The pharmacokinetics of midazolam in patients with congestive heart failure. Br J Clin Pharmacol 29: 565–569

Pearson A A, Gaffney T E, Walle T, Privitera P J 1989 A stereoselective central hypotensive action of atenolol. J Pharmacol Exp Ther 250: 759–763

Pepine C J 1989 New concepts in the pathophysiology of acute myocardial infarction. Am J Cardiol 64: 2B–8B

Prasad K, Kalra J, Chan W P, Chaudhary A K 1989 Effect of oxygen free radicals on cardiovascular function at organ and cellular levels. Am Heart J 117: 1196

Raby K E, Goldman L, Greager M A et al 1989 Correlation between preoperative ischemia and major cardiac events after peripheral vascular surgery. N Engl J Med 321: 1296–1300

Rich S, Brundage B H 1989 Pulmonary hypertension: a cellular basis for understanding the pathophysiology and treatment. J Am Coll Cardiol 14: 545–550

Riska H, Sovijarvi A R A, Ahonen A, Salorinne Y, Sundberg S, Stenius-Aarniala B 1990 Effects of captopril on blood pressure and respiratory function compared to verapamil in patients with hypertension and asthma. J Cardiovasc Pharmacol 15: 57–61

Robbins G R, Wynands J E, Whalley D G 1990 Pharmacokinetics of alfentanil and clinical responses during cardiac surgery. Can J Anaesth 37: 52–57

Rocci M L Jr, Valiquett T, Sirgo M A 1989 Effects of age on the elimination of labetalol. Clin Pharmacokinet 17: 452–457

Rocha E, Paramo J A, Fernandez F J et al 1989 Clotting activation and impairment of fibrinolysis in malignancy. Thromb Res 54: 699–707

Rossi M, Marti G, Ricordi L et al 1989 Cardiac autonomic dysfunction in obese subjects. Clin Sci 76: 567–572

Rouan G W, Lee T H, Cook E F, Brand D A, Weisberg M C, Goldman L 1989 Clinical characteristics and outcome of acute myocardial infarction in patients with initially normal or nonspecific electrocardiograms (A report from the Multicenter Chest Pain Study). Am J Cardiol 64: 1087–1092

Routledge P A, Stargel W W, Barchowsky A, Wagner G S, Shand D G 1989 Factors affecting free (unbound) lignocaine concentration in suspected acute myocardial infarction. Br J Clin Pharmacol 28: 593–597

Saini V, Carr D B, Verrier R L 1989 Comparative effects of the opioids fentanyl and buprenorphine on ventricular vulnerability during acute coronary artery occlusion. Cardiovasc Res 23: 1001–1006

Sanders M H, Keller F A 1989 Chronotropic effects of progressive hypoxia and hypercapnia. Respiration 55: 1–10

Saour J N, Sieck J O, Mamo L A R, Gallus A S 1990 Trial of different intensities of anticoagulation in patients with prosthetic heart valves. N Engl J Med 322: 428–432

Scherrer U, Vissing S, Morgan B J, Hanson P, Victor R G 1990 Vasovagal syncope after infusion of a vasodilator in a heart-transplant recipient. N Engl J Med 322: 602–604

Schlueter W A, Batlle D C 1989 Renal effects of antihypertensive drugs. Drugs 37: 900–925

Schnaper H W 1989 Practical issues in drug selection and dosing. Am J Cardiol 63: 27B–31B

Schoors D F, Vercruysse I, Musch G, Massart D L, Dupont A G 1990 Influence of nicardipine on the pharmacokinetics and pharmacodynamics of propranolol in healthy volunteers. Br J Clin Pharmacol 29: 497–501

Schwartz A 1989 Calcium antagonists: review and perspective on mechanism of action. Am J Cardiol 64: 3I–9I

Schwartz L B, Bissell M G, Murphy M, Gewertz B L 1988 Renal effects of dopamine in vascular surgical patients. J Vasc Surg 8: 367–374

Schwartzman M L, Martasek P, Rios A R et al 1990 Cytochrome P450-dependent arachidonic acid metabolism in human kidney. Kidney Int 37: 94–99

Shaw P J, Bates D, Cartlidge N E F et al 1989 An analysis of factors predisposing to neurological injury in patients undergoing coronary bypass operations. Q J Med 267: 633–646

Shub C 1989 Heart failure and abnormal ventricular function—pathophysiology and clinical correlation (part 1). Chest 96: 636–640

Silverstein M N, Petitt R M, Solberg L A Jr, Fleming J S, Knight R C, Schacter L P 1988 Anagrelide: a new drug for treating thrombocytosis. N Engl J Med 318: 1292–1294

Smith F, Lee R, Haindl W 1989 Hypoxic cardiomyopathy: acute myocardial dysfunction after severe hypoxia. Aust NZ J Med 19: 488–492

Sudhir K, Jennings G L, Bruce A 1989 Cardiovascular-risk reduction: initial diuretic therapy compared with calcium-antagonist (felodipine) therapy for primary hypertension. Med J Aust 151: 277–279

Sumimoto T, Takayama Y, Iwasaka T et al 1989 Oxygen delivery, oxygen consumption and hemoglobin-oxygen affinity in acute myocardial infarction. Am J Cardiol 64: 975–979

The Xamoterol in Severe Heart Failure Study Group 1990 Xamoterol in severe heart failure. Lancet 336: 1–6

Thomas P, Dixon M S, Winterton S J, Sheridan D J 1990 Acute haemodynamic effects of cromakalim in patients with angina pectoris. Br J Clin Pharmacol 29: 325–331

Topaz O, Perin E, Cox M, Mallon S M, Castellanos A, Myerburg R J 1989 Young adult survivors of sudden cardiac arrest: analysis of invasive evaluation of 22 subjects. Am Heart J 118: 281–287

Travis S, Wray R, Harrison K 1989 Perioperative anticoagulant control. Br J Surg 76: 1107–1108

Tresch D D, Thakur R K, Hoffmann R G, Aufderheide T P, Brooks H L 1990 Comparison of outcome of paramedic-witnessed cardiac arrest in patients younger and older than 70 years. Am J Cardiol 65: 453–457

Ueno M, Seferynska I, Beckman B, Brookins J, Nakashima J, Fisher J W 1989 Enhanced erythropoietin secretion in hepatoblastoma cells in response to hypoxia. Am J Physiol 257: C743–749

Usui A, Kato K, Abe T, Murase M, Tanaka M, Takeuchi E 1989 Beta-enolase in blood plasma during open heart surgery. Cardiovasc Res 23: 737–740

Vallance P, Collier J, Moncada S 1989 Effects of endothelium-derived nitric oxide on peripheral arteriolar tone in man. Lancet II: 997–999

Van Der Poll T, Buller H R, Cate H T, Wortel C H et al 1990 Activation of coagulation after administration of tumor necrosis factor to normal subjects. N Engl J Med 322: 1622–1627

Vane J R, Anggard E E, Botting R M 1990 Regulatory functions of the vascular endothelium. N Engl J Med 323: 27–36

Van Lente F, Martin A, Ratliff N B, Kazmierczak S C, Loop F D 1989 The predictive value of serum enzymes for perioperative myocardial infarction after cardiac operations. An autopsy study. J Thorac Cardiovasc Surg 98: 704–710

v der Leyen H, Schmitz W, Scholz H, Scholz J 1989 New positive inotropic agents acting by phosphodiesterase inhibition or alpha$_1$-adrenergic stimulation. Pharmacol Res 21: 329–337

Van Zwieten P A 1989 Drugs interacting with alpha adrenoceptors. Cardiovasc Drugs Ther 3: 121–133

Vaughan Williams E M 1970 Classification of antiarrhythmic drugs. In: Sandoe E, Flendsted-Jensen E, Olsen K (eds) Symposium on Cardiac Arrhythmias. Sweden AB Astra, Sodertalje, 449

Venter J C, Fraser C M, Kerlavage A R, Buck M A 1989 Molecular biology of adrenergic and muscarinic cholinergic receptors. Biochem Pharmacol 38: 1197–1208

Vinik A, Moattari A R 1989 Use of somatostatin analog in management of carcinoid syndrome. Dig Dis Sci 34 (March 1989 suppl): 145–275

Wahbha M M A E, Morley C A, Al-Shamma Y M H, Hainsworth R 1989 Cardiovascular reflex responses in patients with unexplained syncope. Clin Sci 77: 547–553

Wakefield T W, Ucros I, Kresowik T F, Hinshaw D B, Stanley J C 1989 Decreased oxygen consumption as a toxic manifestation of protamine sulfate reversal of heparin anticoagulation. J Vasc Surg 9: 772–777

Waldemar G, Paulson O B 1989 Angiotensin converting enzyme inhibition and cerebral circulation—a review. Br J Clin Pharmacol 28 (suppl 2): 177S–182S

Walls J T, Schuder J C, Curtis J J, Stephenson H E Jr, McDaniel W C, Flaker G C 1989 Adverse effects of permanent cardiac internal defibrillator patches on external defibrillation. Am J Cardiol 64: 1144–1147

Weisel R D, Mickle D A G, Finkle C D, Tumiati L C, Madonik M M, Ivanov J 1989 Delayed myocardial metabolic recovery after blood cardioplegia. Ann Thor Surg 48: 503–507

Zaloga G P, Hughes S S 1990 Oliguria in patients with normal renal function. Anesthesiology 72: 598–602

2. Medicine relevant to anaesthesia (2)

L. Kaufman

RESPIRATION

Physiology

Control of respiration

Van Lunteren (1988) has reviewed many of the factors involved in respiratory muscle coordination including the diaphragm, the muscles of the rib cage as well as the accessory muscles of respiration. The abdominal muscles are involved in expiration, especially the transverse abdominis. The muscles of the nose, tongue and pharynx and larynx are concerned with speech and protection of the respiratory tract, but they are intimately involved in the physiology of breathing and function as a valve which influences air flow during expiration (Bartlett 1989). The vocal cords begin to separate before the onset of contraction of the diaphragm and even the cricothyroid muscle can be considered to be an accessory muscle of respiration (Woodson 1989). Animal studies show that the nerves to the posterior cricoarytenoid muscle (the abductor of the vocal cord) is always active during inspiration; expiratory activity may occur as well, being enhanced by hypercapnia and inhibited by hypoxia (Zhou et al 1989).

Fifty percent of respiratory resistance is found in the nasal cavity during quiet respiration. The airflow resistance is directly related to the sympathetic tone of the capacitance vessels. The blood supply to the nasal mucosa is controlled by the adrenergic (alpha-2, alpha-1, and beta-2 receptors) and non-adrenergic mechanisms involving neuropeptide-Y (NPY) (Lacroix 1989). Most of the studies on blood supply of the lung have been restricted to measurement of the total bronchial blood flow, with very little interest on circulation of the airway mucosa which in fact has much of the blood distributed to it. The blood flow ranges from $30-95 \, \mathrm{ml \, min}^{-1}/100 \, \mathrm{g}$ wet tissue. Blood flow is influenced by the inspired air, airway and vascular pressure and autonomic transmitters (Wanner 1989).

Factors affecting the endogenous control of bronchomotor tone have been reviewed by Leff (1988), indicating that tone is influenced by calcium released post-synaptically, acting on smooth muscle. The pathogenesis of airway hyper-responsiveness is discussed; it may be allergic, neurogenic or even myogenic. Vasoactive peptides may relax the airway in vitro but have little action in vivo. Substance P, neurokinins and calcitonin, gene-related peptides, may be involved in asthma. It has also been suggested that neuropeptides may be involved in the transmission of non-adrenergic and non-cholinergic nerves (Barnes 1987).

Ciliac activity

Ciliary epithelium is present in the upper and lower respiratory tract down to the respiratory bronchioles. It is estimated that the surface of each cell contains 200 cilia which beat in two layers of fluid, the periciliary fluid and the mucus. Ciliary activity may be impaired due to loss of ciliary epithelium and changes in the mucus and periciliary fluid. Thus ciliary activity may be impaired due to chronic bronchitis while smoking inhibits ciliary activity completely. Other inhibiting factors include viral and bacterial infection, asthma and allergic rhinitis (Wilson 1988). Nasal ciliary activity is inhibited by local anaesthetics, antihistamines and propranolol while cholinergic agents and beta-adrenergic drugs increase ciliary activity (Hermens & Merkus 1987).

The propulsion of mucus by cilia is affected by anaesthesia, in that the inhalation of dry gases readily inhibits ciliary activity. Sleigh et al (1988) have reviewed many of the factors affecting mucociliary transport which depends on the cilia, mucus and the periciliary fluid. Clearance of mucus appears to be more related to factors that stimulate secretion and pH change rather than changes of ciliary activity. The secretion of mucus appears to stimulate ciliary beating. The liquid collected from the airway surface which is a mixture of periciliary fluid and mucus gland secretion is hyperosmolar. Albumin can be actively secreted into the lumen of the trachea, especially in the presence of salbutamol (Widdicombe 1989).

Surfactant

The hormonal regulation of pulmonary surfactant has been reviewed by Ballard (1989) indicating its synthesis, composition, storage and regulation. At least three surfactants have been identified (SP-A, SP-B, SP-C). Glucocorticoids are advocated in conditions where surfactant may be expected to be deficient, but it appears that glucocorticoids both stimulate and inhibit the synthesis of SP-A while only stimulating SP-B and SP-C. This leads to the possibility that prolonged treatment with glucocorticoids may lead to deficiency in SP-A.

Endocrine function

The lungs have a non-respiratory metabolic function, including the metabolism of vasoactive hormones. Hietanen et al (1988) found the plasma concentrations of adrenaline and angiotensin II were reduced in patients who have undergone resection of the lung, or those with obstructive or fibrotic lung disorders. There was an inverse relationship between post-exercise renin levels and the size of the total pulmonary vascular bed.

It is often forgotten that the lung has a large endothelial surface and receives the whole of the cardiac output. The lung is capable of metabolizing 5-hydroxytryptamine (5-HT), noradrenaline and prosta-glandins. Other compounds metabolized in the lung include enkephalins, vasoactive intestinal peptide (VIP), ATP, ADP, adenosine, atrial natriuretic peptide (ANP), insulin, progesterone, prolactin and gluco-corticoids. Tricyclics inhibit the pulmonary 5-HT uptake (Camus & Jeannin 1988).

Smoking

The pharmacology of nicotine is discussed in detail by Benowitz (1988), outlining the mode and sites of action of the drug on the autonomic ganglia, the adrenal medulla, the neuromuscular junction and the brain. It has an action on mood, reducing tension and stress but increases cardiac output and causes peripheral vasoconstriction. It increases the circulating levels of catecholamines, vasopressin, growth hormone, ACTH, cortisol, prolactin, neurophysin I and beta-endorphin. The pH of cigarette smoke is alkaline, and nicotine being in an un-ionized state is readily absorbed through the mouth. The blood concentration rises rapidly as absorption from the small airways is quick irrespective of pH. Nicotine is rapidly metabolized in the liver, having a half-life of approximately 2 h. Smoking constitutes a major risk factor for patients with possible coronary artery or peripheral vascular disease and the progression of hypertension is accelerated. Although nicotine itself does not produce cancer, it forms nitrosonornicotine and related compounds which are carcinogenic. Smoking accelerates the metabolism of drugs such as lignocaine, propranolol and theophylline while by reducing the blood flow in superficial tissue, the absorption of insulin may be delayed. Antacids and H_2 blockers are less effective in smokers in the treatment of peptic ulcers.

There are possible dangers for non-smokers exposed to tobacco smoke which contains oxides of nitrogen, nicotine, carbon monoxide and possible carcinogens. It is estimated that non-smokers exposed to cigarette smoke inhale the equivalent of 0.1 to 1 cigarette a day. There have been reports of diminished lung function, chronic respiratory symptoms and malignancy as a result of involuntary smoking (Fielding & Phenow 1988). Studies on aircraft indicate that passengers in non-smoking areas are not effectively protected from circulating smoke as assessed by nasal and eye irritation and measurement of urinary cotinine levels (Mattson et al 1989). The effects of smoking on carboxyhaemoglobin have been studied by Kirkham et al

(1988), indicating that smoking produces acute changes in ventilation/perfusion.

Smoking as a major cause of post-operative pulmonary complications has been discussed by Jones (1984). Patients should be discouraged from smoking even for 24 h before operation to reduce the level of carboxyhaemoglobin. Studies on those who inhaled smoke from fires revealed an increase in polymorphonuclear leucocytes and macrophages on bronchoalveolar lavage, suggesting that lung damage occurs from the excess release of inflammatory mediators which readily become exhausted and are unable to combat infection (Clark et al 1988). These changes may also occur in response to chronic exposure to cigarette smoke.

Diaphragmatic weakness

Dyspnoea or orthopnoea is a symptom of diaphragmatic weakness or even paralysis. Lung function tests and reduction of maximal inspiratory pressure may reveal restrictive disease. Fluoroscopy may show an elevation of the diaphragm or paradoxical movement. The causes of diaphragmatic weakness or paralysis range from: lesions of the cervical spinal cord or anterior horn cells; neuropathy of the phrenic nerves which may be metabolic, endocrine, toxic or viral; neuromuscular—myasthenia gravis, Lambeth–Eaton syndrome; and myopathies and chest wall abnormalities such as kyphoscoliosis, ankylosing spondylitis. Often the diagnosis is made from biopsy from non-respiratory muscles or nerves, assuming that the abnormality is in the diaphragm (Wilcox & Pardy 1989). The measurements of transdiaphragmatic pressures in response to transcutaneous phrenic nerve stimulation are only of value when the weakness of the diaphragm is severe (Mier et al 1989). In patients with chronic interstitial lung disease, there is reduced inspiratory muscle strength but the neural component of respiration is normal or even increased (Gorini et al 1989).

Breathlessness

The assessment of breathlessness has been reviewed by Cockcroft et al (1989) who attempted to quantify the disability. It is an important symptom of many diseases and the diagnosis of cardiac or respiratory aetiology can still be confusing. Pulmonary function tests may be necessary to differentiate between the two (Staats 1988). Hyperventilation may occur during panic attacks, but the diagnosis may only be confirmed by constant monitoring such as the use of a transcutaneous carbon dioxide sensor (Hibbert & Pilsbury 1988).

Hypercapnia

It has been postulated that ventilatory response to CO_2 differs during rapid eye movement (REM) sleep compared with slow wave sleep, but this has not been confirmed in normal man by Warley et al (1989). The role of abdominal muscles, especially the transverse abdominis has been considered by Arnold et al (1988). They have shown that during hypercapnia the muscle shortens below resting length and during occluded breath it lengthens. This is important probably because expiration is calculated to improve ventilation. During hyperoxia, elimination of excess CO_2 is probably by the effects on blood flow to the brain and also by sensitivity of central chemoreceptors (Chonan et al 1988). The effects of hypercapnia on respiration, acid–base balance, central nervous system and the cardiovascular system are discussed by Weinberger et al (1989).

Disease and lung function

Inflammatory bowel disease

Disorders of pulmonary function occur in patients with inflammatory bowel disease. Bonniere et al (1986) demonstrated that a high proportion of patients had an increased physiological dead space in the upper part of the lung and also showed increased lymphocytes on bronchoalveolar lavage. Heatley et al (1982) noted that 50% of patients with inflammatory bowel disease had reduced pulmonary function while Patwardhan et al (1983) reported three cases of pleuropericarditis. Simple tests of lung function may fail to reveal any abnormality, although recently Wilcox et al (1987) reported two cases with ulcerative colitis, one of whom developed sclerosing peribronchiolitis and the other demonstrated fibrotic obliterative bronchitis affecting the large airways.

It has been claimed that there is no apparent relationship between changes in the lung and those in the bowel, and in fact pulmonary complications have been reported even following colectomy. Recent studies have examined these claims more fully and it was found that reduced gas transfer factor was not related to the severity of the disease. However, increased functional residual capacity and residual volume were associated with active inflammatory bowel disorders and these return to normal during remission (Douglas et al 1989).

Huntington's chorea

It might be expected that there would be significant alterations of respiration in Huntington's chorea due to the choreiform movements of the respiratory muscles. Bollen et al (1988) showed that during sleep, there was no difference between patients affected with the disease and the controls. Although there have been reports of apnoea following the induction of anaesthesia with thiopentone, central mechanisms affecting the respiration appear to be intact.

Pregnancy

In the last few months of pregnancy the functional residual capacity (FRC), expiratory reserve and residual volume decrease, although the total lung capacity is unchanged. The closing volume increases and may even exceed the FRC, resulting in mild hypoxaemia. Tenholder & South-Paul (1989) have discussed the causes of dyspnoea in pregnancy and the possibility that drugs used in the medical management may cross the placental barrier (the critical molecular weight is 1000 daltons). They also outline some specific syndromes which cause apnoea and which complicate pregnancy. These include alpha$_1$-antitrypsin deficiency, cystic fibrosis, sarcoidosis, pulmonary hypertension and also pulmonary thromboembolism which may require treatment with heparin which does not cross the placental barrier. The use of oral anticoagulants is more hazardous and should be discontinued by the 37th week, and in fact not given to the nursing mother. Other possible causes of dyspnoea are amniotic fluid embolism and post-partum pleural effusions. Patients with asthma are improved during pregnancy (Juniper et al 1989).

Parkinson's disease

It had been assumed that in Parkinson's disease, tremor and rigidity were responsible for the diminished pulmonary function. Maximal expiratory and inspiratory flow volumes are sensitive indicators of upper airway obstruction, and Bogaard et al (1989) have confirmed that reduced pulmonary function is associated with upper airway obstruction. The expiratory and inspiratory volumes may also be affected by incoordination or weakness of the respiratory muscles.

Kyphoscoliosis

In kyphoscoliosis, lung volumes are decreased and the respiratory elastance is increased, resulting in rapid and shallow respiration. Patients are able to compensate for the increased elastic load during anaesthesia in a manner similar to that of normal adults (Baydur et al 1989).

Ankylosing spondylitis

Patients with ankylosing spondylitis exhibit a marked reduction of vital capacity without any evidence of air flow obstruction. This is probably due to the rigidity and reduced expansion of the thorax, with compensatory action of the diaphragm. There is also a reduction in maximal trans-respiratory pressure, indicating a decrease in respiratory muscle strength (Vanderschueren et al 1989).

Quadriplegia

Lung compliance was reduced both in acute and chronic quadriplegia, probably due to the decrease in lung volume and also the altered mechanics of the lung. There was a marked distortion of configuration of the abdomen and rib cage during deep inspiration, especially in acute quadriplegia. In the chronic condition, respiratory function is less affected because more use is made of the accessory muscles of respiration. The reduction of ventilation is not necessarily due to muscle paralysis but due to the decreased compliance of the lung and distortion of the chest wall (Scanlon et al 1989). Coughing can still occur as a result of contraction of the clavicular portion of the pectoralis major muscles (Estenne & De Troyer 1990).

Air hunger may develop in mechanically ventilated quadriplegics when the end-tidal P_{CO_2} increases by 10 mmHg above resting levels, probably due to an increase in chemoreceptor afferent stimulation to the sensory cortex as well as the increased discharge from respiratory motor centres (Banzett et al 1989).

Myasthenia gravis

Myasthenia gravis is characterized by weakness and fatigue of the voluntary muscles which may also result in respiratory weakness. Mier-Jedrzejowicz et al (1988) found that there was weakness in the expiratory and inspiratory muscles which readily responded to edrophonium. Vital capacity was not a sensitive indicator of muscle weakness. The more sensitive tests were respiratory mouth pressure and transdiaphragmatic pressure during maximal sniffs but even in the latter, it did not detect diaphragmatic weakness unless it was marked. Peripheral muscle weakness such as that of the quadriceps did not necessarily reflect that of respiratory muscles; the latter were often only mildly affected despite profound respiratory muscle weakness. Although tests are being devised to quantify the tests for respiratory muscle strength, it has been proved more difficult to assess respiratory muscle fatigue which may be a feature in myasthenia gravis (Laroche et al 1989).

Muscular dystrophy

Studies on patients with Duchenne muscular dystrophy showed that they had normal blood gas values when awake. In 50% of the patients, apnoea and hypopnoea occurred with steep falls in oxygen saturation which appeared to be correlated with functional residual capacity (Manni et al 1989). Hypoxaemia occurred during REM sleep and this responded to the inhalation of oxygen, but the use of oxygen therapy for long term treatment still remains to be determined (Smith et al 1989a).

Achondroplasia (dwarfism)

Achondroplasia (dwarfism) is associated with apnoea, tachypnoea, excessive snoring, cor pulmonale and recurrent pneumonia. This has been ascribed to brain stem compression and there was a distinct improvement following craniotomy (Nelson et al 1988).

Hepatic cirrhosis

There have been many studies performed to determine the cause of hypoxaemia in hepatic cirrhosis including hypoxic pulmonary vaso-constriction; however, Melot et al (1989) concluded that hypoxaemia was due to ventilation–perfusion mismatch, and there was no abnormal pulmonary vascular response to hypoxia. Nevertheless, Edell et al (1989) concluded that not only was there mismatching, there was also an increased right-to-left shunt and a possibility of impairment of diffusion.

Coronary artery surgery

Following coronary artery surgery, hypoxaemia can develop and is associated with restriction of ventilation. Reduction of vital capacity, total lung capacity and inspiratory capacity were greater in patients who had an internal mammary artery graft as opposed to a saphenous vein graft. This has been ascribed to the fact that greater trauma results from placing the arterial graft and together with the pleural drain, there is increased pain which may restrict respiratory movement. Excessive analgesia also reduces respiratory function (Jenkins et al 1989).

Pectus excavatum (funnel chest)

Surgical correction of funnel chest is performed for psychological and cosmetic reasons, and it has been assumed that this would be accompanied by improved lung function to increase the anteroposterior chest diameter. However, Derveaux et al (1988) found that following surgery the vital capacity, FEV_1, transpulmonary and transdiaphragmatic pressures were all reduced. The reduction of lung function was due to the extensive surgery on the sternum and the parasternal areas, which involved resection of several rib cartilages, sternophrenolysis and dividing the intercostal muscles in the parasternal area.

Cor pulmonale

In a study of pulmonary vasculature of patients with hypoxic cor pulmonale, there were changes in the intima of the pulmonary arteries including fibrosis and elastosis. There were also changes in the arterioles which were diagnostic of obstructive airway disease. There was no correlation between the pathological findings and the changes in arterial blood gases, pulmonary artery pressure or haematocrit. There was no difference in the outcome whether patients were treated with oxygen or not (Wilkinson et al 1988). There is a need to reexamine the use of continuous oxygen in patients with pulmonary hypertension (Leading article, Lancet 1988b). Abnormal flow patterns are seen in the jugular venous system in pulmonary hypertension due to increased diastolic flow velocity and decreased systolic flow velocity (Ranganathan & Sivaciyan 1989). Patients with chronic bronchitis, emphysema, chronic asthma, fibrosing alveolitis or kyphoscoliosis are all likely to develop pulmonary hypertension. The use of vasodilators has been surprisingly disappointing, although theoretically ACE inhibitors might be effective. Investigations should include assessment of pulmonary haemodynamics and also sleep studies to see whether patients develop nocturnal hypoxia (Peacock 1990). Nifedipine lowered the pulmonary artery pressure in animal experiments, but proved disappointing in clinical practice (Mookherjee et al 1988). Even in systemic hypertension, the pulmonary vessels are hyper-reactive in response to adrenoreceptor stimulation and hypoxia (Guazzi et al 1989).

Cystic fibrosis

In patients with cystic fibrosis, there is a decrease in the rate of water transport through mucosal tissue. They may have problems in inhaling dry air through the mouth which will require the greatest degree of humidification. Although cold air requires less humidification, the availability of water is also reduced. Drying of the mucosa leads to airway irritation with reduced ciliary activity (Primiano et al 1988).

Sarcoidosis

Sarcoidosis affects not only the interstitial tissue of the lung, but may cause obstruction of both the large and small airways. Pulmonary hypertension is known to occur and it has been suggested that diffusion is limited because of thickening of the alveolar wall. Despite being a restrictive as well as an obstructive lung disease, it also showed increased pulmonary vascular resistance and reduced transfer factor. The degree of mismatch of ventilation and perfusion were not marked. However, the difference between calculated and measured Pao_2 indicated a marked diffusion defect, at rest and during exercise (Eklund et al 1989).

Sepsis

Endotoxic shock is a recognized cause of adult respiratory distress syndrome (see Barrowcliffe & Jones 1988). The inhalation of endotoxin decreased gas transfer factor (Rylander et al 1989). In animal studies,

Boczkowski et al (1988) have shown that acute sepsis decreases diaphragmatic strength by affecting contractility as well as reducing its endurance capacity.

Obesity

Although obesity affects the mechanics of respiration, there have been conflicting reports of the effects of overweight on vital capacity or total lung capacity. Surprisingly, obese patients do not have increased maximal respiratory pressures to overcome the restrictions from the weight of the chest wall and reduced compliance (Kelly et al 1988). Patients who had surgical procedures such as banded gastroplasty for refractory obesity, lost weight following the operation which was accompanied by an increase in total lung capacity, expiratory reserve volume and gaseous exchange (Thomas et al 1989).

Drugs and lung function

Theophylline is known to improve diaphragmatic fatigue, especially in patients with chronic obstructive airway disease (Murciano et al 1984, 1989). However, in the doses used it does not appear to increase skeletal muscle strength including the muscles of respiration (Brophy et al 1989). It also increases peripheral ventilation as reflected in the reduction in the volume of trapped gas (Chrystyn et al 1988). However, in the elderly, the renal and metabolic elimination of theophylline is reduced (Shin et al 1988). Pretreatment with aminophylline reduces central depression of ventilation induced by hypoxia, but has little effect on the hyperventilation produced by hyperoxia (Georgopoulos et al 1989, see also Addis 1990, Johnston 1990).

   Diaphragmatic function is surprisingly also improved following an infusion of dopamine, presumably by improving the blood flow to the diaphragm (Aubier et al 1989). Doxapram also improves ventilation centrally by increasing the neuromuscular drive (Okubo et al 1988).

   Diazepam is known to have a central respiratory depressant action in patients with chronic obstructive pulmonary disorders (COPD). Beaupre et al (1988) found that even a single oral dose of 10 mg diazepam resulted in respiratory depression, an effect not seen with zopiclone, a non-benzodiazepine sedative. Nitrazepam or flunitrazepam does not affect oxygenation during sleep in patients on maintenance doses of theophylline (Midgren et al 1989).

Peri-operative pulmonary complications

Respiratory mechanics and the effects of anaesthesia on respiration as well as some other aspects of lung function are discussed in a symposium on the lung (edited by Hull & Jones 1990). Pre-operative evaluation of pulmonary function is discussed in detail by Jackson (1988) with consideration given to factors such as site of surgical incision, pre-existing pulmonary disease, duration of operation, history of smoking and obesity. Pre-operative hypercapnia was considered to be a major hazard. In evaluating patients for lung resection, factors considered to be high risk were as follows: a predicted post-operative FEV_1 less than 1000 ml; severe dyspnoea on exertion and age. Advice is also given regarding the prevention of post-operative pulmonary complications in patients with COPD, including regimes involving chest physiotherapy, bronchodilators, antibiotics, deep breathing manoeuvres and the discontinuing of smoking. The incidence of pulmonary complications was not influenced by the type of anaesthesia, whether it was general or spinal.

Prediction of post-operative respiratory failure in patients undergoing resection for lung cancer was also considered by Nakahara et al (1988). They found that all patients with post-operative $FEV_1 < 30\%$ of predicted, required mechanical ventilation. Markos et al (1989) accepted that a figure of 40% of predicted produced no post-operative mortality but it was felt that below that, the mortality was 50%. It should be noted that during thoracotomy involving one-lung ventilation in the lateral position, end-tidal PCO_2, CO_2 elimination and compliance of the operated side were significantly decreased at the end of the operation (Malmkvist et al 1989).

Vodinh et al (1989) assessed the value of pre-operative lung function tests to predict post-operative pulmonary complications following vascular surgery, when COPD and coronary heart disease are not uncommon. The incidence of PRC (post-operative respiratory complications) was 53% in patients undergoing abdominal aortic surgery. The only risk factors that could be identified were decreases in pre-operative FEV_1/VC and PaO_2. Surprisingly smoking did not appear to affect the outcome while the ASA classification was unable to identify the patients at risk. In contrast to accepted views, Poe et al (1988) indicated that the maximum expiratory flow volume curve and single-breath nitrogen test were significant predictors of post-operative pulmonary complications, but were not specific enough to indicate whether intensive physiotherapy would prevent pulmonary complications. A reduction in FVC was the only indicator of prolonged hospitalization. They found that smoking, old age and obesity carried no additional risk of developing post-operative complications. Despite previous claims that adequate pain relief following abdominal surgery would reduce pulmonary complications, Jayr et al (1988) found that epidural analgesia with bupivacaine and morphine improved patients' comfort, but the post-operative PaO_2 and spirometric studies were similar to the control group given general anaesthesia with post-operative parenteral morphine.

Schwieger et al (1989) have reviewed lung function during anaesthesia and respiratory problems in the post-operative period. They considered changes in lung function due to anaesthesia and surgery, noting that upper abdominal surgery reduced functional residual capacity to 70% of pre-operative levels for up to one week. There were also alterations in the ventilation/perfusion ratio, and alterations in pulmonary gas exchange. Post-operative hypoxaemia may be due to hyperventilation, shunting of blood, reduced cardiac output and increased oxygen consumption due to shivering. The mechanisms leading to post-operative respiratory failure were decreased alveolar ventilation, atelectasis and interstitial lung oedema. When it is impossible to measure mixed venous oxygen, Zetterstrom (1988) has advocated the use of an estimate of venous admixture derived from arterial blood analysis and with the arterio-venous oxygen content difference given a value of 50 ml/l. The ratio of Pao_2 and the inspired oxygen concentration was also a useful index.

Jones et al (1990) confirmed that post-operative hypoxaemia results from impaired gaseous exchange during anaesthesia and in the post-operative period. This is probably due to reduced tone in the muscles of the chest wall and bronchi as well as changes in vasomotor tone. In addition, there are episodic periods of obstructive apnoea which may be related to sleep pattern and analgesia. There is an early phase of post-operative hypoxaemia due to sedation and also a late phase which may last for a week and is associated with a reduction of the functional residual capacity (FRC).

Gas exchange during anaesthesia is also discussed by Hedenstierna (1990) who agreed that perfusion of blood through the atelectatic zone is the major cause of impaired gaseous exchange. The reasons for atelectasis are still unknown and are less prominent during ketamine anaesthesia. Wheatley et al (1990) demonstrated the high incidence of post-operative hypoxaemia using pulse oximetry following lower abdominal surgery, and this was particularly noticeable in patients with extradural diamorphine. Pre-operative monitoring may predict the risk of patients developing post-operative hypoxaemia.

Selsby & Jones (1990) discussed the relative merits of techniques of chest physiotherapy to reduce post-operative pulmonary complications. The 'forced expiratory technique' with postural drainage was superior to both coughing and postural drainage with percussion and vibration (PDPV); this however may produce bronchospasm and hypoxaemia in some patients (Selsby & Jones 1990).

Compensatory growth of lung occurs following pneumonectomy, and this process appears to be associated with hyperplasia as opposed to hypertrophy. Evidence for this is based on pulmonary function studies, the results of which are still incomplete (Cagle & Thurlbeck 1988). Measurement of gas tensions in the pneumonectomy space has been undertaken by Simonsen et al (1989), who showed that the equilibrium difference between arterial Po_2 and the pneumonectomy space Po_2 was a sensitive method of detecting bronchopleural fistula.

The infusion of doxapram 2 mg/min in saline for 6 h in the immediate post-operative period and repeated the next day led to a significant reduction of post-operative pulmonary complications, and an increase in Pao_2 level (Jansen et al 1990).

Sleep apnoea syndrome (SAS)

The sleep apnoea syndrome (SAS) was reviewed in detail by Partridge in *Review 2* (1984). Sleep apnoea was defined by Guilleminault et al (1978) as an absence of air flow at the nose and mouth lasting for at least 10 s, and occurring more than 30 times during a 'seven-hour sleep'.

Sleep apnoea may be divided into three groups: obstructive, central and mixed (obstructive and central). In the obstructive group, air flow ceases but there are still abdominal and thoracic inspiratory movements. In the central group, air flow ceases and there are no respiratory efforts. In the mixed group, there are both obstructive and central components. Since the review by Partridge (1984), there have been repeated references to some of the problems which occur such as cardiac arrhythmias and even cardiac arrest. It is said to be associated with obesity, hypertension and even the intermittent hypoxia during sleep may lead to polycythaemia. Anaesthetists should be aware that patients with SAS are at risk if sedated, or given total intravenous anaesthesia without attempting to ensure that the airway is secure. The clinical features of SAS have been summarized by Whyte et al (1989) in a review of 80 patients. Snoring and somnolence were features at least once a day when the subjects were not in bed. Ten reported falling asleep whilst flying or driving. Restless sleep was also a feature while a quarter of patients had nocturnal choking attacks. More than a quarter of subjects had ankle swelling or were hypertensive. Golding-Wood et al (1990) reported the difficulty of identifying simple snorers or those likely to develop SAS. They advocated the correction of possible nasal obstruction, reduction in weight and less consumption of alcohol.

During sleep there is an increase in upper airway resistance, and also marked activity of the genioglossus, especially during hypoxaemia. Despite the increased sub-atmospheric pressure created by the diaphragm, the patency of the pharynx is maintained by the genioglossus (Parisi et al 1988). Thus imbalance between the factors which constrict the upper airway such as negative pressure generated by the diaphragm, and dilatation of the upper airway due to the genioglossus may lead to SAS, especially during REM sleep (Issa et al 1988). This view is confirmed by Smith et al (1988) who concluded that the upper airway is like a Starling resistor with a collapsible segment. However, Hudgel & Hendricks (1988) considered the site of narrowing in the upper airway during sleep was at the level of palate or hypopharynx. The narrowest section of the pharyngeal airspace was in the region posterior to the soft palate and this was the site of the obstruction (Horner et al 1989). There may be a critical occlusion pressure when the nasal pressure is below this level (Schwartz et al 1988). Pharyngeal tone may depend on sensitive information arising from receptors in the pharynx and larynx, as studies have shown that when local anaesthesia is applied to the pharynx and glottis, the pharyngeal patency is reduced (DeWeese & Sullivan 1988). Hudgel et al (1988) re-affirmed that the limitation of flow in the upper airway was within the pharynx and not in the nose. Flow rate in the upper airway may differ when the patients are awake and is not necessarily indicative of events during sleep. In fact there is a marked variation in the ability of the upper airway to collapse during sleep (Wiegand et al 1989). Glottic movements during quiet respiration may affect functional abnormalities in pulmonary disorders (Yanai et al 1989), while the cross-sectional area of the glottis is reduced in SAS (the obstructive type), especially in man (Rubinstein et al 1989).

Griggs et al (1989) have demonstrated that there was impaired contractility of the respiratory muscles. Excessive daytime somnolence, a feature of SAS, is thought to be due to disturbed sleep and not to hypoxaemia (Roehrs et al 1989). Series et al (1989a) found that the patency of the pharynx was more sensitive to the decrease of central respiratory drive. Abnormal speech may help to identify the SAS patients (Fox et al 1989). The awake hypoxic ventilatory drive is inversely related to the degree of oxygen saturation during sleep, but this does not apply to the hypercapnic ventilatory drive (Kunitomo et al 1989). Lung volume influences the period of apnoea and the resulting oxygen desaturation (Series et al 1989b). If the lung volume is increased, the period of apnoea is prolonged (Hamilton et al 1988). The less the lung volume, the greater the oxygen saturation falls during apnoea. The mixed venous oxygen saturation plays a substantial part in determining the fall of arterial oxygen saturation (Fletcher et al 1989). A rapid fall in cardiac output may decrease uptake from the lung oxygen stores, leading to a fall in oxygen saturation while in a situation of chronic reduced cardiac output, the rate of desaturation will increase during apnoea (Findley 1989).

Despite the high incidence of cardiac arrhythmias with sleep apnoea, Gonzalez-Rothi et al (1988) were unable to demonstrate polysomnographically (continuous oxygen saturation, oral and nasal air flows, abdominal chest wall movement, EEG, oculogram, ECG) the increased incidence of mortality compared with the control group. Those related to SAS had the highest incidence of car accidents presumably due to somnolence. On the other hand, He et al (1988) found that the mortality was greater in those patients with an apnoea index > 20 (apnoea index = the mean number of apnoeas per hour of sleep). None of the patients treated with tracheostomy or nasal continuous positive airway pressure (CPAP) died. In patients with mild to moderate obstructive apnoea undergoing surgery to improve the upper airway, many have reported subjective improvements which were not necessarily confirmed by polysomnography (Regestein et al 1988).

During sleep there is a biphasic ventilatory response which increases initially and is followed by marked depression under mild hypoxic conditions (Chin et al 1989). In congestive heart failure an abnormal pattern of sleep occurs (Cheyne–Stokes respiration) even during light sleep, despite the fact that oxygen saturation is normal when patients are awake (Hanly et al 1989a). Hypertension may occur in obstructive sleep apnoea patients (Partinen & Guilleminault 1990). Correction of the nocturnal hypoxaemia with oxygen therapy may reduce the incidence of Cheyne–Stokes respiration (Hanly et al 1989b); nasal continuous positive airway pressure is effective in patients with chronic congestive heart failure with sleep apnoea syndrome, resulting in reduction of dyspnoea and improvement in left ventricular function (Takasaki et al 1989). Patients with interstitial pulmonary disease who have insufficient ventilatory response to hypercapnia have marked falls in oxygen desaturation during sleep (Tatsumi et al 1989). Nasal obstruction leads to reduced $P\text{CO}_2$ during sleep (Tanaka & Honda 1989). SAS may be associated with other medical disorders, e.g. chronic uraemia, but the symptoms resolve in response to weight loss and haemodialysis (Tardif et al 1988).

Stradling & Warley (1988) described the bilateral diaphragmatic paralysis resulting in hypoxaemia and hypercapnia during REM sleep but not initially during the day, suggesting that REM sleep factor initiates hypoventilation and apnoea.

There is a possible link with hypertension, although the results may be influenced by complex interactions involving chemical, mechanical and autonomic responses (Coccagna et al 1988). Despite the fact that there are theoretical grounds for a possible relationship between sleep apnoea and systemic hypertension, Stradling (1989) felt that the link was tenuous. In the obstructive type, pulmonary hypertension, hypoxaemia and hypercapnia may develop even during the day (Krieger et al 1989a).

SAS causes reversible decreased levels of plasma insulin-like growth factor, testosterone and sex hormone-binding globulin (Grunstein et al 1989). These hormone levels may be suitable markers of the severity of the disease, as they are closely related to the levels of arterial oxygen desaturation.

Sleep loss is not uncommon in respiratory disease and even in normal adults prolonged sleep loss leads to a reduction in inspiratory muscle endurance, although the FEV_1 and FVC are unaffected (Chen & Tang 1989).

Treatment

Block (1988) commented on the place of drugs in the management of SAS. Progesterone (Provera) stimulates respiration but has little effect in SAS (obstructive). Protriptyline (Vivactil) reduces the amount of REM sleep while oxygen therapy is effective when there is desaturation. Acetazolamide

(Diamox) stimulates respiration by producing metabolic acidosis. There appears to be no place for the use of drugs such as strychnine, nicotine or almitrine. Effects of alcohol and benzodiazepines are deleterious in that they relax the pharyngeal musculature during sleep, accentuating the obstructive element.

Severe hypoxaemia reduces ATP levels with resultant increased adenosine production. Serum adenosine fell in patients who had been successfully treated (Findley et al 1988).

Nasal intermittent positive pressure ventilation (nCPAP) had little effect on spirometric studies, although exercise tolerance improved (Carroll & Branthwaite 1988). Better results were obtained by Aubert-Tulkens et al (1989) who combined nCPAP with weight loss. Plasma levels of ANP rise during acute hypoxia in normal subjects (Kawashima et al 1989) and it is also raised during sleep in obstructive sleep apnoea (OSA) and may reflect the increased loss of water, sodium and chloride. There is also an increase in potassium loss. However, these effects can be reduced by nCPAP, restoring the ANP secretion to normal (Krieger et al 1988, 1989b).

Asthma

Holgate & Finnerty (1988) have reviewed some of the factors explaining the pathogenesis and clinical implications of asthma. The disease is characterized by reversible limitation of air flow. It may be subdivided into extrinsic and intrinsic categories, depending on whether there is an external precipitating factor. The bronchi are hyper-responsive and there is a possible inter-relationship between inhalants and the environmental factors that produce attacks. The early reaction in asthma involves the activation of mast cells which release histamine, and also mobilize arachidonic acid leading to prostaglandins and leukotrienes. The later reaction is also described, with limitation of air flow which is difficult to reverse with beta-2 adrenoceptor agonists.

The eicosanoids and airway smooth muscle is discussed in more detail by Gardiner (1989). The 'eicosanoids' include the prostanoids comprising prostaglandins and thromboxane TXA_2 (produced by the enzyme cyclo-oxygenase), and the leukotrienes (produced by 5-lipoxygenase). The prostanoids and the leukotrienes are not stored but are synthesized in response to the appropriate stimulus. The prostanoids are capable of producing bronchodilatation or bronchoconstriction, and were at one time thought to have a physiological role in maintaining the tone of the bronchi. However, the leukotrienes always cause bronchoconstriction. Another factor is the phospholipid mediator, platelet activating factor (PAF) which may be responsible for bronchoconstriction, hyper-responsiveness and inflammation. PAF, which can readily produce features of bronchial asthma has led to the search for antagonists; BN 52063, a PAF antagonist, does not have any beneficial effects on pulmonary function but does provide some relief from exercise-induced bronchoconstriction (Wilkens et al 1990). Other PAF antagonists are being developed which so far have been shown only to affect the skin responses to allergens (Chung & Barnes 1988). Human mast cells are resistant to endogenous opioid peptides and substance P (Miadonna et al 1988).

Nocturnal asthma may have a vagal component as it can be reversed with intravenous atropine ($30\,\mu g/kg$) (Morrison et al 1988). Aspirin and other non-steroidal anti-inflammatory drugs may precipitate attacks of asthma (Picado et al 1989). Inhaled naloxone has little effect on resting bronchial muscle tone, but modulates bronchoconstriction induced by exercise in asthmatic patients. It has been suggested that this is due to antagonism of the endogenous opioids released during exercise (Popa & Rients 1989). Surprisingly, inhaled frusemide also appears to be effective against bronchoconstrictor challenge (Bianco et al 1989). Asthmatics have a higher incidence of gastro-oesophageal reflux, but there is no evidence suggesting possible inhalation precipitated wheezing (Nagel et al 1988).

Asthma continues to be a major respiratory disorder and it appears that the severity, prevalence, morbidity and mortality are on the increase. There are inflammatory changes in the airways, with infiltration of eosinophils and lymphocytes. The bronchi are hyper-responsive to different stimuli resulting in bronchoconstriction. The mast cells release histamine but it is of interest that although beta-adrenergic agonists stabilize these cells, they have little effect on bronchial irritability. Steroids have little effect on mast cells but inhibit bronchial irritability. The macrophages may be involved in the late response to allergens and these are again inhibited by steroids but not by beta-adrenergic agonists. It has been suggested that asthma is a chronic inflammatory disorder with eosinophilic bronchitis. Beta-adrenergic agonists and theophylline have no effect on eosinophils, although steroids are effective. Prostaglandin D_2 and leukotrienes increase bronchial irritability leading to bronchoconstriction, leakage of protein in the small vessels and mucous secretion. PAF increases the number of eosinophils in the lung adhering to the vascular endothelium. Acetylcholine causes bronchoconstriction while the neuropeptides such as substance P and neurokinin are also bronchoconstrictors.

Beta-adrenergic agonists and theophylline inhibit the leakage of fluid in the small vessels, although the former does stabilize the mast cells. Beta-2 adrenergic receptors activate adenylate cyclase leading to increased cyclic AMP. They have little effect on the late response to allergens and the subsequent bronchial irritability. Acute exacerbations of asthma can be treated by inhalation of beta-adrenergic agonists. Theophylline acts by inhibiting the production of phosphodiesterase, allowing cyclic AMP to increase. It does inhibit the late response to allergens. The side effects include cardiac arrhythmias.

Anticholinergic agents such as ipratropium inhibit muscarinic receptors in the airways, resulting in bronchodilatation. They have little effect on the mast cells and are usually given in combination with a beta-adrenergic agonist.

The mode of action of steroids is still unknown. Although they have little effect on mast cells, they inhibit the release of possible allergens from macrophages and eosinophils. They are effective if given by inhalation and reduce microvascular leakage.

The mechanism of the use of sodium cromoglycate is still uncertain, but it inhibits the late response and bronchial hyper-irritability. There is little effect, not as originally thought, on the mast cells. The antihistamines have been singularly disappointing (see Barnes 1989).

The management of acute asthma is considered by Cottam & Eason (Ch. 3).

Chronic obstructive pulmonary disease (COPD)

Patients with chronic obstructive pulmonary disease are likely to develop respiratory failure, even without being subjected to sedation or anaesthesia. Response to exercise is often used as a guide to the extent of disability. However, Ries et al (1988) found that spirometry and carbon monoxide diffusing capacity were unreliable indicators in identifying patients who were likely to develop exercise-induced hypoxaemia. The technique of measurement may influence the response of transfer factor of salbutamol in patients with COPD (Chinn et al 1988). Two-thirds of the patients with COPD developed metabolic acidosis during exercise which may contribute to dyspnoea. Sue et al (1988) suggested that these patients may benefit from exercise training. Hypoxaemia can develop during air travel in patients with COPD, and preflight ground levels of Pao_2 and FEV_1 may predict which patient will develop hypoxaemia when exposed to hypobaric conditions during flight (Dillard et al 1989).

During REM sleep, the 'blue bloaters' develop hypoxaemia which may be due to irregular ventilation. There may be a rise in pulmonary arterial pressure and cardiac irregularities. Secondary polycythaemia may also develop. These patients require oxygen at night, and also the use of almitrine which stimulates respiration via the carotid body (Flenley 1988). The patients with a high arterial Pco_2 and reduced functional residual capacity develop oxygen desaturation during REM sleep (Manni et al 1988).

Patients with COPD are advised not to smoke, but the evidence for this advice being beneficial is controversial. Significant falls in peak expiratory flow rate were reduced in smokers and previous heavy smokers, but were much less in those who had advanced chronic bronchitis or emphysema suggesting that other factors are involved in the development of COPD (Nunn & Gregg 1989, Gregg & Nunn 1989).

Beta-agonists and ipratropium have been used in therapy but steroids appear to be effective in some patients, although given by inhalation they are of little value. Antibiotic therapy reduces sputum volume and infection. Cor pulmonale is treated with diuretics and oxygen, and digoxin only when there are signs of left ventricular failure (Anthonisen 1988). Steroids may in fact slow down the progression of the disease (Postma et al 1988, see also Clague & Calverley 1990). Salbutamol also improves the distribution of ventilation to the lung bases (Bell et al 1988). Verapamil may have a place in reducing pulmonary vascular resistance which is often increased due to the concomitant hypoxaemia. It remains to be seen whether this drug will be of any value in the treatment of acute hypoxic pulmonary vasoconstriction and exacerbation of COPD (Treacher et al 1987).

Respiratory failure

The detailed management of respiratory insufficiency following thoracic trauma has been outlined by Pepe (1989), indicating the needs for mechanical ventilation. Severely injured patients are also at risk of developing ARDS, the criteria of which have recently been re-appraised (Rocker et al 1989). A useful marker may be the elastase-complex levels which are related to capillary permeability. Increased levels of hydrogen peroxide can be detected in the expired breath of patients with ARDS, suggesting that oxygen metabolites may contribute to the development of the condition (Sznajder et al 1989, see also Barnard et al 1989). The value of mixed venous oxygen tension results in critically ill patients may be limited in the presence of peripheral oxygen shunting (Carlile & Gray 1989). In hypoxaemia, venous oxygen tension is not a reliable indicator of tissue oxygenation (Gutierrez et al 1989).

The decision of when to ventilate seriously ill patients with ARDS is debatable but the treatment may carry its own hazards and complications. Pingleton (1988) has extensively reviewed the complications of acute respiratory failure and these are briefly listed as follows:

1. Pulmonary complications—emboli, barotrauma (pneumothorax, tension pneumothorax, mediastinal emphysema) and fibrosis. Pulmonary emboli should be suspected when there is an increased $P(A–a)o_2$ gradient and hypocapnia (Cvitanic & Marino 1989). Systemic gas embolism may be more frequent than previously imagined and may be detected by disturbances in heart rhythm, mental status, seizures, hypotension and localized pain (Marini & Culver 1989).

2. Hazards associated with ventilation and monitoring—insertion of a pulmonary artery catheter may result in pneumothorax, air embolism, arrhythmias, rupture of the vessels, infection or thrombosis. Hazards of intubation include bronchial intubation, pneumothorax, tracheal injury; the use of a ventilator may provoke infection as well as many of the problems associated with disconnection and problems of weaning.

3. Gastrointestinal complications may lead to pneumoperitoneum, changes in gastrointestinal activity and gastrointestinal haemorrhage.

4. Cardiovascular complications include alterations in haemodynamics and arrhythmias.

5. Renal problems include acute renal failure and the failure to maintain proper fluid balance.

6. Infections—these include nosocomial pneumonia and bacteraemia.

7. Nutritional complications include malnutrition and hypercapnia as a result of intravenous elementation.

Transtracheal oxygen has been recommended for patients with chronic hypoxaemia, but this leads to a decrease in minute ventilation as the transtracheal flow increases (Couser & Make 1989). In acute hypoxia, insufflation of oxygen enriched air reduces dead space, tidal volume and minute ventilation without affecting the $Paco_2$; but in chronic hypoxaemia it may reduce $Paco_2$ due to reduction in dead space volume (Bergofsky & Hurewitz 1989). In the UK, it appears that there is only a small place for transtracheal oxygen (Leading article, Lancet 1988a). The use of a transtracheal catheter with a reservoir may be of value when an oxygen concentrator is used (Collard et al 1989), while Jackson et al (1990) have advocated the use of an implanted tunnelled catheter. The use of a pulsed oxygen delivery system, in contrast to continuous oxygen, appears to give satisfactory Pao_2 levels in patients with chronic respiratory disease (Senn et al 1989).

In man there is a biphasic ventilatory response to hypoxia. The initial change in ventilation is due to the effect on chemoreceptors. This effect may be activated by calcium while the late response, which might be central, could be influenced by serotonin acting as a neurotransmitter. However, methysergide and verapamil have little effects on the hypoxic responses (Long et al 1989).

Prolonged oxygen therapy

Prolonged oxygen therapy may result in oxygen toxicity and animal experiments have demonstrated the value of N-acetylcysteine (NAC). NAC affects pulmonary vascular resistance, arterial $Paco_2$, delays the development of V/Q abnormalities and reduces alveolar and interstitial oedema (Wagner et al 1989).

Artificial ventilation

Conventional mechanical ventilation is still the mainstay of providing artificial ventilation, although the introduction of high frequency ventilation is less clear. High frequency ventilation may be classified as high frequency positive pressure ventilation (HFPPV), high frequency jet ventilation (HFJV) and high frequency forced diffusion or oscillatory ventilation (HFOV). Much of the equipment available at the moment involves the use of HFJV. It is of use in laryngeal surgery, repairing of tracheal injury and also during thoracic surgery (see Mapleson et al 1989). The transport of gases appears to be related to pendelluft flow during HFOV (Ultman et al 1988). HFPPV and HFJV can maintain normal blood gases in the short term treatment of respiratory failure without any major differences in their action on cardiovascular system (Courtney et al 1989). Slutsky (1988, see also Guenard et al 1989) considers the place of 'unconventional' methods of ventilation in neonates with IRDS and in the management of bronchopleural fistula. There have been suggestions that positive end-expiratory pressure (PEEP) influences hormonal secretion such as AVP and recent studies have confirmed that ANF was reduced, both in conditions where cardiac function was normal and during left ventricular failure. Plasma ANF concentrations were related to transmural left ventricular end-diastolic pressure, and during PEEP ventilation atrial distension diminished reducing ANF release (Hevroy et al 1989). There is increased clearance of radiolabelled technetium in high surface tension pulmonary oedema in the newborn, and this effect is enhanced by both conventional and high frequency oscillation ventilation (Jefferies et al 1988). High elevation pulmonary oedema may be protected by the use of PEEP (Dreyfuss et al 1988).

Auto-PEEP occurs when the alveolar pressure does not decrease to zero at the end of expiration, possibly due to airway closure or inadequate expiratory time. This can easily be measured in patients who are breathing spontaneously, and Hoffman et al (1989) advise the use of respiratory inductive plethysmography.

The problems of weaning patients from ventilators have been outlined by Browne (1988a, 1988b), indicating that not only should ventilatory failure be considered as a cause of respiratory problems, but cardiovascular, neurological and metabolic abnormalities may also contribute to the problem. Weaning may involve simple techniques such as disconnecting the patient from the ventilator and using a T-piece adaptor attached to a constant flow of oxygen enriched humidified air, to intermittent mandatory ventilation and mandatory volume ventilation. Gay et al (1989) were critical of CPAP or PEEP in weaning, although in patients with expiratory flow limitation it was possible to demonstrate hyperinflation with the application of PEEP. Weaning patients who are also being treated for left ventricular failure may require the use of a diuretic, otherwise they may suffer relapse (see Permutt 1988).

Thus weaning still requires clinical judgement. Murciano et al (1988) have shown that problems can still arise from respiratory muscle fatigue even though the arterial blood gas samples are satisfactory. They developed a technique by occluding the trachea for 0.1 s to assess the inspiratory muscular drive. The high occlusion pressure was associated with electromyographic evidence of diaphragmatic fatigue (also see Sassoon et al 1988). In patients on assisted ventilation, diaphragmatic activity was measured by

EMG continued after the ventilator had been triggered. This ceased when the ventilator-assisted volume approached the patient's spontaneous tidal volume, but even high flow rates may not rest the work of the diaphragm (Flick et al 1989).

Elliott et al (1990) have advocated the use of intermittent positive pressure ventilation through a well fitted nasal mask, and demonstrated that oxygen tension rose and carbon dioxide tension fell in patients with acute exacerbation of chronic respiratory disorders. There may also be a place for home mechanical ventilation, especially in patients with external hypoxaemia (Peters & Viggiano 1988).

DIABETES

There is a general consensus of opinion that diabetes is an autoimmune disorder in genetically susceptible patients. There appears to be an environmental stimulus, either viral or chemical leading to beta cell destruction. Mandrup-Poulsen (1988) has studied the cellular and humoral immune responses and found that the process is complex, in that it is unlikely that islet cell antibodies are responsible. Interleukin I, which is secreted by macrophages and natural killer cells, leads to the formation of intracellular free radicals, resulting in the destruction of beta cells. The control of blood sugar involves not only the pancreas, but also the adrenal medulla and liver. Insulin secreted by beta cells lowers blood sugar while glucagon secreted by the alpha cells increases blood sugar (see Niijima 1989). The role of activation of cyclic AMP phosphodiesterase is discussed by Smoake & Solomon (1989).

Somatostatin released by the D cells inhibits both insulin and glucagon, and may exert fine control on other pancreatic endocrine hormones. The use of somatostatin analogues in the treatment of diabetics has been disappointing, and is accompanied by adverse effects on the gastrointestinal tract such as diarrhoea (Osei et al 1989).

Diabetes may occur as a result of chronic pancreatitis in which there is decreased insulin secretion and also low glucagon levels. The response to insulin-induced hypoglycaemia is reduced, consequently hypoglycaemia may be less readily recognized. There are increased levels of amino acids, a decrease in insulin requirements and a resistance to ketosis. Care is required in maintaining blood glucose levels as chronic pancreatitis behaves like a brittle diabetic (Sjoberg & Kidd 1989).

Hypoglycaemia

Hypoglycaemia may occur in normal individuals and has been labelled as 'functional hypoglycaemia'. Hypoglycaemic symptoms occur but they are not necessarily related to the level of blood sugar which ranges from 3.7 mmol/l to 7.5 mmol/l. The accepted level of blood sugar for hypoglycaemia should be less than 2.8 mmol/l (Snorgaard & Binder 1990). In patients, with normal glucose tolerance and hyperinsulinaemia, there is an increased risk of coronary artery disease (Zavaroni et al 1989).

Treatment of hypoglycaemia which is said to occur in 3% of insulin treated patients may range from oral carbohydrate to intravenous dextrose. Glucagon 0.5 to 1 mg may also be administered. Animal studies suggest that there may be a place for the use of fructose 1-6 diphosphate (Farias et al 1989).

Insulin

There has been a move to transfer patients from porcine insulin to human insulin to avoid untoward allergic responses, but there are reports of an increased incidence of hypoglycaemia with patients being unaware of the complication, as the manifestations of hypoglycaemia are less or even absent. The potency of both types of insulin are identical although porcine insulin is more lipophilic. The sympathetic response to hypoglycaemia was more evident with porcine insulin, but there was no difference in neurological symptoms such as headache, dizziness, tiredness, anxiety and visual disturbances (Heine et al 1989). Gale (1989) concluded that there was no real evidence to support the view that hypoglycaemia was more common in patients on human insulin, or that it was responsible for the increase in sudden death in diabetics. However he indicated that unless there is a valid reason, patients should not be transferred from animal to human insulin.

The formulations of insulin have recently been outlined by MacPherson & Feely (1990) and were considered in *Anaesthesia Review 7* (Kaufman 1990, p. 26). They felt that the place for human insulin was only for the newly diagnosed patients, and for those who have developed lipoatrophy or allergy to insulin. When a change is necessary, the dose of human insulin should be reduced by 10% in those taking less than 0.9 U/kg and 25% in those on higher doses.

Antiglycaemic agents

The pharmacology of oral antiglycaemic agents is outlined by Gerich (1989), who showed that sulfonylureas stimulate the release of insulin by increasing the beta cell sensitivity to glucose, but they do not increase the synthesis of insulin. They may have extrapancreatic actions, and may also decrease plasma total cholesterol. Although sulfonylureas cause gastro-intestinal upsets, haemolytic anaemia and dermatitis have also been reported. The commonest cause of complications of oral antiglycaemic agents is hypoglycaemia.

Biguanides do not affect the stimulation of insulin secretion, but appear to act by reducing basal hepatic glucose production. Phenformin is no longer available because of the high incidence of lactic acidosis, although metformin still has a place. Other antiglycaemic agents currently under-going clinical investigation include alpha-2 adrenergic antagonists, and intestinal glycosidase inhibitors which delay the absorption of carbohydrate.

Associated medical disorders

Patients with diabetes are potentially liable to develop cardiovascular and renal disease. As well as retinopathy and neuropathy, there are also respiratory problems.

Respiration

Williams et al (1984) noted that there was reduced sensitivity to hypoxaemia and hypercapnia in diabetics. Hansen et al (1989) reported the case of an insulin-dependent diabetic who developed bronchial obstruction as a result of fungal infection which responded to amphotericin B. Hansen et al (1989) also reviewed the literature on pulmonary complications in patients with diabetes and these are as follows:

Infections—zygomycosis, mycobacterioses, bacterial infections, viral infections.

Physiologic changes—reduced elastic recoil of the lungs, reduced diffusing capacity of the lungs for carbon monoxide, diminished bronchial reactivity and elevated arterial oxygen tension.

Disordered breathing—central hypoventilation, sleep apnoea, cardiorespiratory arrest.

Miscellaneous—pulmonary oedema, pneumomediastinum, pneumo-thorax, plugging of airways with mucus, aspiration pneumonia, pulmonary xanthogranulomatosis, and respiratory failure caused by electrolyte imbalance.

Cardiovascular system

There is an increased incidence of sudden unexpected death in diabetics, and this may be due to the reduction in the ventricular fibrillation threshold rather than ischaemic changes (Fusilli et al 1989). There is also an increase in resting platelet noradrenaline release in type 1 diabetic patients which may result in increased platelet aggregation, promoting changes in the vessel wall and arterial thrombosis (Smith et al 1989b). Zarich & Nesto (1989) have presented evidence that there is a distinct cardiomyopathy in diabetes, apart from the enhanced coronary atherosclerosis seen in diabetic patients.

There is a highly significant increase in autonomic neuropathy in diabetes, and this was reflected in the marked decrease in heart rate and blood pressure during induction of anaesthesia. Thirty-five percent of diabetes require intra-operative vasopressors (Burgos et al 1989). Neuropathy may not be confined to the vagus nerve (Kennedy et al 1989). The measurement of heart rate during deep breathing is a sensitive test for cardiac vagal denervation. The QT interval is often decreased. Diabetic autonomic neuropathy is common but the symptoms are surprisingly rare (Watkins 1990).

Hypertension. Hypertension and diabetes are closely associated. It had been suggested that patients with hypertension developed diabetes during the course of treatment. Trost (1989) suggested a simple treatment regime including a calcium antagonist or an ACE inhibitor. If the blood pressure is not under control, an alpha-1 blocker, a beta-blocker (cardioselective) or a diuretic is advocated. If treatment is unsuccessful the drugs may be given in combination.

Neuropathy

The aetiology of peripheral nerve damage is still unresolved. Decreased nerve conduction can be restored by normoglycaemia and suppression of aldose reductase. This enzyme is involved in the reduction of glucose to sorbitol, the accumulation of which may be a factor. There may also be hypoxia of the nerve tissue due to microvascular changes.

Neuropathy is often insidious in onset, it may be diffuse or affect individual nerves such as the median nerve, the lateral popliteal nerve or even the cranial nerves, especially the ophthalmic nerve. Neuropathy may lead to ulceration of the foot (Ward 1989). There is impaired neuro-muscular transmission and decreased response to tetanic stimulation (Schiller & Rahamimoff 1989).

Restoring insulin function by pancreatic transplantation halts the progress of diabetic polyneuropathy (Kennedy et al 1990). Thermo-regulatory sweating test may reveal a distal loss of sweating which is often associated with neuropathy, and is another useful diagnostic aid (Fealey et al 1989).

Nephropathy

The pathophysiology of this complication is not completely understood and accounts for 25% of the new cases of end-stage renal disease each year. There is thickening of the basement membranes of the glomerular capillaries and renal tubules. Treatment involves the control of blood pressure and restriction of protein intake. Fasting levels of blood glucose should be between 5.6–7.8 mmol/l. Other possible lines of treatment include aldose reductase inhibitors and antiplatelet therapy, as well as the reduction in lipid which may be toxic to the endothelium of the renal cells. The management of end-stage renal disease can involve dialysis and renal transplantation (Reddi & Camerini-Davalos 1990). Glucose control appears to limit renal damage whereas the duration of diabetes is of more importance in the aetiology of retinopathy (Chase et al 1989). No cases of retinopathy or microalbuminuria were found if the glycohaemoglobin value was just 1.1 times the upper limit of normal, but if it were 1.5 times the upper limit, 30% of patients had microalbuminuria and retinopathy. Insulin decreases sodium excretion by an action on the proximal renal tubules (Skott et al 1989). Insulin also increases plasma renin activity and angiotensin II but decreases aldosterone (Trovati et al 1989). An increase in plasma renin activity may be due to the reduction of plasma potassium concentration.

The osmotic release of AVP is normal in diabetics but if there is autonomic neuropathy, release is impaired in response to stretching of the cardiovascular receptors (Reid et al 1989).

Gastric emptying

In diabetic patients, there may be delayed gastric emptying and this may have implications for the absorption of oral drugs used to control blood sugar levels. Groop et al (1989a) found that hyperglycaemia inhibited the absorption of glipizide (a sulphonylurea drug) when the plasma glucose level rose above 7 mmol/l. When the concentration reached 11 mmol/l, the levels of plasma glipizide were reduced by 50%. Erythromycin acts as a motilin agonist and improves gastrointestinal motility (Janssens et al 1990).

Insulin resistance

Insulin resistance has been ascribed to insulin-binding antibodies, insulin receptor defects or excessive destruction of insulin. It may occur during major surgical procedures due to the release of hormones that raise the level of blood sugar. Extensive burns and sepsis also produce syndromes which are said to cause insulin resistance. These are usually measured as a response to blood glucose, but Jahoor et al (1989) found that there was no reduction in the effectiveness of insulin to suppress protein breakdown. Peripheral glucose uptake is also reduced in sepsis (Shangraw et al 1989).

Insulin resistance may occur in liver fat and muscle tissues. The role of insulin in skeletal muscles is discussed by Beck-Nielsen (1989), indicating the place of insulin in stimulating pyruvate dehydrogenase in skeletal muscles and there may be a defect in the enzyme to account for insulin resistance. It is interesting to note that references are made to the fact that in non-insulin dependent diabetic patients, the liver is insulin resistant.

Insulin dependent diabetes mellitus (IDDM)

Insulin dependent diabetes mellitus (IDDM) is thought to be due to an autoimmune mechanism which destroys the beta cells. Shah et al (1989) postulated that the function of beta cells promotes the process that hastens their own destruction. An experimental group of patients received four times greater insulin than the conventionally treated group using an external artificial pancreas, demonstrating that suppression of endogenous insulin in the first two weeks after the diagnosis of IDDM had been made may improve beta cell function during the subsequent year (Shah et al 1989).

Non-insulin dependent diabetes mellitus (NIDDM)

Type II diabetes (non-insulin dependent diabetes, NIDDM), affects approximately 5% of adults in the United Kingdom and America, although in some Pacific Islands it may reach 20–35%. At the time the diagnosis is made there is deficiency in both secretion and action of insulin (Leading article, Lancet 1989a). Oral antidiabetic drugs have a high incidence of failure in the management of diabetes, and this could not be explained in 50% of patients being treated (Groop et al 1989b). Non-diabetic patients with insulin resistance are likely to develop NIDDM later. There may be a defect in insulin-mediated glycogen synthesis by skeletal muscles (Bogardus & Lillioja 1990).

Diabetic ketoacidosis

The management of diabetic ketoacidosis has been reviewed by Sanson & Levine (1989), who drew attention to the fact that 20 to 30% of patients present with diabetic ketoacidosis as the first indication of diabetes. Treatment is concerned with restoring plasma volume and electrolyte imbalance, reversing acidosis and treating any precipitating cause of the disease. Careful monitoring is essential in the management of diabetic ketoacidosis. Therapy involves the administration of low dose intravenous insulin infusion with fluid replacement including potassium as required. Bicarbonate is reserved for patients whose pH falls below 7.0 to 7.1. Fluid replacement is almost always necessary as deficits may vary between 4–10 l in an average adult. The laboratory investigations should involve not only blood glucose, but electrolytes including bicarbonate and phosphate, blood urea nitrogen and creatinine, serum ketones, arterial blood gas analysis, urinalysis, ECG and chest X-ray. Initial treatment may be an intravenous bolus of 0.1–0.2 U/kg insulin, followed by continuous infusion of $0.1\,U\,kg^{-1}/h$. Despite adequate levels of insulin, ketones are cleared at a slower rate than glucose. Initially, fluid should consist of 0.9% saline but when the serum glucose falls to 13.9 mmol/l, dextrose may be added to avoid potential hypoglycaemia. Potassium is given at a rate of 20–30 mmol/h initially.

The dangers of bicarbonate therapy are hypokalaemia, cerebral oedema and hypoxaemia of the peripheral tissues. The regime advocated by

Kitabchi (1989) advised against the use of bicarbonate which might cause intracellular acidosis by the Bohr effect, and felt that there seemed to be no particular indication to use phosphate supplements to accelerate the re-generation of 2,3-DPG (see also Wright 1989). However, Riley et al (1989) criticized these conclusions as the study was based on a small number of cases and maintained the need for alkali therapy. In fact the metabolic acidosis may persist after recovery from ketonaemia (Oh et al 1990).

Rosenbloom (1990) recorded 69 cases of intracerebral complications of diabetic ketoacidosis resembling cerebral oedema. Episodes of increased intracranial pressure leading to respiratory arrest were noted and the cause may be related to basilar oedema, haemorrhage, thrombosis or infection. In 50% of the patients, there were premonitory signs of development of cerebral oedema such as headache, incontinence, changes in behaviour, pupil size and blood pressure, fits, bradycardia or fluctuations in temperature. Despite early intervention the recovery rate was only 50%.

Hyperglycaemic hyperosmolar non-ketotic syndrome (HHNS)

This syndrome is characterized by hyperglycaemia without ketosis, with a marked increase in serum osmolality and evidence of dehydration. Precipitating factors include burns, parenteral feeding, peritoneal dialysis or haemodialysis. It may be produced by drugs such as diuretics, steroids, beta-blockers, phenytoin or diazoxide. Loss of water exceeds that of sodium resulting in dehydration and also hypertonicity. Electrolytes especially potassium are also depleted. Blood sugar is often greater than 33.3 mmol/l and osmolality greater than 350 mosm/l. Potassium loss is similar to that seen in diabetic ketoacidosis. Treatment involves the use of sodium chloride, either 0.9% or 0.45% with insulin 10–15 units, followed by an infusion of $0.1\,U\,kg^{-1}/h$. The mortality varies between 10 to 60% (Levine & Sanson 1989).

CNS

Trigeminal neuralgia

The treatment of trigeminal neuralgia is hampered by the fact that no model has yet been constructed to fully represent all the clinical features of the condition. However, many of the drugs appear to be effective in the management of this particular type of pain. Fromm (1989) has set up an experimental model, showing that carbamazepine affects the segmental or afferent inhibition of stimuli to the trigeminal nucleus neurons. Baclofen has a similar action to carbamazepine and phenytoin, and the L isomer, is five times more effective than the racemic mixture. Intrathecal baclofen is also effective in the management of spasticity (see Leading article, Lancet 1989b). The endorphin system is not involved in the production of trigeminal neuralgia.

Parkinson's disease

Marden (1990) has reviewed the mechanisms that are likely to cause Parkinson's disease; striatal dopamine deficiency as a cause led to the use of levodopa, decarboxylase inhibitors and drugs such as bromocriptine which stimulate dopamine receptors centrally. Another view is that neurotoxins such as tetrahydropyridine (MPTP) destroy the substantia nigra. Deprenyl, a selective monoamine oxidase inhibitor (type B) prolongs the action of dopamine in the brain, and appears to delay the onset of disabilities associated with Parkinson's disease (The Parkinson Study Group 1989). It may not be widely appreciated that long term treatment with levodopa leads to psychiatric side effects such as confusion, hallucinations, disorientation and paranoia. These have led to the possible use of antipsychotic drugs, and Wolters et al (1989) has advocated the use of clozapine, a benzodiazepine derivative with strong antipsychotic and sedative actions. A major side effect is agranulocytosis. In a review of the clinical pharmacology of antipsychotic drugs, Lader (1989) also refers to the use of chlorpromazine in Parkinson's disease (see also Bakheit 1990).

Head injuries

Head injury is a major result of trauma leading to 150 000 admissions per annum in the UK, but only 4% of patients are referred to neurosurgical units. Primary brain damage may be diffuse or focal and is not usually amenable to treatment, but secondary brain damage can be prevented and treated. Hypoxaemia, pulmonary complications and hypotension may develop as well as the effects of brain damage due to compression by haematoma, and brain swelling due to venous engorgement.

Mendelow (1990) has reviewed the pathophysiology of head injury involving assessment of patency of the airway, respiration and the circulation. The transfer of patients, even within a hospital for specialist investigations such as CT scan and magnetic resonance imaging may result in secondary injuries. Andrews et al (1990) emphasizes the need for prior resuscitation. Transferring patients to neurosurgical units also has its hazards as hypoxaemia or hypertension may occur leading to a poor outcome. Nearly 50% of comatose patients were transported without adequate supervision of the airway (Gentleman & Jennett 1990). Monitoring of all patients with head injuries should include blood gas analysis, expecially as some patients in coma who appear to be breathing adequately are hypoxaemic when the Pao_2 blood samples are measured. Pulse oximetry may fail to detect hypoxaemia if the peripheral circulation is inadequate.

In the neurosurgical unit, intracranial pressure is monitored and cerebral perfusion pressure calculated. Treatment must ensure that there is adequate ventilation while increased intracranial pressure may require the use of mannitol or dexamethasone, although treatment with barbiturates has proved disappointing. It may be necessary to remove a haematoma (Mendelow 1990). Hypoventilation and ischaemia lead to marked alterations in cerebral blood flow and cerebral energy metabolism, with a decrease in cerebral tissue pH due to the accumulation of lactic acid (Andersen et al 1988).

Hyperglycaemia may result as part of the stress response to injury, and is a significant marker of the extent of the cerebral injury and may predict the outcome (Young et al 1989). A serum glucose concentration of less than 10 mmol/l leads to a more favourable outcome, while a level in the region of 15 mmol/l predicts a fatal outcome. No correlation between the levels of hyperglycaemia and acute stroke could be demonstrated (Woo et al 1988).

Peripheral nerve injury

Methylprednisolone in a dose of 30 mg/kg followed by infusion of 5.4 mg kg^{-1}/h for 23 h led to improved neurological recovery following acute spinal injury, provided medication was started within the first 8 h after injury. Naloxone was without effect (Bracken et al 1990). In a review of the causes of lumbar arachnoiditis by Bourne (1990), many of the causes were due to spinal operation and drugs injected into the CSF. There were 36 cases where the cause was due to injection of contrast media, but only two incidences involving anaesthetic agents and two episodes of 'bloody tap'.

Sleep

Borbely & Tobler (1989) have prepared an extensive review on endogenous substances that promote sleep. Various hormones may be implicated but the results are difficult to interpret in view of the effects on REM and NREM sleep. Prostaglandin D_2 produces NREM sleep while VIP enhances REM sleep in some animals and has the opposite effect in others. Growth hormone levels increase after the onset of sleep. Insulin infusion enhances NREM sleep but again arginine vasotocin (AVT) has different effects depending on the species. Other hormones implicated are pro-opiomelanocortin-derivatives, serotonin and tryptophan which is considered by some to be the hormone that results in natural sleep. Also involved may be adenosine, acetylcholine, catecholamines, melatonin, steroids, calcium, and interleukin I which have circadian patterns that affect sleep.

Treatment of insomnia depends on the cause which may be anxiety, pain and sleep disorders following operation. Insomnia may result from the withdrawal of hypnotic drugs such as benzodiazepines. Insomnia may be short term or long term, the latter being associated with psychiatric disorders, alcohol abuse and medical problems such as hypertension, hyperthyroidism and Parkinson's disease (Gillin & Byerley 1990).

Barbiturates are seldom used for night sedation and these have been replaced by benzodiazepines which may be short-acting (e.g. triazolam, midazolam), intermediate-acting (oxazepam, lorazepam, temazepam) and long-acting (diazepam, clonazepam). The side effects of these drugs are partially dose-dependent. Other drugs in use are antihistamines, tricyclics which are claimed to be safe in patients with sleep apnoea, and tryptophan which unfortunately has side effects including eosinophilia and myalgia. However, a feature of tricyclic antidepressants appears to be the anti-arrhythmic action on the heart (Manoach et al 1989).

Sleep deprivation may lead to delirium especially in the elderly, although delirium may be a feature of myocardial infarction or even pneumonia. It may be drug-induced, e.g. pethidine, or may result from drug withdrawal (see Lipowski 1989).

Neuromuscular problems

The respiratory manifestations of neuromuscular disorders are considered in the section on respiration.

The relationship between muscle power developed during exercise and fatigue and muscle pain is still inexact (Jones et al 1989). Hypocarbia promotes fatigue of the diaphragm but improvement was noted with theophylline. Respiratory effort is noted when diaphragm fatigue develops, but surprisingly it is not related to the intensity of diaphragmatic contractions (Ward et al 1988). During exercise the arterial plasma potassium concentration rises, but there is no evidence to suggest that changes in potassium have any effect on ventilation via the chemoreceptors (Paterson et al 1989).

Brahams (1989) reported a medico-legal inquiry in a patient with myotonic dystrophy who died following surgery; sedation administered for pain appeared to be the main cause of death and was not related to the operation. There was also inadequate post-operative monitoring. There may be other causes of death in myotonic dystrophy such as cardiomyopathy, falling temperature which may promote weakness and which is associated with a marked uptake of potassium by the fatigued muscle (Moxley et al 1989). Respiratory failure and pulmonary infection are major causes of morbidity and mortality in muscular dystrophy. Assessment of the capacity to cough may be readily reflected in the maximum expiratory pressure generated at mouth level using a simple anaeroid manometer. If the pressure was greater than 60 cm H_2O, then it was concluded that the patients had adequate capacity for coughing and clearing secretions (Szeinberg et al 1988).

These observations had previously been noted by Kaufman (1962). Patients with muscular dystrophy underventilate during sleep and this has been successfully treated by IPPV via nasal mask (Heckmatt et al 1990). Besides muscular dystrophy, neuromuscular involvement may occur in other diseases such as primary hyperparathyroidism (Turken et al 1989).

Myasthenia gravis

The natural course of myasthenia gravis has been reviewed by Oosterhuis (1989) and Fonseca & Havard (1990). It appears that the disease reaches its maximum intensity in the first seven years during which time 25% will succumb and 20% will have spontaneous transitory remissions. The outlook is less favourable in patients with a thymoma.

Cerebral circulation

The use of revascularization techniques to improve cerebral blood flow in atherosclerotic conditions have proved to be singularly disappointing. However, Onesti et al (1989) have indicated that bypass grafting still appears to have a place in progressive vascular disorders of unknown origin, such as Moya Moya disease and intracranial aneurysms.

Anaesthetic techniques for the management of patients undergoing surgery for cerebral aneurysm often involves hypotensive anaesthesia. Lagerkranser et al (1989) have shown that continuous infusions of adenosine produced satisfactory hypotension without affecting cerebral oxygenation; it may even have a protective effect by reducing cerebral oxygen demand. Following a period of hypotension, there was an increase in cerebral blood flow secondary to the increase in arterial blood pressure, but this was not considered to be detrimental to the patients.

Posture may affect the intracranial pressure during neurosurgical procedures. In the supine position, venous hypertension resulting from PEEP was transmitted to the brain but without causing an increase in intracranial hypertension. This effect did not occur in the sitting position; however, in patients with increased intracranial pressure, head flexion or rotation with institution of PEEP resulted in a dangerous increase in intracranial pressure (Lodrini et al 1989). Neurological complications may also occur following cardiopulmonary bypass surgery (Shaw et al 1987).

Despite the advances in pharmacology, drug therapy in 'cerebral resuscitation' has proved disappointing, especially in the use of barbiturates. A recent discovery has been that of the N-methyl-D-aspartate (NMDA) type of glutamate receptors; there exists the possibility that antagonists may be of value in the management of cerebral ischaemia (Rogers & Kirsch 1989).

Nimodipine, a calcium antagonist and a cerebral vasodilator, reduces cerebral infarction and improves prognosis following subarachnoid haemorrhage (Pickard et al 1989). Other drugs on trial include infusions of dextran 40, glycerol, naftidrofuryl, beta-blockers, steroids and prostacyclin (Lowe 1990).

There is a general acceptance that patients suffering from brain death may have their organs retrieved to benefit others, but the definition of brain death and its ethic considerations appear to limit the number of organs available for transplantation (Younger et al 1989).

Alcohol

Charness et al (1989) have reviewed the effects of alcohol on the central nervous system, indicating how ethanol and its metabolites, including acetaldehyde, damage the nervous system. Blood levels of ethanol above 5.4 mmol/l are associated with mild intoxication and above this level, there are signs of vestibular and cerebellar dysfunction including nystagmus, diplopia, dysarthria and ataxia. Ethanol potentiates GABA activity by affecting the ion flux at chloride channels. Associated complications include Wernicke's encephalopathy which is associated with thiamine deficiency, dementia, cerebellar degeneration, pontine myelinolysis, neuropathy and myopathy. Withdrawal of alcohol in chronic alcoholic leads to tremor, autonomic hyperactivity, nausea, vomiting, confusion and hallucination. These respond readily to beta-adrenergic antagonists or even alpha-2 adrenergic receptor agonists. Gamma-hydroxybutyric acid also appears to be effective in reducing withdrawal symptoms (Gallimberti et al 1989).

HISTAMINE

Histamine antagonists

Histamine receptor antagonists have been classified into H_1- and H_2-receptor antagonists; the former decreasing vascular permeability and relaxing smooth muscle whereas the latter are involved in decreasing gastric acid secretion. A H_3-receptor antagonist has been described, e.g. thiopramide which appears to be involved in the feedback mechanism controlling histamine synthesis and release. The clinical pharmacology of H_1-receptor antagonists has been reviewed by Simons (1989) indicating the use of H_1-receptor antagonists in conditions such as allergic rhinitis, urticaria, asthma, upper respiratory tract infections and anaphylaxis. Simons (1989) draws attention to the possible danger of using H_1-receptor antagonists during pregnancy, and also to the fact that there is less efficacy in these first generation drugs which cause pronounced sedation.

Cimetidine and ranitidine are advocated for reducing gastric acid contents and increasing pH, especially prior to obstetric anaesthesia. Ewart et al (1990) demonstrated that omeprazole was more consistent than ranitidine at maintaining gastric pH greater than 3.5. However, Scarr et al (1989) found that clear fluids could be given until 3 h prior to surgery, without any attempt to block acid secretion except in emergency cases or in obstetrics.

Although central effects with H_2-receptor antagonists are rare, Berlin (1989) has drawn attention to the possibility of mental confusion, agitation, depression, hallucination and even extrapyramidal effects.

Omeprazole is a prodrug and its metabolites have specific and irreversible effects on the H^+K^+-ATPase in the parietal cells of the stomach, which are responsible for the final phase of gastric acid secretion. A dose of 40 mg would be expected to reduce gastric acid secretion.

VOMITING AND ANTIEMETICS

Brizzee (1990) studied the mechanics of vomiting in animals, showing that the act of vomiting is preceded by abnormal peristaltic activity of the small bowel with inhibition of peristalsis in the stomach. In the upper bowel there is antiperistalsis with reflux into the stomach. There are cyclic phases of oesophageal dilatation, gastric emptying, gastric reflux and oesophageal collapse. The expulsive forces are due to sustained abdominal contraction, but there is no active contraction of the stomach or oesophagus.

Metoclopramide, a dopamine-2 receptor antagonist is widely used as an antiemetic, but the incidence of side effects appears to be understated. Miller & Jankovic (1989) reported Parkinsonism, tardive dystonia and akathisia. The side effects are more common in women, with a ratio of 3 to 1. Involuntary movements usually stop when the drug is discontinued, but they have been known to continue indefinitely. Bateman et al (1989) reported extrapyramidal symptoms following the use of metoclopramide and prochlorperazine, the actions being greater with the former drug in patients under 30 years, while the latter drug is more likely to affect patients over the age of 60. Metoclopramide releases catecholamines and increases blood pressure, especially in patients with essential hypertension and these effects can be reduced by pirenzepine, a tricyclic anticholinergic agent (Syvalahti et al 1988).

The control of vomiting produced by cytotoxic drugs may involve the use of a combination of antiemetics (Marin et al 1990).

The recently introduced antiemetic ondansetron, an antagonist of T3 serotonin receptors (5-HT3), is particularly effective against nausea and vomiting produced by the cytotoxic agent cisplatin which increases the excretion of 5-HIAA (Cubeddu et al 1990). Marty et al (1990) confirmed that ondansetron was more effective than metoclopramide and was without its extrapyramidal side effects.

REFERENCES

Addis G J 1990 Theophylline in the management of airflow obstruction—1. Much evidence suggests that theophylline is valuable. Br Med J 300: 928–929
Andersen B J, Unterberg A W, Clarke G D, Marmarou A 1988 Effect of posttraumatic hypoventilation on cerebral energy metabolism. J Neurosurg 68: 601–607
Andrews P J D, Piper I R, Dearden N M, Miller J D 1990 Secondary insults during intrahospital transport of head-injured patients. Lancet 335: 327–330
Anthonisen N R 1988 Chronic obstructive pulmonary disease. Can Med Assoc J 138: 503–510
Arnold J S, Haxhiu M A, Cherniack N S, van Lunteren E 1988 Transverse abdominis length changes during eupnea, hypercapnia, and airway occlusion. J Appl Physiol 64: 658–665
Aubert-Tulkens G, Culee C, Rodenstein D O 1989 Cure of sleep apnea syndrome after long-term nasal continuous positive airway pressure therapy and weight loss. Sleep 12: 216–222
Aubier M, Murciano D, Menu Y, Boczkowski J, Mal H, Pariente R 1989 Dopamine effects on diaphragmatic strength during acute respiratory failure in chronic obstructive pulmonary disease. Ann Intern Med 110: 17–23
Bakheit A M O 1990 Drug treatment of Parkinson's disease. Hosp Update 16: 497–504

Ballard P L 1989 Hormonal regulation of pulmonary surfactant. Endocr Rev 10: 165–181
Banzett R B, Lansing R W, Reid M B, Adams L, Brown R 1989 "Air hunger" arising from increased PCO_2 in mechanically ventilated quadriplegics. Respir Physiol 76: 53–68
Barnard J W, Patterson C E, Hull M T, Wagner W W Jr, Rhoades R A 1989 Role of microvascular pressure in reactive oxygen-induced lung edema. J Appl Physiol 66: 1486–1493
Barnes P J 1987 Neuropeptides in human airways: function and clinical implications. Am Rev Respir Dis 136: S77–S83
Barnes P J 1989 A new approach to the treatment of asthma. N Engl J Med 321: 1517–1527
Barrowcliffe M, Jones J G 1988 The pathophysiology and treatment of adult respiratory distress syndrome (ARDS). In: Kaufman L (ed) Anaesthesia Review 5. Churchill Livingstone, Edinburgh, pp 182–195
Bartlett D Jr 1989 Respiratory functions of the larynx. Physiol Rev 69: 33–57
Bateman D N, Darling W M, Boys R, Rawlins M D 1989 Extrapyramidal reactions to metoclopramide and prochlorperazine. Q J Med 71: 307–311
Baydur A, Swank S M, Stiles C M, Sassoon C S H 1989 Respiratory elastic load compensation in anesthetized patients with kyphoscoliosis. J Appl Physiol 67: 1024–1031
Beaupre A, Soucy R, Phillips R, Bourgouin J 1988 Respiratory center output following zopiclone or diazepam administration in patients with pulmonary disease. In: Duron B, Levi-Valensi P (eds) Sleep Disorders and Respiration. John Libbey Eurotext Ltd, Colloque INSERM, Vol 168, pp 123–124
Beck-Nielsen H 1989 Insulin resistance in skeletal muscles of patients with diabetes mellitus. Diabetes Metab Rev 5: 487–493
Bell D, Kirby T P, Nicoll J J, Brash H M, Connaughton J J, Muir A L 1988 Regional distribution of ventilation in chronic obstructive lung disease and the effect of salbutamol. Respiration 54: 179–189
Benowitz N L 1988 Pharmacologic aspects of cigarette smoking and nicotine addiction. N Engl J Med 319: 1318–1329
Bergofsky E H, Hurewitz A N 1989 Airway insufflation: physiologic effects on acute and chronic gas exchange in humans. Am Rev Respir Dis 140: 885–890
Berlin R G 1989 Effects of H_2-receptor antagonists on the central nervous system. Drug Dev Res 17: 97–108
Bianco S, Pieroni M G, Refini R M, Rottoli L, Sestini P 1989 Protective effect of inhaled frusemide on allergen-induced early and late asthmatic reactions. N Engl J Med 321: 1069–1073
Block A J 1988 Drugs, sleep and breathing. In: Duron B, Levi-Valensi P (eds) Sleep Disorders and Respirations. John Libbey Eurotext Ltd, Colloque INSERM, Vol 168, pp 91–103
Boczkowski J, Dureuil B, Branger C et al 1988 Effects of sepsis on diaphragmatic function in rats. Am Rev Respir Dis 138: 260–265
Bogaard J M, Hovestadt A, Meerwaldt J, Meche F G A, Stigt J 1989 Maximal expiratory and inspiratory flow-volume curves in Parkinson's disease. Am Rev Respir Dis 139: 610–614
Bogardus C, Lillioja S 1990 Where all the glucose doesn't go in non-insulin-dependent diabetes mellitus. N Engl J Med 322: 262–263
Bollen E L, Den Heijer J C, Ponsionen et al 1988 Respiration during sleep in Huntington's chorea. J Neurol Sci 84: 63–68
Bonniere P, Wallaert B, Cortot A et al 1986 Latent pulmonary involvement in Crohn's disease: biological, functional, bronchoalveolar lavage and scintigraphic studies. Gut 27: 919–925
Borbely A A, Tobler I 1989 Endogenous sleep-promoting substances and sleep regulation. Physiol Rev 69: 605–670
Bourne I H J 1990 Lumbo-sacral adhesive arachnoiditis: a review. J Roy Soc Med 83: 262–265
Bracken M B, Shepard M J, Collins W F, Holford T R, Young W, Baskin D S et al 1990 A randomized, controlled trial of methylprednisolone or naloxone in the treatment of acute spinal-cord injury. Results of the second National Acute Spinal Cord Injury Study. N Engl J Med 322: 1405–1411
Brahams D 1989 Postoperative monitoring in patients with muscular dystrophy. Lancet II: 1053–1054
Brizzee K R 1990 Mechanics of vomiting: a minireview. Can J Physiol Pharmacol 68: 221–229

Brophy C, Mier A, Moxham J, Green M 1989 The effect of aminophylline on respiratory and limb muscle contractility in man. Eur Respir J 2: 652–655

Browne D R G 1988a Weaning patients from ventilators: 1. Hosp Update 14: 1809–1818

Browne D R G 1988b Weaning patients from ventilators: 2. Hosp Update 14: 1898–1906

Burgos L G, Ebert T J, Asiddao C, Turner L A, Pattison C Z, Wang-Cheng R, Kampine J P 1989 Increased intraoperative cardiovascular morbidity in diabetics with autonomic neuropathy. Anesthesiology 70: 591–597

Cagle P T, Thurlbeck W M 1988 Postpneumonectomy compensatory lung growth. Am Rev Respir Dis 138: 1314–1326

Camus P H, Jeannin L 1988 The lung and drugs: mutual influences. Eur Respir J 1: 85–92

Carlile P V, Gray B A 1989 Effect of opposite changes in cardiac output and arterial PO_2 on the relationship between mixed venous PO_2 and oxygen transport. Am Rev Respir Dis 140: 891–898

Carroll N, Branthwaite M A 1988 Control of nocturnal hypoventilation by nasal intermittent positive pressure ventilation. Thorax 43: 349–353

Charness M E, Simon R P, Greenberg D A 1989 Ethanol and the nervous system. N Engl J Med 321: 442–454

Chase H P, Jackson W E, Hoops S L, Cockerham R S, Archer P G, O'Brien D 1989 Glucose control and the renal and retinal complications of insulin-dependent diabetes. JAMA 261: 1155–1160

Chen H-I, Tang Y-R 1989 Sleep loss impairs inspiratory muscle endurance. Am Rev Respir Dis 140: 907–909

Chin K, Ohi M, Hirai M, Kuriyama T, Sagawa Y, Kuno K 1989 Breathing during sleep with mild hypoxia. J Appl Physiol 67: 1198–1207

Chinn D J, Askew J, Rowley L, Cotes J E 1988 Measurement technique influences the response of transfer factor (TICO) to salbutamol in patients with airflow limitation. Eur Respir J 1: 15–21

Chonan T, ElHefnawy A M, Simonetti O P, Cherniack N S 1988 Rate of elimination of excess CO_2 in humans. Respir Physiol 73: 379–394

Chrystyn H, Mulley B A, Peake M D 1988 Dose response relation to oral theophylline in severe chronic obstructive airways disease. Br Med J 297: 1506–1510

Chung K F, Barnes P J 1988 PAF antagonists—Their potential therapeutic role in asthma. Drugs 35: 93–103

Clague J E, Calverley P M A 1990 Management of chronic obstructive pulmonary disease. Hosp Update 16: 20–32

Clark C J, Pollock A J, Reid W H, Campbell D, Gemmell C 1988 Role of pulmonary alveolar macrophage activation in acute lung injury after burns and smoke inhalation. Lancet II: 872–874

Coccagna G, Lugaresi E, Cirignotta F 1988 Sleep apnea syndrome and systemic hypertension. In: Duron B, Levi-Valensi P (eds) Sleep Disorders and Respiration. John Libbey Eurotext Ltd, Colloque INSERM, Vol 168, pp 155–169

Cockcroft A, Adams L, Guz A 1989 Assessment of breathlessness. Q J Med 72: 669–676

Collard P H, Wautelet F, Delwiche J P, Prignot J, Dubois P 1989 Improvement of oxygen delivery in severe hypoxaemia by a reservoir cannula. Eur Respir J 2: 778–781

Courtney S E, Spohn W A, Weber K R, Miles D S, Gotshall R W, Wong R C 1989 Cardiopulmonary effects of high frequency positive-pressure ventilation versus jet ventilation in respiratory failure. Am Rev Respir Dis 139: 504–512

Couser J I Jr, Make B J 1989 Transtracheal oxygen decreases inspired minute ventilation. Am Rev Respir Dis 139: 627–631

Cubeddu L X, Hoffman I S, Fuenmayor N T, Finn A L 1990 Efficacy of ondansetron (GR 38032F) and the role of serotonin in cisplatin-induced nausea and vomiting. N Engl J Med 322: 810–816

Cvitanic O, Marino P L 1989 Improved use of arterial blood gas analysis in suspected pulmonary embolism. Chest 95: 48–51

Derveaux L, Ivanoff I, Rochette F, Demedts M 1988 Mechanism of pulmonary function changes after surgical correction for funnel chest. Eur Respir J 1: 823–825

DeWeese E L, Sullivan T Y 1988 Effects of upper airway anesthesia on pharyngeal patency during sleep. J Appl Physiol 64: 1346–1353

Dillard T A, Berg B W, Rajagopal K R, Dooley J W, Mehm W J 1989 Hypoxemia during air travel in patients with chronic obstructive pulmonary disease. Ann Intern Med 111: 362–367

Douglas J G, McDonald C F, Leslie M J, Gillon J, Crompton G K, McHardy G J R 1989 Respiratory impairment in inflammatory bowel disease: does it vary with disease activity? Respir Med 83: 389–394

Dreyfuss D, Soler P, Basset G, Saumon G 1988 High inflation pressure pulmonary edema. Am Rev Respir Dis 137: 1159–1164

Edell E S, Cortese D A, Krowka M J, Rehder K 1989 Severe hypoxemia and liver disease. Am Rev Respir Dis 140: 1631–1635

Eklund A, Broman L, Broman M, Holmgren A 1989 V/Q and alveolar gas exchange in pulmonary sarcoidosis. Eur Respir J 2: 135–144

Elliott M W, Steven M H, Phillips G D, Branthwaite M A 1990 Non-invasive mechanical ventilation for acute respiratory failure. Br Med J 300: 358–360

Estenne M, De Troyer A 1990 Cough in tetraplegic subjects: an active process. Ann Intern Med 112: 22–28

Ewart M C, Yau G, Gin T, Kotur C F, Oh T E 1990 A comparison of the effects of omeprazole and ranitidine on gastric secretion in women undergoing elective Caesarean section. Anaesthesia 45: 527–530

Farias L A, Sun J, Markov A K 1989 Improved brain metabolism with fructose 1-6 diphosphate during insulin-induced hypoglycemic coma. Am J Med Sci 297: 294–299

Fealey R D, Low Phillip A, Thomas J E 1989 Thermoregulatory sweating abnormalities in diabetes mellitus. Mayo Clin Proc 64: 617–628

Fielding J E, Phenow K J 1988 Health effects of involuntary smoking. N Engl J Med 319: 1452–1460

Findley L J 1989 Nocturnal hypoxemia in sleep apnea. Chest 96: 716

Findley L J, Boykin M, Fallon T, Belardinelli L 1988 Plasma adenosine and hypoxemia in patients with sleep apnea. J Appl Physiol 64: 556–561

Flenley D C 1988 Hypoxia during sleep in COPD patients. In: Duron B, Levi-Valensi P (eds) Sleep Disorders and Respiration. John Libbey Eurotext Ltd, Colloque INSERM, Vol 168, pp 251–260

Fletcher E C, Costarangos C, Miller T 1989 The rate of fall of arterial oxyhemoglobin saturation in obstructive sleep apnea. Chest 96: 717–722

Flick G R, Bellamy P E, Simmons D H 1989 Diaphragmatic contraction during assisted mechanical ventilation. Chest 96: 130–135

Fonseca V, Havard C W H 1990 The natural course of myasthenia gravis. Br Med J 300: 1409–1410

Fox A W, Monoson P K, Morgan C D 1989 Speech dysfunction of obstructive sleep apnea—a discriminant analysis of its descriptors. Chest 96: 589–595

Fromm G H 1989 Review: The pharmacology of trigeminal neuralgia. Clin Neuropharmacol 12: 185–194

Fusilli L, Lyons M, Patel B, Torres R, Hernandez F, Regan T 1989 Ventricular vulnerability in diabetes and myocardial norepinephrine release. Am J Med Sci 298: 207–214

Gale E A M 1989 Hypoglycaemia and human insulin. Lancet II: 1264–1266

Gallimberti L, Canton G, Gentile N et al 1989 Gamma-hydroxybutyric acid for treatment of alcohol withdrawal syndrome. Lancet II: 787–789

Gardiner P J 1989 Eicosanoids and airway smooth muscle. Pharmacol Ther 44: 1–62

Gay P C, Rodarte J R, Hubmayr R D 1989 The effects of positive expiratory pressure on isovolume flow and dynamic hyperinflation in patients receiving mechanical ventilation. Am Rev Respir Dis 139: 621–626

Gentleman D, Jennett B 1990 Audit of transfer of unconscious head-injured patients to a neurosurgical unit. Lancet 335: 330–334

Georgopoulos D, Holtby S G, Berezanski D, Anthonisen N R 1989 Aminophylline effects on ventilatory response to hypoxia and hyperoxia in normal adults. J Appl Physiol 67: 1150–1156

Gerich J E 1989 Oral hypoglycemic agents. N Engl J Med 321: 1231–1245

Gillin J C, Byerley W F 1990 The diagnosis and management of insomnia. N Engl J Med 322: 239–248

Golding-Wood D G, Brockbank M J, Swanston A R, Croft C B 1990 Assessment of chronic snorers. J R Soc Med 83: 363–367

Gonzalez-Rothi R J, Foresman G E, Block A J 1988 Do patients with sleep apnea die in their sleep? Chest 94: 531–538

Gorini M, Spinelli A, Ginanni R et al 1989 Neural respiratory drive and neuromuscular coupling during CO_2 rebreathing in patients with chronic interstitial lung disease. Chest 96: 824–830

Gregg I, Nunn A J 1989 Peak expiratory flow in symptomless elderly smokers and ex-smokers. Br Med J 298: 1071–1072

Griggs G A, Findley L J, Suratt P M, Esau S A, Wilhoit S C, Rochester D F 1989 Prolonged relaxation rate of inspiratory muscles in patients with sleep apnea. Am Rev Respir Dis 140: 706–710

Groop L C, Luzi L, DeFronzo R A, Melander A 1989a Hyperglycaemia and absorption of sulphonylurea drugs. Lancet II: 129–130

Groop L, Schalin C, Franssilla-Kallunki A, Widen E, Ekstrand A, Eriksson J 1989b Characteristics of non-insulin-dependent diabetic patients with secondary failure to oral antidiabetic therapy. Am J Med 87: 183–190

Grunstein R R, Handelsman D J, Lawrence S J, Blackwell C, Caterson I D, Sullivan C E 1989 Neuroendocrine dysfunction in sleep apnea: reversal by continuous positive airways pressure therapy. J Clin Endocrinol Metab 68: 352–358

Guazzi M D, Berti M, Doria E et al 1989 Enhancement of the pulmonary vasconstriction reaction to alveolar hypoxia in system high blood pressure. Clin Sci 76: 589–594

Guenard H, Cros A M, Boudey C 1989 Variations in flow and intra-alveolar pressure during jet ventilation: theoretical and experimental analysis. Respir Physiol 75: 235–246

Guilleminault C, Van den Hoed J, Mitler M M 1978 In: Guilleminault C, Dement W C (eds) Sleep Apnoea Syndromes. Liss, New York, pp 1–12

Gutierrez G, Lund N, Acero A L, Marini C 1989 Relationship of venous PO_2 to muscle PO_2 during hypoxemia. J Appl Physiol 67: 1093–1099

Hamilton R D, Winning A J, Horner R L, Guz A 1988 The effect of lung inflation on breathing in man during wakefulness and sleep. Respir Physiol 73: 145–154

Hanly P J, Millar T W, Steljes D G, Baert R, Frais M A, Kryger M H 1989a Respiration and abnormal sleep in patients with congestive heart failure. Chest 96: 480–488

Hanly P J, Millar T W, Steljes D G, Baert R, Frais M A, Kryger M H 1989b The effect of oxygen on respiration and sleep in patients with congestive heart failure. Ann Intern Med 111: 777–782

Hansen L A, Prakash U B S, Colby T V 1989 Pulmonary complications in diabetes mellitus. Mayo Clin Proc 64: 791–799

He J, Kryger M H, Zorick F J, Conway W, Roth T 1988 Mortality and apnea index in obstructive sleep apnea—experience in 385 male patients. Chest 94: 9–14

Heatley R V, Thomas P, Prokipchuk E J, Gauldie J, Sieniewicz D J, Bienenstock J 1982 Pulmonary function abnormalities in patients with inflammatory bowel disease. Q J Med New Series L1 203: 241–260

Heckmatt J Z, Loh L, Dubowitz V 1990 Night-time nasal ventilation in neuromuscular disease. Lancet 335: 579–582

Hedenstierna G 1990 Gas exchange during anaesthesia. Br J Anaesth 64: 507–514

Heine R J, Van Der Heyden E A P, Van Der Veen E A 1989 Responses to human and porcine insulin in healthy subjects. Lancet II: 946–948

Hermens W A J J, Merkus F W H M 1987 The influence of drugs on nasal ciliary movement. Pharm Res 4: 445–449

Hevroy O, Klow N E, Forsdahl K, Mjos O D 1989 Plasma concentrations of atrial natriuretic factor during positive end-expiratory pressure ventilation in dogs with normal or impaired left ventricular function. Acta Anaesthesiol Scand 33: 549–553

Hibbert G, Pilsbury D 1988 Hyperventilation in panic attacks—Ambulant monitoring of transcutaneous carbon dioxide. Br J Psychiatry 153: 76–80

Hietanen E, Marniemi J, Liippo K, Seppanen A, Hartiala J, Viinamakis O 1988 Role of pulmonary diseases and physical condition in the regulation of vasoactive hormones. Clin Physiol 8: 581–590

Hoffman R A, Ershousky P, Krieger B P 1989 Determination of auto-PEEP during spontaneous and controlled ventilation by monitoring changes in end-expiratory thoracic gas volume. Chest 96: 613–616

Holgate S T, Finnerty J P 1988 Recent advances in understanding the pathogenesis of asthma and its clinical implications. Q J Med 66 (No 249): 5–19

Horner R L, Shea S A, McIvor J, Guz A 1989 Pharyngeal size and shape during wakefulness and sleep in patients with obstructive sleep apnoea. Q J Med 72: 719–735

Hudgel D W, Hendricks C 1988 Palate and hypopharynx—sites of inspiratory narrowing of the upper airway during sleep. Am Rev Respir Dis 138: 1542–1547

Hudgel D W, Hendricks C, Hamilton H B 1988 Characteristics of the upper airway pressure-flow relationship during sleep. J Appl Physiol 64: 1930–1935

Hull C J, Jones J G (eds) 1990 Symposium on the lung. Br J Anaesth 65: 1–152

Issa F G, Edwards P, Szeto E, Lauff D, Sullivan C 1988 Genioglossus and breathing responses to airway occlusion: effect of sleep and route of occlusion. J Appl Physiol 64: 543–549

Jackson Maj C V 1988 Preoperative pulmonary evaluation. Arch Intern Med 148: 2120–2127

Jackson M, King M, Hockley S, Wells F, Shneerson J M 1990 Early experience with an implantable intratracheal oxygen catheter. Br Med J 300: 909–910

Jahoor F, Shangraw R E, Miyoshi H, Wallfish H, Herndon D N, Wolfe R R 1989 Role of insulin and glucose oxidation in mediating the protein catabolism of burns and sepsis. Am J Physiol 257: E323–E331

Jansen J E, Sorensen A I, Naesh O, Erichsen C, Pedersen A 1990 Effect of doxapram on postoperative pulmonary complications after upper abdominal surgery in high-risk patients. Lancet 335: 936–938

Janssens J, Peeters T L, Vantrappen G et al 1990 Improvement of gastric emptying in diabetic gastroparesis by erythromycin. N Engl J Med 322: 1028–1031

Jayr C, Mollie A, Bourgain J L et al 1988 Postoperative pulmonary complications: general anesthesia with postoperative parenteral morphine compared with epidural analgesia. Surgery 104: 57–63

Jefferies A L, Kawano T, Mori S, Burger R 1988 Effect of increased surface tension and assisted ventilation of ^{99m}Tc-DTPA clearance. J Appl Physiol 64: 562–568

Jenkins S C, Soutar S, Forsyth A, Keates J R W, Moxham J 1989 Lung function after coronary artery surgery using the internal mammary artery and the saphenous vein. Thorax 44: 209–211

Jones J G 1984 Pulmonary complications following general anaesthesia. In: Kaufman L (ed) Anaesthesia Review 2. Churchill Livingstone, Edinburgh, pp 21–38

Jones D A, Newham D J, Torgan C 1989 Mechanical influences on long-lasting human muscle fatigue and delayed-onset pain. J Physiol 412: 415–427

Jones J G, Sapsford D J, Wheatley R G 1990 Postoperative hypoxaemia: mechanisms and time course. Anaesthesia 45: 566–573

Johnston I D A 1990 Theophylline in the management of airflow obstruction. 2. Difficult drugs to use, few clinical indications. Br Med J 300: 929–931

Juniper E F, Daniel E E, Roberts R S, Kline P A, Hargreave F E, Newhouse M T 1989 Improvement in airway responsiveness and asthma severity during pregnancy. A prospective study. Am Rev Respir Dis 140: 924–931

Kaufman L 1962 Disordered respiration in dystrophia myotonica. M.D. thesis, Edinburgh University

Kaufman L (ed) 1990 Medicine relevant to anaesthesia (2). In: Anaesthesia review 7. Churchill Livingstone, Edinburgh, p 26

Kawashima A, Kubo K, Hirai K, Yoshikawa S, Matsuzawa Y, Kobayashi T 1989 Plasma levels of atrial natriuretic peptide under acute hypoxia in normal subjects. Respir Physiol 76: 79–92

Kelly T M, Jensen R L, Elliott C G, Crapo R O 1988 Maximum respiratory pressures in morbidly obese subject. Respiration 54: 73–77

Kennedy W R, Navarro X, Sakuta M, Mandell H, Knox C K, Sutherland D E R 1989 Physiological and clinical correlates of cardiorespiratory reflexes in diabetes mellitus. Diabetes Care 12: 399–408

Kennedy W R, Navarro X, Goetz F C, Sutherland D E R, Najarian J S 1990 Effects of pancreatic transplantation on diabetic neuropathy. N Engl J Med 322: 1031–1037

Kirkham A J T, Guyatt A R, Cumming G 1988 Acute effect of smoking on rebreathing carbon monoxide, breath-hold carbon monoxide and alveolar oxygen. Clin Sci 75: 371–373

Kitabchi A E 1989 Low-dose insulin therapy in diabetic ketoacidosis: fact or fiction. Diabetes Metab Rev 5: 337–363

Krieger J, Imbs J-L, Schmidt M, Kurtz D 1988 Renal function in patients with obstructive sleep apnea—effects of nasal continuous positive airway pressure. Arch Intern Med 148: 1337–1340

Krieger J, Sforza E, Apprill M, Lampert E, Weitzenblum E, Ratomaharo J 1989a Pulmonary hypertension, hypoxemia, and hypercapnia in obstructive sleep apnea patients. Chest 96: 729–737

Krieger J, Laks L, Wilcox I et al 1989b Atrial natriuretic peptide release during sleep in patients with obstructive sleep apnoea before and during treatment with nasal continuous positive airway pressure. Clin Sci 77: 407–411

Kunitomo F, Kimura H, Tatsumi K et al 1989 Abnormal breathing during sleep and chemical control of breathing during wakefulness in patients with sleep apnea syndrome. Am Rev Respir Dis 139: 164–169

Lacroix J S 1989 Adrenergic and non-adrenergic mechanisms in sympathetic vascular control of the nasal mucosa. Acta Physiol Scand 136 (suppl 581): 5–63

Lader M 1989 Clinical pharmacology of antipsychotic drugs. J Int Med Res 17: 1–16

Lagerkranser M, Bergstrand G, Gordon E et al 1989 Cerebral blood flow and metabolism during adenosine-induced hypotension in patients undergoing cerebral aneurysm surgery. Acta Anaesthesiol Scand 33: 15–20

Laroche C M, Moxham J, Green M 1989 Respiratory muscle weakness and fatigue. Q J Med New Series 71, 71: 373–397

Leading article 1988a Transtracheal oxygen. Lancet II: 22–24

Leading article 1988b Pulmonary hypertension: new information from necropsy-based studies. Lancet II: 1315–1316

Leading article 1989a Type 2 diabetes or NIDDM: looking for a better name. Lancet I: 589–591

Leading article 1989b Spasticity. Lancet II: 1488–1490

Leff A R 1988 Endogenous regulation of bronchomotor tone. Am Rev Respir Dis 137: 1198–1216

Levine S N, Sanson T H 1989 Treatment of hyperglycaemic hyperosmolar non-ketotic syndrome. Drugs 38: 462–472

Lipowski Z J 1989 Delirium in the elderly patient. N Engl J Med 320: 578–582

Lodrini S, Montolivo M, Pluchino F, Borroni V 1989 Positive end-expiratory pressure in supine and sitting positions: its effects on intrathoracic and intracranial pressures. Neurosurgery 24: 873–877

Long G R, Filuk R, Balakumar M, Easton P A, Anthonisen N R 1989 Ventilatory response to sustained hypoxia: effect of methysergide and verapamil. Respir Physiol 75: 173–182

Lowe G D O 1990 Drugs in cerebral and peripheral arterial disease. Br Med J 300: 524–528

MacPherson J N, Feely J 1990 Insulin. Br Med J 300: 731–736

Malmkvist G, Fletcher R, Nordstrom L, Werner O 1989 Effects of lung surgery and one-lung ventilation on pulmonary arterial pressure, venous admixture and immediate postoperative lung function. Br J Anaesth 63: 696–701

Mandrup-Poulsen T 1988 On the pathogenesis of insulin-dependent diabetes mellitus. Dan Med Bull 35: 438–460

Manni R, Cerveri I, Brushi C, Zoia C, Tartara A 1988 Sleep and oxyhemoglobin desaturation patterns in chronic obstructive pulmonary diseases. Eur Neurol 28: 275–278

Manni R, Ottolini A, Cerveri I et al 1989 Breathing patterns and $HbSaO_2$ changes during nocturnal sleep in patients with Duchenne muscular dystrophy. J Neurol 236: 391–394

Manoach M, Varon D, Neuman M, Erez M 1989 The cardio-protective features of tricyclic antidepressants. Gen Pharmacol 20: 269–275

Mapleson W W, Smith G, Sykes M K (eds) 1989 Symposium on high frequency ventilation. Br J Anaesth 63 (suppl 1): 1S–115S

Marin J, Ibanez M C, Arribas S 1990 Therapeutic management of nausea and vomiting. Gen Pharmacol 21: 1–10

Marini J J, Culver B H 1989 Systemic gas embolism complicating mechanical ventilation in the adult respiratory distress syndrome. Ann Intern Med 110: 699–703

Markos J, Mullan B P, Hillman D R et al 1989 Preoperative assessment as a predictor of mortality and morbidity after lung resection. Am Rev Respir Dis 139: 902–910

Marsden C D 1990 Parkinson's disease. Lancet 335: 948–952

Marty M, Pouillart P, Scholl S et al 1990 Comparison of the 5-hydroxytryptamine$_3$ (serotonin) antagonist ondansetron (GR 38032F) with high-dose metoclopramide in the control of cisplatin-induced emesis. N Engl J Med 322: 816–821

Mattson M E, Boyd G, Byar D et al 1989 Passive smoking on commercial airline. JAMA 261: 867–872

Melot C, Naeije R, Dechamps P, Hallemans R, Lejeune P 1989 Pulmonary and extrapulmonary contributors to hypoxemia in liver cirrhosis. Am Rev Respir Dis 139: 632–640

Mendelow A D 1990 Management of head injury. Hosp Update March: 195–206

Miadonna A, Leggieri E, Tedeschi A, Lorini M, Froldi M, Zanussi C 1988 Study of the effect of some neuropeptides and endogenous opioid peptides on in vitro histamine release from human lung mast cells and peripheral blood basophils. Agents Actions 25: 11–16

Midgren B, Hansson L, Skeidsvoll H, Elmqvist D 1989 The effects of nitrazepam and flunitrazepam on oxygen desaturation during sleep in patients with stable hypoxemic nonhypercapnic COPD. Chest 95: 765–768

Mier A, Brophy C, Moxham J, Green M 1989 Twitch pressures in the assessment of diaphragm weakness. Thorax 44: 990–996

Mier-Jedrzejowicz A K, Brophy C, Green M 1988 Respiratory muscle function in myasthenia gravis. Am Rev Respir Dis 138: 867–873

Miller L G, Jankovic J 1989 Metoclopramide-induced movement disorders. Clinical findings with a review of the literature. Arch Intern Med 149: 2486–2492

Mookherjee S, Ashutosh K, Dunsky M et al 1988 Nifedipine in chronic cor pulmonale: acute and relatively long-term effects. Clin Pharmacol Ther 44: 289–296

Morrison J F J, Pearson S B, Dean H G 1988 Parasympathetic nervous system in nocturnal asthma. Br Med J 296: 1427–1429

Moxley R T III, Ricker K, Kingston W J, Bohlen R 1989 Potassium uptake in muscle during paramyotonic weakness. Neurology 39: 952–955

Murciano D, Aubier M, Lecocguic Y, Pariente R 1984 Effects of theophylline on diaphragmatic strength and fatigue in patients with chronic obstructive pulmonary disease. N Engl J Med 311: 349–353

Murciano D, Boczkowski J, Lecocguic Y, Emili M, Pariente R, Aubier M 1988 Tracheal occlusion pressure: a simple index to monitor respiratory muscle fatigue during acute respiratory failure in patients with chronic obstructive pulmonary disease. Ann Intern Med 108: 800–805

Murciano D, Auclair M-H, Pariente R, Aubier M 1989 A randomized, controlled trial of theophylline in patients with severe chronic obstructive pulmonary disease. N Engl J Med 320: 1521–1525

Nagel R A, Brown P, Perks W H, Wilson R S E, Kerr G D 1988 Ambulatory pH monitoring of gastro-oesophageal reflux in "morning dipper" asthmatics. Br Med J 297: 1371–1373

Nakahara K, Ohno K, Hashimoto J et al 1988 Prediction of postoperative respiratory failure in patients undergoing lung resection for lung cancer. Ann Thorac Surg 46: 549–552

Nelson F W, Hecht T, Horton W A, Butler I J, Goldie W D, Miner M 1988 Neurological basis of respiratory complications in achondroplasia. Ann Neurol 24: 89–93

Niijima A 1989 Neural mechanisms in the control of blood glucose concentration. J Nutr 119: 833–840

Nunn A J, Gregg I 1989 New regression equations for predicting peak expiratory flow in adults. Br Med J 298: 1068–1070

Oh M S, Carroll H J, Uribarri J 1990 Mechanism of normochloremic and hyperchloremic acidosis in diabetic ketoacidosis. Nephron 54: 1–6

Okubo S, Konno K, Ishizaki T, Suganuma T, Takubo T, Takizawa T, Tanaka M 1988 Serum doxapram and respiratory neuromuscular drive in normal man. Eur J Clin Pharmacol 34: 55–59

Onesti S T, Solomon R A, Quest D O 1989 Cerebral revascularization: a review. Neurosurgery 25: 618–629

Oosterhuis H J G H 1989 The natural course of myasthenia gravis: a long term follow up study. J Neurol Neurosurg Psychiatry 52: 1121–1127

Osei K, O'Dorisio T M, Malarkey W B, Craig E L, Cataland S 1989 Metabolic effects of long-acting somatostatin analogue (Sandostatin) in type 1 diabetic patients on conventional therapy. Diabetes 38: 704–709

Parisi R A, Santiago T V, Edelman N H 1988 Genioglossal and diaphragmatic EMG responses to hypoxia during sleep. Am Rev Respir Dis 138: 610–616

Partinen M, Guilleminault C 1990 Daytime sleepiness and vascular morbidity at seven-year follow-up in obstructive sleep apnea patients. Chest 97: 27–32

Partridge M R 1984 Sleep apnoea syndromes. In: Kaufman L (ed) Anaesthesia Review 2. Churchill Livingstone, Edinburgh, pp 10–20

Paterson D J, Friedland J S, Oliver D O, Robbins P A 1989 The ventilatory response to lowering potassium with dextrose and insulin in subjects with hyperkalaemia. Respir Physiol 76: 393–398

Patwardhan R V, Heilpern R J, Brewster A C, Darrah J J 1983 Pleuropericarditis: an extraintestinal complication of inflammatory bowel disease. Arch Intern Med 143: 94–96

Peacock A 1990 Pulmonary hypertension due to chronic hypoxia. Br Med J 300: 763

Pepe P E 1989 Acute post-traumatic respiratory physiology and insufficiency. Surg Clin N Am 69: 157–173

Permutt S 1988 Circulatory effects of weaning from mechanical ventilation: the importance of transdiaphragmatic pressure. Anesthesiology 69: 157–160

Peters S G, Viggiano R W 1988 Home mechanical ventilation. Mayo Clin Proc 63: 1208–1213

Picado C, Castillo J A, Montserrat J M, Agusti-Vidal A 1989 Aspirin-intolerance as a precipitating factor of life-threatening attacks of asthma requiring mechanical ventilation. Eur Respir J 2: 127–129

Pickard J D, Illingworth M R, Shaw M D M et al 1989 Effect of oral nimodipine on cerebral infarction and outcome after subarachnoid haemorrhage: British aneurysm nimodipine trial. Br Med J 298: 636–642

Pingleton S K 1988 Complications of acute respiratory failure. Am Rev Respir Dis 137: 1463–1493

Poe R H, Kallay M C, Dass T, Celebic A 1988 Can postoperative pulmonary complications after elective cholecystectomy be predicted? Am J Med Sci 295: 29–34

Popa V, Rients P 1989 The effect of inhaled naloxone on resting bronchial tone and exercise-induced asthma. Am Rev Respir Dis 139: 702–709

Postma D S, Peters I, Steenhuis E J, Sluiter H J 1988 Moderately severe chronic airflow obstruction. Can corticosteroids slow down obstruction? Eur Respir J 1: 22–26

Primiano F P Jr, Saidel G M, Montague F W Jr, Kruse K L, Green C G, Horowitz J G 1988 Water vapour and temperature dynamics in the upper airways of normal and CF subjects. Eur Respir J 1: 407–414

Ranganathan N, Sivaciyan V 1989 Abnormalities in jugular venous flow velocity in pulmonary hypertension. Am J Cardiol 63: 719–724

Reddi A S, Camerini-Davalos R A 1990 Diabetic nephropathy. Arch Intern Med 150: 31–43

Regestein Q R, Ferber R, Johnson T S, Murawski B J, Strome M 1988 Relief of sleep apnea by revision of the adult upper airway—a review of clinical experience. Arch Otolaryngol Head Neck Surg 114: 1109–1113

Reid W, Ewing D J, Lightman S L et al 1989 Vasopressin secretion in diabetic subjects with and without autonomic neuropathy: responses to osmotic and postural stimulation. Clin Sci 77: 589–597

Ries A L, Farrou J T, Clausen J L 1988 Pulmonary function tests cannot predict exercise-induced hypoxemia in chronic obstructive pulmonary disease. Chest 93: 454–459

Riley L J Jr, Cooper M, Narins R G 1989 Alkali therapy of diabetic ketoacidosis: biochemical, physiologic, and clinical perspectives. Diabetes Metab Rev 5: 627–636

Rocker G M, Wiseman M S, Pearson D, Shale D J 1989 Diagnostic criteria for adult respiratory distress syndrome: time for reappraisal. Lancet 1: 120–123

Roehrs T, Zorick F, Wittig R, Conway W, Roth T 1989 Predictors of objective level of daytime sleepiness in patients with sleep-related breathing disorders. Chest 95: 1202–1206

Rogers M C, Kirsch J R 1989 Current concepts in brain resuscitation. JAMA 261: 3143–3147

Rosenbloom A L 1990 Intracerebral crises during treatment of diabetic ketoacidosis. Diabetes Care 13: 22–33

Rubinstein I, England S J, Zamel N, Hoffstein V 1989 Glottic dimensions in healthy men and women. Respir Physiol 77: 291–299

Rylander R, Bake B, Fischer J J, Helander I M 1989 Pulmonary function and symptoms after inhalation of endotoxin. Am Rev Respir Dis 140: 981–986

Sanson T H, Levine S N 1989 Management of diabetic ketoacidosis. Drugs 38: 289–300

Sassoon C S H, Mahutte C K, Te T T, Simmons D H, Light R W 1988 Work of breathing and airway occlusion pressure during assist-mode mechanical ventilation. Chest 93: 571–576

Scanlon P D, Loring S H, Pichurko B M et al 1989 Respiratory mechanics in acute quadriplegia—Lung and chest wall compliance and dimensional changes during respiratory maneuvers. Am Rev Respir Dis 139: 615–620

Scarr M, Maltby J R, Jani K, Sutherland L R 1989 Volume and acidity of residual gastric fluid after oral fluid ingestion before elective ambulatory surgery. Can Med Assoc J 141: 1151–1154

Schiller Y, Rahamimoff R 1989 Neuromuscular transmission in diabetes: response to high-frequency activation. J Neurosci 9: 3709–3719

Schwartz A R, Smith P L, Wise R A, Gold A R, Permutt S 1988 Induction of upper airway occlusion in sleeping individuals with subatmospheric nasal pressure. J Appl Physiol 64: 535–542

Schwieger I, Gamulin Z, Suter P M 1989 Lung function during anesthesia and respiratory insufficiency in the postoperative period: physiological and clinical implications. Acta Anaesthesiol Scand 33: 527–534

Selsby D, Jones J G 1990 Some physiological and clinical aspects of chest physiotherapy. Br J Anaesth 64: 621–631

Senn S, Wanger J, Fernandez E, Cherniack R M 1989 Efficacy of a pulsed oxygen delivery device during exercise in patients with chronic respiratory disease. Chest 96: 467–472

Series F, Cormier Y, Desmeules M, La Forge J 1989a Effects of respiratory drive on upper airways in sleep apnea patients and normal subjects. J Appl Physiol 67: 973–979

Series F, Cormier Y, Lampron N, La Forge J 1989b Influence of lung volume in sleep apnoea. Thorax 44: 52–57

Shah S C, Malone J I, Simpson N E 1989 A randomized trial of intensive insulin therapy in newly diagnosed insulin-dependent diabetes mellitus. N Engl J Med 320: 550–554

Shangraw R E, Jahoor F, Miyoshi H et al 1989 Differentiation between septic and postburn insulin resistance. Metabolism 38: 983–989

Shaw P J, Bates D, Cartlidge N E F et al 1987 Neurologic and neuropsychological morbidity following major surgery: comparison of coronary artery bypass and peripheral vascular surgery. Stroke 18: 700–707

Shin S-G, Juan D, Rammohan M 1988 Theophylline pharmacokinetics in normal elderly subjects. Clin Pharmacol Ther 44: 522–530

Simons F E R 1989 H_1-receptor antagonists: clinical pharmacology and therapeutics. J Allergy Clin Immunol 84: 845–861

Simonsen L, Halkier E, Christensen B, Gothgen I H, Krasnik M 1989 Changes in pneumonectomy-space gas tensions. Scand J Clin Lab Invest 49: 109–112

Sjoberg R J, Kidd G S 1989 Pancreatic diabetes mellitus. Diabetes Care 12: 715–724

Skott P, Hother-Nielsen O, Bruun N E et al 1989 Effects of insulin on kidney function and sodium excretion in healthy subjects. Diabetologia 32: 694–699

Sleigh M A, Blake J R, Liron N 1988 The propulsion of mucus by cilia. Am Rev Respir Dis 137: 726–741

Slutsky A S 1988 Nonconventional methods of ventilation. Am Rev Respir Dis 138: 175–183

Smith P L, Wise R A, Gold A R, Schwartz A R, Permutt S 1988 Upper airway pressure-flow relationships in obstructive sleep apnea. J Appl Physiol 64: 789–795

Smith P E M, Edwards R H T, Calverley P M A 1989a Oxygen treatment of sleep hypoxaemia in Duchenne muscular dystrophy. Thorax 44: 997–1001

Smith C C T, Wilson A P, Prichard B N C, Betteridge D J 1989b Platelet efflux of noradrenaline in patients with type 1 diabetes mellitus. Clin Sci 76: 603–607

Smoake J A, Solomon S S 1989 Insulin control of cyclic AMP phosphodiesterase. Life Sci 45: 2255–2268

Snorgaard O, Binder C 1990 Monitoring of blood glucose concentration in subjects with hypoglycaemic symptoms during everyday life. Br Med J 300: 16–18

Staats B A 1988 Dyspnea—heart or lungs? Int J Cardiol 19: 13–17

Stradling J R 1989 Sleep apnoea and systemic hypertension. Thorax 44: 984–989

Stradling J R, Warley A R H 1988 Bilateral diaphragm paralysis and sleep apnoea without diurnal respiratory failure. Thorax 43: 75–77

Sue D Y, Wasserman K, Moricca R B, Casaburi R 1988 Metabolic acidosis during exercise in patients with chronic obstructive pulmonary disease. Chest 94: 931–938

Syvalahti E K G, Ylitalo A, Scheinin M, Tarvonen S, Lauren L 1988 Comparison of the effects of metoclopramide on sympathetic and muscarinic responses after pretreatment with atropine and pirenzepine. Int J Clin Pharmacol Ther Toxicol 26: 16–21

Szeinberg A, Tabachnik E, Rashed N et al 1988 Cough capacity in patients with muscular dystrophy. Chest 94: 1232–1235

Sznajder J I, Fraiman A, Hall J B et al 1989 Increased hydrogen peroxide in the expired breath of patients with acute hypoxemic respiratory failure. Chest 96: 606–612

Takasaki Y, Orr D, Popkin J, Rutherford R, Liu P, Bradley T D 1989 Effect of nasal continuous positive airway pressure on sleep apnea in congestive heart failure. Am Rev Respir Dis 140: 1578–1584

Tanaka Y, Honda Y 1989 Nasal obstruction as a cause of reduced PCO_2 and disordered breathing during sleep. J Appl Physiol 67: 970–972

Tardif C, Nouvet G, Verdure-Poussin A 1988 Sleep apnea syndrome and metabolic acidosis: a coincidental association? In: Duron B, Levi-Valensi P (eds) Sleep Disorders and Respiration. John Libbey Eurotext Ltd, Colloque INSERM, Vol 168, pp 191–192

Tatsumi K, Kimura H, Kunitomo F, Kuriyama T, Honda Y 1989 Arterial oxygen desaturation during sleep in interstitial pulmonary disease—correlation with chemical control of breathing during wakefulness. Chest 95: 962–967

Tenholder Col M F, South-Paul Maj J E 1989 Dyspnea in pregnancy. Chest 96: 381–388

The Parkinson Study Group 1989 Effect of deprenyl on the progression of disability in early Parkinson's disease. N Engl J Med 321: 1364–1371

Thomas P S, Owen E R T C, Hulands G, Milledge J S 1989 Respiratory function in the morbidly obese before and after weight loss. Thorax 44: 382–386

Treacher D F, Douglas A, Jones A, Bateman N T, Bradley R D, Cameron I R 1987 The acute haemodynamic effects of intravenous verapamil in patients with chronic obstructive airways disease. Q J Med 66: 941–952

Trost B N 1989 Hypertension in the diabetic patient—selection and optimum use of antihypertensive drugs. Drugs 38: 621–633

Trovati M, Massucco P, Anfossi G et al 1989 Insulin influences the renin-angiotensin-aldosterone system in humans. Metabolism 38: 501–503

Turken S A, Cafferty M, Silverberg S J et al 1989 Neuromuscular involvement in mild, asymptomatic primary hyperparathyroidism. Am J Med 87: 553–557

Ultman J S, Shaw R G, Fabiano D C, Cooke K A 1988 Pendelluft and mixing in a single bifurcation lung model during high-frequency oscillation. J Appl Physiol 65: 146–155

Vanderschueren D, Decramer M, Van Den Daele P, DeQueker J 1989 Pulmonary function and maximal transrespiratory pressures in ankylosing spondylitis. Ann Rheum Dis 48: 632–635

Van Lunteren E 1988 Respiratory muscle coordination. J Lab Clin Med 112: 285–300

Vodinh J, Bonnet F, Touboul C, Lefloch J P, Becquemin J P, Harf A 1989 Risk factors of postoperative pulmonary complications after vascular surgery. Surgery 105: 360–365

Wagner P D, Mathieu-Costello O, Bebout D E, Gray A T, Natterson P D, Glennow C 1989 Protection against pulmonary O_2 toxicity by N-acetylcysteine. Eur Respir J 2: 116–126

Wanner A 1989 Circulation of the airway mucosa. J Appl Physiol 67: 917–925

Ward J D 1989 Cause and treatment of peripheral nerve damage in diabetes. Hosp Update December: 891–898

Ward M E, Eidelman D, Stubbing D G, Bellemare F, Macklem P T 1988 Respiratory sensation and pattern of respiratory muscle activation during diaphragm fatigue. J Appl Physiol 65: 2181–2189

Warley A, Clarke M, Phillips T, Stradling J 1989 Ventilatory response to an inhaled constant CO_2 load and added dead space in healthy men, awake and asleep. Respir Physiol 75: 183–192

Watkins P J 1990 Diabetic autonomic neuropathy. N Engl J Med 322: 1078–1079

Weinberger S E, Schwartzstein R M, Weiss J W 1989 Hypercapnia. N Engl J Med 321: 1223–1230

Wheatley R G, Somerville I D, Sapsford D J, Jones J G 1990 Postoperative hypoxaemia—comparison of extradural, i.m. and patient-controlled opioid analgesia. Br J Anaesth 64: 267–275

Whyte K F, Allen M B, Jeffrey A A, Gould G A, Douglas N J 1989 Clinical features of the sleep apnoea/hypopnoea syndrome. Q J Med 72: 659–666

Widdicombe J G 1989 Airway mucus. Eur Respir J 2: 107–115

Wiegand L, Zwillichy C W, White D P 1989 Collapsibility of the human upper airway during normal sleep. J Appl Physiol 66: 1800–1808

Wilcox P G, Pardy R L 1989 Diaphragmatic weakness and paralysis. Lung 167: 323–341

Wilcox P, Miller R, Miller G et al 1987 Airway involvement in ulcerative colitis. Chest 92: 18–22

Wilkens J H, Wilkens H, Uffman J, Bovers J, Fabel H, Frolich J C 1990 Effects of a PAF-antagonist (BN 52063) on bronchoconstriction and platelet activation during exercise induced asthma. Br J Clin Pharmacol 29: 85–91

Wilkinson M, Langhorne C A, Heath D, Barer G R, Howard P 1988 A pathophysiological study of 10 cases of hypoxic cor pulmonale. Q J Med 66: 65–85

Williams J G, Morris A, Hayter R C, Ogilvie C M 1984 Respiratory responses of diabetics to hypoxia, hypercapnia, and exercise. Thorax 39: 529–530

Wilson R 1988 Secondary ciliary dysfunction. Clin Sci 75: 113–120

Wolters E Ch, Hurwitz T A, Peppard R F, Calne D B 1989 Clozapine: an antipsychotic agent in Parkinson's disease. Clin Neuropharmacol 12: 83–90

Woo E, Ma J T C, Robinson J D, Yu Y L 1988 Hyperglycemia is a stress response in acute stroke. Stroke 19: 1359–1364

Woodson G E 1989 Effects of recurrent laryngeal nerve transection and vagotomy on respiratory contraction of the cricothyroid muscle. Ann Otol, Rhinol Laryngol 98: 373–378

Wright A D 1989 Diabetic emergencies in adults. Prescribers' J 29: 147–154

Yanai M, Sekizawa K, Sasaki H, Takishima T 1989 Control of the larynx in patients with obstructive and restrictive pulmonary impairment. Eur Respir J 2: 31–35

Young B, Ott L, Dempsey R, Haack D, Tibbs P 1989 Relationship between admission hyperglycemia and neurologic outcome of severely brain-injured patients. Ann Surg 210: 466–473

Younger S J, Landefeld S, Coulton C J, Juknialis B W, Leary M 1989 "Brain death" and organ retrieval. A cross-sectional survey of knowledge and concepts amongst health professionals. JAMA 261: 2205–2210

Zarich S W, Nesto R W 1989 Diabetic cardiomyopathy. Am Heart J 118: 1000–1012

Zavaroni I, Bonora E, Pagliara M et al 1989 Risk factors for coronary artery disease in healthy persons with hyperinsulinemia and normal glucose tolerance. N Engl J Med 320: 702–706

Zetterstrom H 1988 Assessment of the efficiency of pulmonary oxygenation. The choice of oxygenation index. Acta Anaesthesiol Scand 32: 579–584

Zhou D, Huang Q, St John W M, Bartlett D Jr 1989 Respiratory activities of intralaryngeal branches of the recurrent laryngeal nerve. J Appl Physiol 67: 1171–1178

3. The intensive care management of acute asthma

S. Cottam   J. Eason

This article addresses the problem of identifying those acute asthmatics who are most likely to benefit from admission to an intensive care unit (ICU) and offers suggestions concerning their medical management following such an admission. To put the matter in context: asthma, defined as acute reversible airways obstruction, has a prevalence of between 1.5 and 5% in the UK, although it has been claimed that as many as 20% of the population will become wheezy at some period in their lives (Gregg 1977). Precise estimation of the prevalence of asthma is made difficult by the need to exclude other causes of wheezing: neoplasia, bronchiectasis, tuberculosis, chronic obstructive airways disease, acute left ventricular failure, polyarteritis nodosa and related conditions can all mimic asthma, as can cystic fibrosis and inhalation of a foreign body in children.

Advances in our understanding of the pathophysiology of asthma separate the acute increase in airways resistance into two phases—an *initial*, acute bronchospastic phase and a *delayed*, sustained, inflammatory response. Contraction of bronchial smooth muscle gives rise to the sensation of tightness within the chest and often responds to the administration of bronchodilator drugs, such as the beta-agonists and theophyllines. The prolonged secondary response at which steroid therapy is directed results from the release of a variety of inflammatory mediators, and leads to bronchial oedema, accompanied by hypersecretion of viscid mucus. This produces the widespread mucus plugging which is the pathological hallmark of all but the most hyperacute cases of fatal asthma.

Theoretically, asthma is classified as *intrinsic* or *extrinsic*, depending on whether an external precipitant can be identified. A clinically more useful distinction is drawn between juvenile onset asthma (characterized by acute usually allergic episodes, separated by long periods of normal lung function) and the late onset variety (typically chronic, non-allergic and relatively intractable). The juvenile onset group, although larger, carries a much better prognosis and does not show the remorseless deterioration which is a feature of late onset asthma.

Diagnosis of asthma relies on the demonstration of a greater than 20% improvement in peak expiratory flow rate (PFR) following the administration of a bronchodilator, although this may exclude otherwise typical late onset cases.

Currently about 2000 people are certified as dying from asthma each year in England and Wales, despite apparent improvements in drug therapy. This suggests that in fatal cases, medical treatment is either ineffective or inadequately administered, or that treatment is commenced too late to affect outcome. Approximately half of asthma deaths occur in patients aged 65 years and over, and on investigation, many of these turn out to have suffered from smoking-induced chronic obstructive airways disease. Smoking and asthma are not mutually exclusive, but most epidemiological studies of asthma mortality confine their attention to younger asthmatics who are non-smokers. Consequently their conclusions cannot be generalized to all asthma deaths. Nevertheless, there remain about a 1000 'pure' asthmatics whose deaths are widely believed to be avoidable (British Thoracic Association 1982, Johnson et al 1984, Rea et al 1986, Eason & Markowe 1987): indeed there is disturbing evidence that the condition is increasing in both prevalence and severity in the 18–34-year age group.

The majority of asthma deaths occur outside hospital (British Thoracic Association 1982). Prompt investigation and diagnosis, appropriate prophylactic therapy and home monitoring of PFR, awareness of the special risks to which patients who experience dramatic nocturnal falls in airway calibre (nocturnal dippers) are exposed, aggressive treatment of acute episodes, improved patient education, and ready access to hospital are all factors which have been repeatedly identified as areas where improved management should reduce mortality. This research should not blind us to the fact that a significant number of deaths (perhaps as many as a third) still occur after admission to hospital (Eason & Markowe 1987, Rothwell et al 1987). There is a widely held view that such deaths should be prevented by better investigation, monitoring and treatment

WHICH ASTHMATICS NEED INTENSIVE CARE?

A district general hospital can expect to treat several acute asthmatics each day. They will all be impressively dyspnoeic, with a tachycardia and a greatly reduced PFR, but most will respond to first-line treatment with a nebulized bronchodilator such as salbutamol. This phenomenon—an apparently life threatening condition in a young patient which usually improves dramatically with treatment—may hold the key to many hospital asthma deaths. A junior doctor will have seen relatively few severe asthmatics—one cannot but sympathize with the inexperienced casualty officer, unfamiliar with the deceptive presentation of life threatening asthma, who, although he may have been thoroughly frightened by the first case he had to deal with, has quickly learnt that all asthmatics, no matter how distressed they appear, soon get better after treatment with a nebulizer. As a result, he may fail to identify, and consequently will underestimate and undertreat, severe cases some of whom will die.

There are no prospective, controlled studies of the indications for and the technical aspects of elective ventilation for severe asthma. This is because relatively few severe cases occur in any one institution and in any event the ethical and methodological problems of denying some patients intensive care and/or ventilation are insurmountable. Proposed indications for ICU admission and for elective ventilation at present amount to no more than clinical common sense, backed up by a number of retrospective studies (Scoggin et al 1977, Santiago & Klaustermeyer 1980, Picado et al 1983, Dales & Munt 1984, Higgins et al 1986, Luksza et al 1986).

There is no argument that cardiac or respiratory arrest during an asthmatic attack constitute absolute indications for ventilation. An unconscious asthmatic demands immediate intubation. In less extreme circumstances, the situation is not so clearcut. Hypoxia, hypercapnia and an unrecordable PFR are markers of a severe attack; these signs must be sought actively, and if present mean that the patient is a candidate for ventilation. However, the most important factor in deciding upon elective intubation and ventilation must be the patient's response to treatment,

Table 3.1   Suggested indications for intervention

Intubate immediately if:
Cardiac/respiratory arrest
Unconsciousness
Inappropriate bradycardia or hypotension

Admit to intensive care unit
If any of the following fail to respond to O_2 nebulized beta-agonists within 20 min:
Pulse > 120/min
Paradox > 25 mmHg (remembering that paradox is effort related)
Pao_2 < 80 mmHg (despite O_2)
$Paco_2$ > 45 mmHg
pH < 7.30
Tachypnoea > 50/min
PFR < 100 l/min
Or any patient with a poor previous history (i.e. a previous respiratory arrest, IPPV, known to deteriorate very rapidly, or with a recent history of nocturnal dipping, and recent hospital admission with asthma)

Intubate electively
Bearing in mind that response to treatment is more important than absolute values, if the patient shows any two of the following:
Pulse > 150/min or ventricular dysrhythmia
Gross paradox (i.e. pulse disappears on inspiration)
Pao_2 < 60 mmHg despite O_2
$Paco_2$ > 60 mmHg
pH < 7.20
Intolerable respiratory distress, exhaustion, inappropriate bradypnoea (< 10/min), 'silent chest' or inability to speak more than single words
Unrecordable PFR

which can be impressive. Patients who are having an acute attack must be watched carefully while salbutamol, nebulized in 100% oxygen, is administered. Since sudden deterioration may occur at any stage, drugs and equipment for emergency intubation should be made ready and kept with the patient while the bronchodilator is being given. If there is no improvement, as assessed clinically and by objective measurement of arterial blood gases and PFR, the patient should be intubated electively.

It is difficult to define absolute criteria for intubation in cases of acute asthma. Signs of a severe attack which suggest intubation are detailed in Table 3.1, but the decision to intervene must take into account the patient's past history. Early intubation may be wise if there is a history of previous rapid deterioration, especially if cardiac arrest has occurred or artificial ventilation was necessary on a previous occasion. Some patients need immediate intubation in the casualty department whilst in other cases the clinician may decide that there is time to transfer the patient to ICU for intensive monitoring and/or elective intubation. In the latter situation, it is mandatory that the patient should be accompanied in transit by medical staff appropriately equipped to perform emergency intubation. Deaths have occurred prior to the implementation of the decision to intubate; such deaths were attributable to delay in organizing ICU admission or to cardiorespiratory arrest occurring in transit of unaccompanied patients (Eason & Markowe 1987). Once it has been decided that an asthmatic needs intubation the doctor concerned is obliged to remain with the patient until the airway has been secured.

One of the most dangerous aspects of acute asthma is the rapidity with which the clinical condition can change. Some patients who initially improve will deteriorate again later on. Patients who exhibit 'nocturnal dipping' with profound falls in airway calibre between 02:00 h and 06:00 h, are especially at risk (Hetzel et al 1977) and require regular objective (PFR and, when appropriate, arterial blood-glas) monitoring. Inadequate clinical assessment and failure to monitor the patient's response to treatment have been repeatedly identified as factors associated with hospital asthma death. In a majority of fatal cases, disease severity was underestimated and consequently undertreated; no acute asthmatic should be discharged from the accident and emergency (A+E) department without prior assessment by an experienced physician, and those with severe attacks must never be left alone in cubicles. As Peter Rothwell puts it, 'young asthmatics who have had life threatening attacks in the past should be accorded the same priority in the A+E department as a 40-year-old with crushing central chest pain' (Rothwell et al 1987).

INTENSIVE CARE MANAGEMENT

Severe asthmatics, that is, those exhibiting the features outlined in Table

3.1, need admission to an ICU so that they can be closely monitored and, if necessary, intubated and ventilated. Those asthmatics who fail to respond to first-line treatment, particularly if they have an adverse past history, define themselves as a group in need of meticulous monitoring which is best provided in an ICU setting. It is worth emphasizing that, no matter how much their distress invites it, sedation must be forbidden as should the use of beta-blocking drugs to treat hypertension and tachycardia (Raine et al 1981, Jackson 1987).

SPECIFIC TREATMENT

Oxygen

All severe asthmatics need oxygen therapy; this should be actively humidified and the inspired oxygen concentration must be monitored. Concern is occasionally expressed over the possibility of causing respiratory depression in an asthmatic who has become dependant on a hypoxic drive to respiration. This may result in the administration of low inspired oxygen concentrations to a patient with severe hypoxia. In the opinion of the authors this practice is to be condemned on the grounds that acquisition of a hypoxic respiratory drive is rare, even amongst chronic bronchitics. Hypoxia, unlike hypercarbia is rapidly fatal, and in any event respiratory depression of this type should be obvious in a properly monitored ICU patient who must be intubated before the $Paco_2$ reaches narcotic levels.

Fluid and electrolytes

Sufferers from acute asthma become dehydrated due to a combination of increased loss of water vapour (as a result of rapid mouth breathing) and diminished intake (resulting from severe dyspnoea and limited mobility). Unfortunately, central venous pressure measurements are not always a reliable guide to the state of the circulation during a severe asthma attack because of pulmonary hyperinflation. Pulmonary capillary wedge pressures (PCWP) can also be misleading as the hyperinflated respiratory unit can act as a static resistor and (in ventilated patients) PCWP may reflect intra-alveolar pressure rather than left atrial pressure. In practice, there is a tendency to overestimate cardiac filling pressures, which is particularly undesirable if ventilation is envisaged, since a major fall in arterial blood pressure is likely to occur on commencing intermittent positive pressure ventilation (IPPV). As a rough guide, otherwise fit patients with acute severe asthma of more than 12 h duration will usually require at least 3 l of fluid and oliguria is more appropriately treated by further volume replacement than a loop diuretic.

A number of drugs act in concert to cause the hypokalaemia which is so typical of acute asthma. Beta-agonists promote cellular potassium influx (Rolf-Smith & Kendall 1984); theophylline and adrenaline also enhance potassium translocation as does the respiratory alkalosis which is an early feature of acute asthma. Although there is no total body potassium deficit, serum hypokalaemia should be corrected lest it summate with other arrythmogenic factors such as hypoxia, hypomagnesaemia, hypercapnia and sympathomimetic drug treatment.

The initial respiratory alkalosis is replaced with a progressive metabolic acidosis as an attack increases in severity. Initially renal bicarbonate excretion is increased, making the later acidosis more severe by reducing the patient's buffering capacity. Lactic acidosis is uncommon (Okrent et al 1987), but if an increased anion gap is found (provided coincident diabetic ketoacidosis is excluded) this indicates very severe asthma and the need for ventilation. If acidosis remains uncorrected, cardiac depression and unresponsiveness to bronchodilators will occur due to down-regulation of beta-receptors.

Physiotherapy

In patients who have not been intubated, physiotherapy should be little and often, taking care to avoid discontinuing the administration of humidified oxygen. Intermittent positive pressure breathing using a pressure cycled device such as the Bird, although in theory ill-advised, can be of value in the hands of an experienced therapist, providing pressure settings are kept low. More important than any of these methods however is the establishment of good rapport between patient and therapist—hypoxia and hypercarbia get worse in a struggling, panicky, tachypnoeic patient: conversely, the establishment of a relaxed controlled pattern of respiration has saved numerous patients from intubation.

In the intubated patient physiotherapy comprises frequent brief episodes of endotracheal suction accompanied by gentle percussion and appropriate positioning. Pulmonary hyperinflation is to be avoided, as is the use of a Waters bag (Mapleson C circuit) because it leads to the application of high levels of positive end expiratory pressure (PEEP). Endotracheal instillation of small volumes (2–5 ml) of *warm* isotonic saline is common practice, in the belief that it loosens inspissated sputum plugs. Other forms of lavage— involving segmental or whole lung washout with saline or bicarbonate and enzyme cocktails, administered via a fibreoptic bronchoscope or double lumen endobronchial tube—have not achieved widespread popularity not-withstanding encouraging case reports. There may be a place for swift and skilful bronchoscopy directed towards a single collapsed lobe in a stable, fully paralysed and sedated patient but even this is unwise in the presence of hypoxia or in patients whose airway pressures exceed $50\,cmH_2O$. An effective mucolytic agent would be of considerable value, but none exists at present.

Drug treatment

Bronchodilators

Beta-2-agonists. All but the most severe cases of asthma should be treated with nebulized beta-2-agonists such as salbutamol or terbutaline, diluted with saline (never water as hyposmolar solutions can exacerbate bronchospasm). Like all vasoactive drugs, beta-agonists inhibit hypoxic pulmonary vasoconstriction (HPV) and can therefore impair ventilation to perfusion matching: for this reason, they should always be given in an oxygen driven nebulizer. There is no place for air driven nebulizers, in home or hospital. New longer acting agents such as salmeterol and formotarol (Wallin et al 1990) are currently being evaluated and may come to replace salbutamol and terbutaline as first-line therapy.

Salbutamol can be given intravenously, as a loading dose of $4\,\mu g/kg$ over one minute followed by an infusion of $2\text{--}20\,\mu g\,kg^{-1}/min$. Compared with nebulization, intravenous administration causes more tachycardia for a given degree of bronchodilation: nevertheless it is appropriate in patients with unrecordable PFR's who may be unable to inhale sufficient salbutamol or terbutaline. Both drugs may also be given subcutaneously or intramuscularly: patients known to be at risk from hyperacute asthma can be given a preloaded syringe for self-administration (Bateman & Clarke 1979).

Prior to the advent of specific beta-2-agents, adrenaline was the bronchodilator of choice in severe asthma. It has largely fallen out of use owing to its arrythmogenic propensities—however, it still has its advocates, particularly in Australia and New Zealand. Although usually given intravenously in a *total* dose of $1\text{--}10\,\mu g/min$ (*not* $\mu g\,kg^{-1}/min$) it can also be nebulized in which case it may usefully inhibit bronchial mucosal oedema.

Theophylline and aminophylline. The mechanism of action of theophylline and its derivatives is not understood. Their low therapeutic index and the need to adjust dosage with respect to body weight, smoking habits, cardiorespiratory status and concurrent drug therapy (Editorial 1983, Jusko et al 1977) have relegated the theophyllines to a second-line role in the treatment of acute asthma, but a majority of chest physicians continue to use them for patients who respond inadequately to nebulized beta-2-agonists. Plasma levels must be monitored ($10\text{--}20\,mg/l$ is the therapeutic range): a loading dose of $5\,mg/kg$ given over 20 min should be followed by an infusion of $0.5\,mg\,kg^{-1}/h$ ($0.9\,mg\,kg^{-1}/h$ in children and adult smokers) (Hendeles & Weinberger 1980). Aminophylline 5 mg is equivalent to theophylline 4 mg. Unless there is time to measure plasma levels before starting treatment, it is wise to omit the loading dose in patients known to be taking oral theophyllines and all doses should be halved in patients receiving drugs which inhibit theophylline metabolism (cimetidine, erythromycin, ciprofloxacin) (Reitberg et al 1981, Reisz et al 1982, Committee on Safety of Medicines 1988). A small number of hospital asthma deaths may be associated with excessive theophylline administration (Hendeles & Weinberger 1980, 1983, Woodcock et al 1983, Eason & Markowe 1989).

Atropinics. Ipratropium bromide exerts an additive bronchodilator effect if given concurrently with beta-2-agonists. The usual dose is 500 μg four hourly conveniently mixed with salbutamol and saline in the same nebulizer. Its beneficial effects are easily overlooked as its maximum action takes 2–3 h to develop. There have been isolated reports of idiosyncratic bronchoconstriction associated with its use (Patel & Tullet 1983).

New bronchodilators. Recent research has emphasized the importance of a delayed inflammatory response which follows the initial bronchoconstrictor response of acute asthma. Terfenadine and azelastine are new selective H_1 antihistamines, which inhibit the initial bronchoconstrictor response to antigen challenge. Leukotriene antagonists (such as LY 171883) may act similarly, whereas the mediators of delayed bronchial inflammation—which include platelet activating factor (PAF) and PAF-acether—may be usefully inhibited by compounds such as BN 52022 and BN 52063, nebulized vasoactive intestinal polypeptide and the thiosulphinates, a group of naturally occurring compounds present in plants of the onion family.

Steroids

Glucocorticoids constitute an essential part of the treatment of acute asthma, although this has been questioned. The authors use hydrocortisone six hourly for as long as the acute phase of the condition lasts. As the patient improves, this can be replaced by a reducing course of oral prednisolone. The evidence for additional benefit from higher steroid dosage (Tanaka et al 1982) is unconvincing and this practice increases the risk of infection, fluid retention, hyperglycaemia, steroid myopathy and psychosis.

Antibiotics

Treating asthma with antibiotics when bronchodilators and steroids are required has been repeatably and rightly condemned. Nevertheless, their use is indicated in a majority of cases severe enough to require ICU admission. Bacterial secondary infection is almost universal after 2–3 days of mechanical ventilation. Whether it is better to await the results of sputum culture or to administer broad-spectrum antibiotics is a matter of debate. The role of selective parenteral and antisepsis regimes (SPEAR) in this group of patients requires evaluation but it may reduce the incidence of endogenous infection to which these patients are certainly prone, whilst the parenteral component (cefotaxime) allows treatment of primary bacterial infection (if present) (Inglis 1990). If erythromycin (Reisz et al 1982) or ciprofloxacin (Committee on Safety of Medicines 1988) have to be used then aminophylline dosage must be reduced.*

Prevention of gastrointestinal bleeding

Stress ulceration and gastrointestinal bleeding are common in ventilated asthmatics. This may be related to steroid and excessive aminophylline administration in some cases (Eason & Markowe 1989). The choice of prophylactic agents lies between sucralfate and the H_2 receptor antagonists. Sucralfate has theoretical advantages in minimizing changes in intragastric pH and hence preserving the patient's defence against infection. Available studies suggest that it is as effective as H_2 receptor antagonists in the prevention of stress ulceration (Editorial 1989). Of the H_2 receptor antagonists, ranitidine is preferable to cimetidine, owing to the latter's extensive interactions (especially with aminophylline whose elimination half-life doubles) (Reitberg ct al 1981).

Intubation

The indications for elective intubation have already been discussed and are summarized in Table 3.1. In the UK there remains a small minority of physicians who perceive intubation of asthmatics as a treatment of last resort, an opinion reinforced, in those who hold it, by the experience of death occurring at intubation or, by degrees, as multi-organ failure supervenes on the ICU. Asthmatics intubated in response to cardio-respiratory arrest have a poor prognosis, when compared to the patients intubated electively. If one only treats the moribund, then the view that it is futile to ventilate asthmatics becomes a self-fulfilling prophecy. Complications, especially myocardial infarction (which is known to occur silently during acute severe asthma) (Chappell 1984) and ischaemic brain damage are minimized by intervention before the patient has deteriorated to a point where hypoxic cardiac and cerebral damage is actually taking place.

Having made the decision to intubate an asthmatic electively, continuous ECG, invasive arterial pressure and oxygen saturation monitoring should be instituted, intravenous access secured and the patient preoxygenated for five minutes with a close fitting facemask whilst appropriate drugs and equipment are assembled (see Table 3.2). Theoretically there is a choice of techniques for induction of anaesthesia. If an inhalational induction is chosen then halothane or isoflurane in 100% oxygen can be used. Despite

---

*Note that the dose of theophylline should be reduced in the presence of erythromycin, and not increased as wrongly stated in *Anaesthesia Review 7*, p. 48.

Table 3.2 Checklist of drugs and equipment for elective intubation

Drugs	Equipment

Inhalational induction
  Oxygen and halothane or enflurane
  or isoflurane
 	
Intravenous induction
  Etomidate ($\pm$ lignocaine,
  $\pm$ fentanyl)
  or Diazemuls
  or Ketamine ($\pm$ Diazemuls)
 	
Optional muscle relaxant
  Suxamethonium or pancuronium
 	
Supplementary Drugs
Atropine
Adrenaline (1 in 100 000)
Aminophylline
	Working ventilator suitably adjusted
	for patient
	Working suction apparatus
	Two working laryngoscopes, one with
	long blade
	Selection of ET tubes, cut to appropriate
	lengths
	Lubricated ETT introducing stylet (plus
	oesophageal bougie or similar for difficult
	intubations)
	ETT cuff inflating syringe
	Tie/tape to secure ETT
	Catheter mount

its well known contraindications we would advocate halothane as the drug of first choice in this situation. Intravenous techniques require a relatively non-cardiodepressant agent with minimal histamine releasing properties; this limits choice to etomidate, ketamine or diazepam. Once consciousness is lost then a muscle relaxant is essential; although this presupposes an experienced operator confident in his intubation skills. Inept attempts to intubate will precipitate vomiting and possibly aspiration. Even mild laryngeal trauma may provoke intense bronchospasm. A number of deaths have occurred at this time. Suxamethonium, although it can cause histamine release and bradycardia, provides the best intubating conditions and has the great advantage of a rapid onset of action; pancuronium, which does not release histamine or cause bradycardia, inevitably leads to a situation in which it becomes necessary to ventilate the patient manually, which may prove impossible in the presence of severe airway obstruction. The authors favour fentanyl, atropine and lignocaine (to minimize pain on injection) followed by etomidate and suxamethonium.

Ventilation

Once a (low pressure, high volume) cuffed endotracheal tube is in place, paralysis can be maintained by pancuronium or vecuronium. An opiate–benzodiazepine cocktail usually provides satisfactory sedation—typically fentanyl or phenoperidine combined with diazepam or midazolam. Ketamine infusions are a popular alternative (Fisher 1977, Rajanna et al 1982, Strube & Hallam 1986); used as an induction agent the drug has been reported to lower airway resistance dramatically although this is unpredictable and in our hands has been disappointing. Ketamine is hallucinogenic and can lead to undesirable cardiovascular stimulation. Low

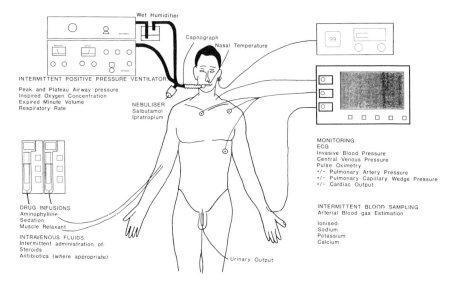

Fig. 3.1 Monitoring of the ventilated asthmatic.

concentrations of isoflurane have been administered for sedation (Kong et al 1989) although the remote risks of fluoride accumulation, immunosuppression and impairment of HPV exist. Tube placement must be confirmed by auscultation—right endobronchial intubation or undiagnosed pneumothorax are likely to prove fatal in severe asthma. Initially, airway pressures will be very high and initiation of IPPV may lead to an acute fall in blood pressure, due to the combined effects of peripheral vasodilatation and cardiac depression (as a result of the anaesthetic drugs) and a decrease in venous return and hence cardiac output (due to high intrathoracic pressure, acute pulmonary hypertension and cardiac tamponade by over-inflated lungs and a vertically stretched pericardium). Arterial blood-gas tensions will dictate an appropriate inspired oxygen concentration. A chest radiograph should be obtained as soon as possible to confirm correct tube placement and to exclude acute lung pathology. Once the patient is stable from a cardiovascular viewpoint and sedated, a nasogastric tube, central venous pressure line and urinary catheter can be inserted (Fig. 3.1).

Choice of ventilator

One of the reasons why ventilation of asthmatics is historically associated with a dismal outcome is that the ventilator technology of the 1950s and 1960s was unequal to the task of ventilating patients with high but fluctuating airway resistance. A powerful flow generator, volume preset and time cycled, with a variable inspiratory to expiratory (I:E) ratio and adjustable inspiratory pressure limits should be used. Ports for humidification, drug nebulization and volatile anaesthetic administration are necessary. Suitable devices include the Siemens-Elema 900 series, the Engstrom Erica, the Bourne Bear, the Puritan-Bennet 7200 and the Ohmeda CPU-1. To attempt to ventilate a severe asthmatic whose airway pressure will commonly exceed $70\,cmH_2O$ on an unsophisticated ventilator is to invite hypotension and pneumothorax.

Dialectics of ventilation

The interaction between a sophisticated ventilator and the deranged haemodynamics and pulmonary mechanics of an acute asthmatic is a uniquely difficult area of pathophysiology. There is no consensus on the degree to which high inflation pressures are transmitted to the alveolar gas spaces and the pulmonary capillaries. Some authors stress the need to reduce peak inspiratory pressure by selecting a rapid respiratory rate with small tidal volumes, even going so far as to advocate intravenous bicarbonate therapy to counteract the resultant respiratory acidosis (Eissa & Pereira 1989). Others, including the authors, favour slower ventilatory rates with larger tidal volumes. This lowers CO_2 more effectively, while generating higher peak (though often lower mean) intrathoracic pressures. Much has been written about the dangers of rapidly reducing a markedly elevated $Paco_2$—the point being that a sudden fall in CO_2 may abruptly terminate sympathetic overactivity and lead to hypotension. In practice, it is rarely possible to achieve sufficient alveolar minute volume in a severe asthmatic to drop CO_2 dangerously fast, except perhaps in a patient whose airway resistance dramatically normalizes itself on initiating ventilation— usually those whose initial deterioration was equally rapid—so the problem is largely academic.

Respiratory mechanics

Spasm of bronchial smooth muscle, oedema of bronchial mucosa and hypersecretion of viscid mucus which plugs the bronchial lumen, combine to increase airway resistance in severe asthma. Asthmatics try to overcome this by increased inspiratory effort; intrapleural pressures as low as $-50\,cmH_2O$ have been recorded during acute asthma (Stalcup & Mellins 1977). In the early stage of an asthma attack, increased respiratory effort leads to pulmonary hyperinflation, which benefits the patient by exerting radial traction on the narrowed airways, so keeping them open. However, as lung volumes increase it becomes harder and harder to inhale an adequate tidal breath and expiration, normally passive, becomes an active process. The patient experiences difficulty in breathing in and out; attempts to empty the lungs are frustrated as the positive intrapleural pressures dynamically compress the airways through which the patient is trying to breathe out. Pulsus paradoxus (arterial hypotension during inspiration) parallels increases in lung volume; it is a useful measure of severity in acute asthma although, since it is effort related, its sudden 'improvement' may indicate impending respiratory arrest. The fight to breathe eventually exhausts even the strongest asthmatic, resulting in carbon dioxide retention and respiratory failure.

The institution of IPPV radically alters lung mechanics in asthma. Ventilators may be required to generate very high inflation pressures— approaching or exceeding $100\ cmH_2O$—in order to force an adequate tidal volume through obstructed airways into hyperinflated lungs. If the extent of airway narrowing was homogeneous throughout the lungs there would be a progressively falling pressure gradient from trachea to alveolus as the energy supplied by the ventilator was used up in overcoming airway resistance. In reality, airway calibre varies regionally and so some areas of lung (particularly where there is a lung cyst or patch of emphysematous tissue), may be exposed to high intra-alveolar pressures. This can lead to pneumothorax, pneumo-mediastinum or in extreme cases pulmonary venous gas embolism. Compression of pulmonary capillaries is reflected by increases in pulmonary artery pressure which can lead to acute right heart failure. Surprisingly, pneumothorax is not all that common in reported series of ventilated asthmatics (Scoggin et al 1977, Santiago & Klaustermeyer 1980, Picado et al 1983, Dales & Munt 1984, Higgins et al 1986, Luksza et al 1986) and circulatory collapse is only seen in patients who are hypovolaemic or have pre-existing heart disease.

In a paralysed asthmatic on a ventilator, expiration is passive. To prevent progressive pulmonary hyperexpansion, the longest possible expiratory period should be provided, to permit as large a proportion as possible of the tidal volume to be exhaled through the narrowed airways, hence our preference for a slow respiratory rate (8–10 breaths/min) with relatively large tidal volumes (10–12 ml/kg—a certain degree of compression within the ventilator tubing and the patient's lungs will reduce the effective tidal volume). This pattern keeps dead space ventilation, mean (but not peak) intrathoracic pressure and total inspiratory time to a minimum, at the price of relatively high peak airway pressures. We have not found it necessary to employ deliberate hypoventilation and bicarbonate therapy (Eissa & Pereira 1989) and have no experience of the use of a low pressure chamber (Lenggenhager 1985) or induced hypothermia. Pulmonary artery catheterization is useful in severe cases as it enables monitoring of pulmonary artery pressures, cardiac output and mixed venous oxygen saturation. This allows optimal volume loading and the use of inotropes where required to optimize oxygen delivery.

Positive end expiratory pressure (PEEP)

PEEP increases lung volume and shifts the tidal volume above functional residual capacity thereby preventing small airway closure, and improving pulmonary gas exchange. This may help to avoid the use of potentially toxic inspired oxygen concentrations. The lungs of asthmatics, however, are already hyperinflated and PEEP, by further distending the lungs, compromises the circulation (by raising mean intrathoracic pressure) and increases the risk of barotrauma. For this reason PEEP is not employed in ventilated asthmatics. There are several reports of dramatic resolution of severe airway obstruction following the application of high ($25\,cmH_2O$) level PEEP in asthmatics (Qvist et al 1982, Shivarum et al 1987). Perhaps PEEP complements the pulmonary hyperexpansion so characteristic of asthma and holds open partly occluded airways. Although the idea is intriguing, there is insufficient evidence to recommend the practice and in our opinion even low levels of PEEP are best avoided in asthmatics.

Management of complications

Straightforward cases, in which the history is short (less than 24 h) and there is no bacterial chest infection may require only a few hours' ventilation. Some patients improve so dramatically that they can be extubated within minutes. A large number of asthmatics, however, will need days or weeks on a ventilator and develop all the problems to which ICU patients are prone. Secondary bacterial infection and acute gastric or duodenal ulceration have already been mentioned, and other common complications include line-related sepsis, pressure sores and steroid myopathy. If airway pressures remain grossly elevated for a long period, in the absence of an underlying chest infection, it is important to exclude other causes of increased airway resistance, such as undiagnosed broncho-pulmonary aspergillosis, polyarteritis nodosa, or pulmonary eosinophilia.

Extubation

Asthmatics are defined by their hyperreactive airways. Acute rises in airway pressure are commonly precipitated by endotracheal suction or by nursing procedures which disturb the patient, even when adequate doses of sedatives and relaxants are employed. This problem is particularly trying at the time of extubation, when sedation is discontinued in an attempt to re-establish spontaneous ventilation. Extubation will only be contemplated once airway pressures have fallen to an acceptable level (30–$35\,cmH_2O$) but a combination of discomfort due to the endotracheal tube, fear and possibly drug withdrawal effects often produce a recurrence of the bronchospasm. Such patients can often be extubated whilst lightly anaesthetized with an inhalational agent such as isoflurane (halothane and ether have also been used) or intravenous propofol or etomidate infusion. Skilful airway maintenance and a readiness to reintubate if required are essential for successful extubation, and in all patients a nerve stimulator must be used to demonstrate full recovery of neuromuscular transmission.

Anticholinesterase drugs are contraindicated due to their propensity to produce bronchorrhea and bronchospasm.

'Total bronchospasm'

There are a small number of asthmatics whom it is impossible to ventilate after intubation, or who develop catastrophically high airway resistance after endotracheal suction or other forms of stimulation. This extreme 'total bronchospasm' may also occur during anaphylactic responses to anaesthetic drugs or antibiotics. Airway pressures exceed $100\,cmH_2O$, and the patient becomes rapidly cyanosed and gas exchange is impossible. Induction of general anaesthesia with an inhalational agent such as ether (Robertson et al 1985), halothane (Bayliff et al 1985), enflurane or isoflurane (Revell et al 1988) may break the bronchospasm but may further depress the circulation and worsen the hypoxia by impairing ventilation and perfusion relationships. Ketamine does not impair HPV and has been reported to be of value in this situation. Alternatively, manual chest compression may be employed: the patient should be inflated with 100% oxygen, the endotracheal tube should be disconnected from the gas source and the patient's chest should be squeezed firmly for 10–15 s until the expiratory wheeze subsides and the lungs have deflated perceptibly. The ventilation–compression cycle is repeated for 5–10 min until the extreme pulmonary hyperinflation has been corrected and manual inflation with an AMBU bag and Rubens valve can be carried out without excessive inspiratory pressures (Eason 1988). The manoeuvre can be lifesaving, particularly in patients whose asthma is of very sudden onset. Patients who have deteriorated gradually have mucus plugging and bronchial oedema which cannot be quickly reversed by this technique.

Follow up

All asthmatics who have been ventilated should be considered at risk of further equally severe attacks. After discharge from the ICU they should be singled out for education in the recognition and treatment of acute episodes and arrangements should be made for their prompt readmission if necessary (Crompton et al 1979). Patients should be issued with peak flow meters and encouraged to record results on a daily basis on diary cards. They should have written instructions on crisis management together with supplies of oral prednisolone for self-medication if their peak flow falls to less than 50% of normal despite bronchodilator treatment. Individuals who are known to suffer from hyperacute attacks may also be given prefilled syringes of terbutaline or adrenaline for intramuscular self-administration in an emergency. Arrangements for priority self admission must be made for these high risk patients at their local hospitals, they should carry warning cards or bracelets, and their family practitioners, if called to attend such a patient in the throes of a severe attack, should administer oxygen-nebulized salbutamol and parenteral hydrocortisone and should personally accompany the patient to the nearest hospital or ideally ICU. In the absence of such a planned strategy young asthmatics will continue to die needlessly.

REFERENCES

Bateman J R M, Clarke S W 1979 Sudden death in asthma. Thorax 34: 40–44
Bayliff C D, Koch J P, Faclier G 1985 The use of halothane in the treatment of status asthmaticus. Drug Intell Clin Pharm 19: 307–309
British Thoracic Association 1982 Death from asthma in two regions of England. Br Med J 285: 1251–1255
Chappell A G 1984 Painless myocardial infarction in asthma. Br J Dis Chest 78: 174–179
Committee on Safety of Medicines 1988 Ciprofloxacin interaction with theophyllines is dangerous. CSM Current problems. No 22
Crompton G K, Grant I W B, Bloomfield P 1979 Edinburgh emergency admission service: a report on ten year's experience. Br Med J ii: 1199–1201
Dales R E, Munt P W 1984 Use of mechanical ventilation in adults with severe asthma. Can Med Assoc J 130: 391–395
Eason J 1988 Ventilating asthmatics. Current Medical Literature (Roy Soc Med)—Reversible obstructive airways disease 2: 57–63
Eason J, Markowe H L J 1987 Controlled investigation of deaths from asthma in hospitals in the North East Thames region. Br Med J 294: 1255–1258
Eason J, Markowe H L J 1989 Aminophylline toxicity—how many hospital asthma deaths does it cause? Respir Med 83: 219–226
Editorial 1983 Theophylline, benefits and difficulties. Lancet ii: 607–608
Editorial 1989 Stress ulcer prophylaxis in critically ill patients. Lancet ii: 1255–1256
Eissa N, Pereira R 1989 Mechanical hypoventilation and bicarbonate therapy in status asthmaticus: appraisal of therapy. Am Rev Respir Dis 17(4): 331
Fisher M M 1977 Ketamine hydrochloride in severe bronchospasm. Anaesthesia 32: 771–772
Gregg I 1977 Epidemiology [of asthma]. In: Clark T J, Godfrey S (eds) Asthma. W B Saunders, Philadelphia, Ch 11
Hendeles L, Weinberger M W 1980 Poisoning patients with intravenous aminophylline. Am J Hosp Pharm 37: 49–50
Hendeles L, Weinberger M 1983 Theophylline, a "state of the art" review. Pharmacotherapy 3: 2–44
Hetzel M R, Clarke T J H, Branthwaite M A 1977 Asthma: analysis of sudden deaths and respiratory arrests in hospital. Br Med J i: 808–811
Higgins B, Greening A P, Crompton G K 1986 Assisted ventilation in severe acute asthma. Thorax 41: 464–467
Inglis T J J 1990 Pulmonary infection in intensive care units. Br J Anaesth 65: 94–106
Jackson D 1987 Beta-blockers in asthma. Br Med J i: 808–811
Johnson A J, Nunn A J, Somner A R et al 1984 Circumstances of death from asthma. Br Med J 288: 1870–1872
Jusko W J, Kroup J R, Vance J W et al 1977 Intravenous theophylline therapy: nomogram guidelines. Ann Int Med 86: 400–404
Kong K L, Willats S M, Prys-Roberts C 1989 Isoflurane compared with midazolam for sedation on the intensive care unit. Br Med J 298: 1277–1280
Lenggenhager K 1985 Treatment of severe bronchial asthma with a low pressure chamber and 100% oxygen. Anesth Analg 64: 551–553
Luksza A R, Smith P, Coakley J et al 1986 Acute severe asthma treated by mechanical ventilation: 10 year's experience from a DGH. Thorax 41: 459–463
Okrent D G, Tessler S, Twersky R A et al 1987 Metabolic acidosis not due to lactic acidosis in patients with severe asthma. Crit Care Med 15: 1098–1101
Patel K R, Tullett W M 1983 Bronchoconstriction in response to ipatropium bromide. Br Med J 286: 1318

Picado C, Montserrat J M, Roca J et al 1983 Mechanical ventilation in severe exacerbation of asthma. Eur J Respir Dis 64: 102–107

Qvist J, Anderson J B, Pemberton M et al 1982 High level PEEP in severe asthma. New Engl J Med 307: 1347–1348

Raine J M, Palazzo M G, Kerr J H et al 1981 Near fatal bronchospasm after oral nadolol in a young asthmatic and response to ventilation with halothane. Br Med J 282: 548–549

Rajanna P, Narayana, Reddy J et al 1982 Ketamine for the relief of bronchospasm during anaesthesia. Anaesthesia 37: 1215

Rea H R, Scragg R, Jackson R et al 1986 A case control study of deaths from asthma. Thorax 41: 833–839

Reisz G R, Ryan P B, Melethil S et al 1982 Erythromycin-induced changes in theophylline kinetics in chronic bronchitis. Am Rev Respir Dis 125 (suppl): 95

Reitberg D P, Bernhard H, Schentag J J 1981 Alteration of theophylline clearance and half life by cimetidine in normal volunteers. Ann Int Med 95: 582–585

Revell S, Greenhalgh D, Absalom S R et al 1988 Isoflurane in the treatment of asthma. Anaesthesia 43: 477–479

Robertson C E, Steedman D, Sinclair C J et al 1985 Use of ether in life threatening acute severe asthma. Lancet i: 187–188

Rolf-Smith S, Kendall H J 1984 Metabolic response to beta-2 stimulants. J R Coll Physicians 18: 190–194

Rothwell R P G, Rea H H, Sears M R et al 1987 Lessons from the national asthma mortality study: deaths in hospital. NZ Med J 100: 189–202

Santiago S M, Klaustermeyer W B 1980 Mortality in status asthmaticus: a 9 year experience in a respiratory ICU. J Asthma Res 17: 75–79

Scoggin C H, Sahn S A, Petty T L 1977 Status asthmaticus: a 9 year experience. JAMA 238: 1158–1162

Shivarum V, Donath J, Khan F et al 1987 Effects of continuous positive airway pressure in acute asthma. Respiration 52: 157–162

Stalcup S A, Mellins R B 1977 Mechanical forces producing pulmonary oedema in acute asthma. New Engl J Med 297: 592–596

Strube P J, Hallam P L 1986 Ketamine by continuous infusion in status asthmaticus. Anaesthesia 41: 1017–1019

Tanaka R M, Santiago S M, Kohn G J et al 1982 Intravenous methyl prednisolone in adults in status asthmaticus. Chest 4: 438–440

Wallin A, Melander B, Rosenhall L et al 1990 Formoterol, a new long acting beta$_2$ agonist for inhalation twice daily, compared with salbutamol in the treatment of asthma. Thorax 45: 259–261

Woodcock A A, Johnson M A, Geddes D M 1983 Theophylline prescribing, serum concentrations and toxicity. Lancet ii: 610–613

4. The role of hypoxia in the control of breathing

D. S. Ward   J. A. Temp

Although the basic elements and organization of the ventilatory controller were understood in the first half of this century and the role of the carotid chemoreceptors was elucidated in the 1920s, much detailed information has only become known in the past decade. Many reflexes and drives determine ventilation, and although oxygen drive does not contribute substantially to normal resting ventilation, the response to hypoxia is an important protective reflex. In the peri-operative period and particularly post-operatively, many factors may induce hypoxaemia, including hypoventilation (particularly with a decreased tidal volume from residual drug effects and from pain associated with breathing), obstructed upper airways, atelectasis and decreased cardiac output. While supplemental oxygen can prevent hypoxaemia in many situations, episodic desaturations can occur even in patients receiving oxygen.

Normally, increased ventilation is thought of in terms of its effect on arterial CO_2, but when hypoxaemia is caused by atelectasis or upper airway obstruction, increased ventilatory drive may help alleviate the hypoxaemia. Thus, the hypoxic ventilatory drive may be an important reflex in the peri-operative period. However, almost every drug administered in the course of anaesthesia alters the control of breathing. In some cases (e.g. muscle relaxants) the result is in clear relation to the drug's intended effect. In most instances, however, the alteration in breathing is an unintended, and usually undesirable, side effect of the drug's primary purpose.

In this chapter, we review the incidence of peri-operative hypoxaemia, the normal ventilatory response to hypoxia, and the effect of anaesthetic drugs on hypoxic control, as well as the phenomenon of hypoxic ventilatory depression.

HYPOXIA IN THE PERI-OPERATIVE PERIOD

In 1962, Nunn and Payne reported a 'surprising' finding made incidentally during their other studies:

> ... the arterial oxygen tension fell rapidly at the conclusion of operation when they began to breathe room air, and remained substantially below normal for at

least twenty-four hours . . . No patient was cyanosed (and) the carbon-dioxide tensions in all patients were never unduly high . . . We have found that postoperative hypoxaemia is, in fact, usual and that it seems to follow even the most trivial surgical procedures under general anaesthesia.

The advent of inexpensive and reliable pulse oximetry in the 1980s has brought a new series of such 'surprising and disturbing' findings throughout the peri-operative period.

The occurrence of intra-operative hypoxia was studied by Raemer et al (1987) in 108 healthy women undergoing anaesthesia for ambulatory gynaecologic procedures. Ten percent of patients had one or more desaturations to less than 90%, and 5% had desaturations to less than 85%. Only 2 of 14 desaturations were recognized by the anaesthetist, emphasizing both that arterial desaturation occurs before the clinical signs and symptoms of hypoxaemia, and that anaesthesia tends to mask those signs.

Tyler et al (1985) monitored 95 healthy ASA I or II adults during transport to the recovery room. All were pre-oxygenated with 100% O_2 for 5 min prior to transport. Thirty-five percent developed hypoxaemia to a saturation of 90% or less during the short course of transport. Twelve percent actually desaturated to 85% or less. Smith & Crul (1988) have essentially duplicated these results. A third of patients will develop hypoxaemia within 3–4 min of breathing room air after operation.

Hypoxaemia in the recovery room has been evaluated with similar results. Canet et al (1989) found 43% of 209 ASA I to III adults were hypoxaemic (O_2 saturation of 90% or less) after breathing room air for 10 min on arrival in the recovery room. Almost 17% were still hypoxaemic on room air after 60 min. Morris et al (1988) found considerably less hypoxaemia. Of 149 inpatients studied, 14% had episodes of desaturation to 90% or less. More surprising, however, was their finding that more patients were hypoxaemic at the time of discharge from the recovery room than at any other measurement time. Both of these studies may underestimate the incidence of hypoxaemia since arterial saturation was measured only intermittently.

The recurring theme throughout these reports is that peri-operative hypoxaemia is a common event, frequently unrecognized by even experienced clinicians. The effect of pain and residual anaesthetic drugs in the post-operative period may also prevent recognition of hypoxaemia.

Assessing the clinical significance of such desaturations is more difficult. Anoxia remains the most common cause of anaesthesia-related preventable deaths. Yet, the degree of morbidity associated with more moderate levels of hypoxia is less clear. While arterial saturations of 70% usually show EEG evidence of CNS dysfunction, various tests of cognitive function are clearly impaired at levels well above 70% (Rebuck et al 1976, Gibson et al 1981). In the words of Nunn & Payne (1962), 'The possibility that in some instances the depopulation of the cerebral cortex may have been accelerated can scarcely be denied.'

Despite the numerous studies cited, no factors consistently predict which patients may become hypoxic. And since few factors reliably predict which patient is likely to be susceptible to a given degree of hypoxia, it is essential that the anaesthetist understands the normal response to hypoxia and the ways in which anaesthetic drugs alter that response.

PHYSIOLOGY OF THE HYPOXIC VENTILATORY RESPONSE

The ventilatory response to hypoxia consists of several interacting reflexes. Figure 4.1 shows diagrammatically the roles of the various elements in controlling ventilation. In order to understand how drugs can affect the hypoxic response, it is first necessary to discuss the normal physiology of the ventilatory response to hypoxia.

The reflex increase in ventilation in response to hypoxia is initiated primarily by the carotid bodies located in the bifurcation of the carotid arteries in the neck. The innervation of the carotid bodies is from a branch of the IX cranial nerve. More than just chemoreception occurs at the carotid body. Neuromodulators, including acetylcholine and dopamine, are involved in processing and transducing the arterial Po_2 into the carotid sinus nerve firing rate (Gronbland 1983).

Until oxygen tension falls below approximately 60–70 mmHg there is

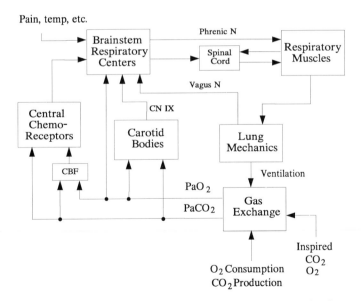

Fig. 4.1 Diagram of the elements of the ventilatory controller. Hypoxaemia effects ventilation through action on the carotid bodies, increasing cerebral blood flow (CBF) which changes the tissue Pco_2 at the central chemoreceptor and by actions (either direct or through neuromodulators) on the central respiratory centres.

little increase in ventilation. However, lower tensions produce a marked increase in ventilation. It is interesting that the ventilatory response occurs at a level of hypoxaemia that clinicians also recognize as a level requiring intervention. The non-linear relationship between the level of hypoxia and ventilation also originates in the carotid bodies but the exact cellular mechanism is unknown. Laboratory and clinical studies on the hypoxic response have used a variety of mathematical descriptions to quantify the response. Such quantification is important in studying a drug effect. For example, the change in the slope and intercept of the hypercapnic ventilatory response is used to characterize a drug's effect on that reflex. The non-linear ventilatory response to hypoxia makes quantification of the hypoxic reflex more difficult. Hyperbolic or exponential functions of end-tidal Po_2 ($P_{ET}o_2$) and a linear function of the haemoglobin oxygen saturation have all been used. Each of these models can describe the data adequately and each has two or three free parameters to estimate from the data. Until the cellular mechanism for the non-linearity is fully understood, it is probably impossible to determine the 'correct' equation for the non-linearity. Due to the breath-to-breath variation in ventilation, one model probably has little superiority over the others, although the hyperbolic model is frequently used in drug studies. A common hypoxic test is to use progressive hypoxia over a 5–10 min period, measuring the breath-by-breath ventilation and $P_{ET}o_2$ data. The hypoxic response is measured by the 'A' parameter, determined by fitting a hyperbolic equation [$V_E = V_0 + A/(P_{ET}o_2 - 32)$ is a commonly used form of the equation] to the breath-by-breath data.

For clinicians the use of a linear equation expressing the increase in ventilation in terms of a decrease in saturation (normal is approximately $0.5-2\,1m^{-1}/\%$ saturation) is perhaps the easiest to interpret. However it must be remembered that the hypoxic response at the carotid body is a function of Pao_2 and not arterial saturation or content. This is most likely the result of the extremely high blood flow relative to the carotid body's metabolism.

Unfortunately this non-linear steady-state response is not the only complex element of the hypoxia ventilatory response. There is a strong interaction between the hypoxic response and the CO_2 level. This interaction takes place in the carotid bodies. Hypercapnia increases ventilation even in hyperoxia through action on the central chemoreceptors; this is the condition in which the hypercapnic response is usually assessed. However, changes in $P_{ET}co_2$ within the normal range causes pronounced changes in the hypoxic sensitivity as well as in the hyperoxic ventilation. An increase in the $P_{ET}co_2$ by only 5 mmHg can more than double the hypoxic sensitivity (measured by the increase in ventilation for a decrease in saturation). This marked sensitivity to asphyxia (hypoxia combined with hypercapnia) is physiologically protective, but it complicates the measurement of the hypoxic response.

If the hypoxic drive is tested by simply giving a subject progressively lower inspired O_2 levels, the increased ventilation will progressively lower Pa_{CO_2} which will then diminish the ventilatory response. Thus, it is extremely important that hypoxic tests be performed under strict isocapnic conditions, since maintaining isocapnia increases the apparent hypoxic sensitivity. In studying drugs, it is important to isolate the drug's effect on the response being studied; thus, when as in many drug studies both the hypercapnic and hypoxic reflexes are altered, the experiment must be carefully designed to determine only the changes in the hypoxic response. This requires that isocapnia be maintained not only during the hypoxic test, but also that the control and drug hypoxic tests must be done at the same CO_2 level. Otherwise, an increase in CO_2 caused by the drug's alteration of the slope or intercept of the hypercapnic response may increase the hypoxic sensitivity and counter any direct depression of the drug on the hypoxic response.

The steady-state response is only one element of the response to hypoxia; the time response to acute imposition of hypoxia is also important and has been receiving increased attention in the physiological literature (Easton et al 1986). The ventilatory response to an isocapnic step decrease in $P_{ET}O_2$ shows a rapid increase to a plateau, with a constant ventilation for 5 to 10 min. Subsequently there is a slow decline to a final value, usually intermediate between the peak hypoxic ventilation and the normoxic ventilation. There is considerable individual variation with some subjects showing very little depression, while others show very little stimulation. At least in adult subjects, the depression does not ordinarily overcome the initial stimulation and the plateau ventilation remains above the pre-hypoxic level. However, in neonates and infants the depression can exceed the stimulation; the resulting total response to hypoxia can be a net decrease in ventilation.

Most studies of hypoxic ventilatory depression have been aimed at increasing understanding of its physiology. Two leading theories have developed: 1. hypoxia increases cerebral blood flow (CBF) and washes out acid metabolites from the area of the central chemoreceptors; and 2. hypoxia alters the balance between central excitatory and inhibitory neural transmitters and a net inhibitory effect results. Neubauer et al (1990) recently published an excellent detailed review of hypoxic ventilatory depression.

Weiskopf & Gabel (1975) were among the earliest to report on hypoxic ventilatory depression in normal humans. Their calculations supported the hypothesis that for a Pa_{O_2} between 40 and 75 mmHg much of the depression can be accounted for by the increase in CBF. However the recent data of Nishimura et al (1987) on the dynamics of the changes in jugular vein P_{CO_2} would seem to indicate that central tissue P_{CO_2} has already decreased to its full extent before the ventilatory depression begins to appear.

While there remains considerable controversy about the relative roles of increased CBF and changes in central neuromodulators in the development of hypoxic ventilatory decline, most investigators ascribe the major role to neuromodulators. Neubauer et al (1990) classified three types of central depression: type I during mild hypoxia and most likely due to the increase in CBF; type II during moderate hypoxia and perhaps caused by alterations in the balance of excitatory and inhibitory neuromodulators; and type III with hypoxia severe enough to cause disruption in the cellular metabolic process. Endogenous opiates, adenosine and GABA have all been studied as possible modulators of type II depression. The role of endogenous opiates was studied by Kagawa et al (1982) who gave a narcotic antagonist, naloxone, to subjects after hypoxic ventilatory depression had developed; there was no increase in ventilation or reversal in the decline. Adenosine has been proposed as an inhibitory central neuromodulator whose levels could increase with hypoxia. This hypothesis has been tested by using aminophylline, a centrally acting antagonist of adenosine, which is known to have multiple effects on the respiratory system, including strengthening the diaphragm and bronchodilation. In adult humans, aminophylline did partially prevent the depression of ventilation (Easton et al 1988). Since some ventilatory depression was still present, adenosine is probably not the sole cause for type II ventilatory decline. The inhibitory neuromodulator GABA is a third possibility for the mediator of hypoxic ventilatory decline. Although there is some data on the respiratory effects of GABA in animals, there is little data on its potential role in mediating hypoxic depression in humans. In animals, activation of CNS GABA receptors results in inhibition of ventilation (Holtman & King 1988). There are two groups of GABA receptors, alpha-receptors and beta-receptors, and activation of either has respiratory effects (Taveira et al 1987).

DRUG EFFECTS

This section will review the effects of drugs commonly used in the practice of anaesthesia on the ventilatory response to acute hypoxia. There are excellent recent reviews covering drug effects on other ventilatory reflexes (Keats 1985, Pavlin & Hornbein 1986). Nearly all studies have focused on the effect of a drug on the ventilation-increasing effects of hypoxia, with little specific information about the role of hypoxic ventilatory decline and drugs on the total hypoxic ventilatory response. Most of the studies have looked at only one drug and have not addressed the possible interactions of the multiple drugs used in current anaesthesia practice. Dose-response and time course data similarly are not available for many drugs. Many drug effect studies have been done in animals and these experiments may allow for more invasive isolation of sites of action. In this review, however, we have tried to focus primarily on human studies where they are available.

Sleep

It may be helpful to compare the changes in hypoxic control of breathing induced by drugs with those 'induced' by normal sleep. Both Berthon-Jones & Sullivan (1982) and Douglas et al (1982) have shown that hypoxic ventilatory response as a function of saturation decreases to two-thirds the awake value during non-REM sleep, and to one-third or one-half the awake value during REM sleep. Far from lulling the anaesthetist into the false security that a given drug decreases hypoxic sensitivity 'no more than in natural sleep,' it must be remembered that anaesthetic drugs, because of alterations in cardiorespiratory physiology, are far more likely to cause hypoxaemia than natural sleep. In addition, hypoxaemia will elicit an arousal response and cause awakening from normal sleep. However, both studies cited above found that up to half the young, healthy, unmedicated research subjects did not awaken from sleep with arterial saturations as low as 70%. The combination of lack of arousal and decreased hypoxic drive

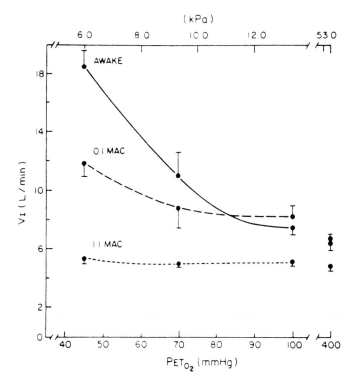

Fig. 4.2 Ventilatory response to four isocapnic oxygen levels in awake, isoflurane sedated (0.1 MAC) and isoflurane anaesthetized (1.1 MAC) subjects. $P_{ET}CO_2$ in the awake and 0.1 MAC groups was approximately 40 mmHg and 44 mmHG in the 1.1 MAC group. (Reproduced with permission from Knill et al 1983).

may contribute to the pathology seen in sleep apnoea patients (Hanning 1989).

Inhalational agents

Knill and associates in a series of studies have convincingly demonstrated that the three fluorinated inhalational agents, isoflurane, enflurane and halothane, all dramatically depress the peripheral chemoreceptors (Knill & Gelb 1978, Knill et al 1979, 1983). The inhalational anaesthetics have multiple effects on respiratory reflexes. Changes in lung and chest wall mechanics induced by anaesthesia also change the ventilatory response. When drugs have many potential sites of action in the ventilatory controller it is difficult to isolate precise mechanisms when studying only the hypoxic ventilatory reflex. However, it is apparent that the hypoxic ventilatory response seems to be uniquely sensitive to inhalational anaesthetics. Anaesthetic levels (1.1 MAC) effectively abolish any response to isocapnic hypoxia (Fig. 4.2). Subanaesthetic levels (0.1 MAC) severely depress the response. In comparison, the response to hypercapnia is unaffected at 0.1 MAC and is still present, although decreased, at 1.1 MAC. Gelb & Knill (1978) concluded that brain tissue levels of halothane remain above the 0.1 MAC level for nearly an hour after a one-hour halothane anaesthetic. If so, then depression of the hypoxic response may persist well into the recovery period.

Interestingly, at anaesthetic levels of halothane (1.1 MAC), ventilation decreased when hypoxia was superimposed on hypercapnia, a startling contrast to the normal synergism between these two stimuli (Knill & Gelb 1978). Whether this is related to the hypoxic depression of ventilation discussed in the previous section is unknown. But, this all presents an ominous warning to the clinician: the very time the patient is most likely to be hypoxaemic is also the time he is least likely to respond to it.

Nitrous oxide

Both Yacoub et al (1976) and Knill & Clement (1982) found that subanaesthetic concentrations of nitrous oxide depress the ventilatory response to isocapnic hypoxia. Although their methods of quantifying the change in the hypoxic response were different, Knill & Clement found that 10–15% nitrous oxide (0.1 MAC) produced a 40% decrease and Yacoub et al found that 30–50% nitrous oxide produced a 65% decrease. These values are consistent with the degree of hypoxic depression found with the fluorinated inhalational agents at the same MAC level.

Yacoub et al (1976) found that nitrous oxide appeared to depress the hypoxic response more than the hypercapnic response, but Knill & Clement (1982) found an equal depression of the hypoxic and hypercapnic responses. Although nitrous oxide is commonly used in combination with inhalational anaesthetics, there is no data on their combined effects.

Barbiturates

The study of the respiratory effects of barbiturates and other intravenous anaesthetics is complicated by the difficulty in obtaining, or even defining, a steady-state condition. Knill et al (1978) approached the problem by administering a bolus dose of thiopentone followed by a variable infusion adjusted to maintain a constant ventilatory pattern, a constant end-tidal CO_2 and either 'sedation' or 'anaesthesia.' Anaesthesia was defined as the loss of eyelid reflex. It should be noted that this method assumes that a steady thiopentone anaesthetic state produces steady respiratory effects, and that these respiratory effects can be used to titrate to the anaesthetic state. It is possible that not all subjects were at the same depth of anaesthesia. However, Knill found thiopentone *sedation* did not alter either the ventilatory response to hypercapnia or to hypoxia. Thiopentone *anaesthesia*, on the other hand, depressed both responses approximately equally.

The hypoxic response of Knill's anaesthetized subjects was actually quite similar to that of awake normocapnic controls, but thiopentone anaesthesia also produced hypercapnia (i.e. elevated resting end-tidal CO_2). This illustrates the potentiation, or synergism, exhibited between hypoxic sensitivity and hypercapnic sensitivity, and the difficulties posed to the respiratory physiologist trying to identify the hypoxic sensitivity alone. Ideal experimental technique calls for strict isocapnic conditions, obtained by artificially elevating the control subject's end-tidal CO_2 to the level of the drug-treated subject. By that measure, thiopentone anaesthesia depresses hypoxic sensitivity, but to a lesser degree than nitrous oxide or the fluorinated inhalational agents.

Hirshman et al (1975a) found that an i.m. injection of pentobarbitone depressed the hypoxic ventilatory response in only five of ten volunteers and did not alter it in the other five. They felt the differences might correlate with levels of physical fitness, but differences in drug absorption, distribution, and metabolism, as well as lean body mass must also be taken into account.

Benzodiazepines

The benzodiazepines also pose problems in defining steady-state conditions and the literature shows highly variable effects on all aspects of respiratory control, including hypoxic control.

Lakshminarayan et al (1976) found diazepam 10 mg i.m. had no effect on resting minute ventilation, resting end-tidal CO_2, or the response to hypercapnia. The response to hypoxia as measured by the 'A' parameter, however, was decreased by 50–60% at 15 to 30 min after the injection.

In contrast, Mora et al (1989) found significant variability in the effects of large i.v. doses of diazepam given for sedation during minor operative procedures (average dose of 100 mg over the average procedure time of 110 min). Two of ten patients actually showed an increase in hypoxic ventilatory response. Since patients who had the longer procedures showed either no change or an increase in the hypoxic response, the authors speculate that a form of acute tolerance to the depressant effects of diazepam may develop. Other considerations include the effects of surgery and pain on repiratory control as well as potential changes in resting end-tidal CO_2 (which were not recorded) and therefore potential changes in the hypercapnic–hypoxic interaction.

Alexander and Gross (1988) studied the effects of sedative doses of midazolam (0.1 mg/kg) on the hypoxic ventilatory response. They chose yet another technique, which might be called the isohypercapnic clamp technique: both midazolam and control runs were performed at a CO_2 level artificially elevated above resting CO_2 (in this case, both were held at 50 mmHg). Hypoxic response was measured as a function of PaO_2 and as V_{90}, the ventilation at 90% saturation. Although they showed a decrease in the hypoxic response under the conditions of their experiment, it is not clear how this relates to clinical practice.

Probably more relevant to the clinician are the findings of Mora et al (1989). They found when patients whose hypoxic ventilatory drive was depressed by diazepam were given flumazenil, a benzodiazepine antagonist, sedation decreased, but the ventilatory response to hypoxia did not return to normal. Similarly, Alexander & Gross (1988) found physostigmine–glycopyrrolate reduced midazolam-induced sedation, but produced no reversal of the measured respiratory depression. Clearly, the use of either flumazenil or physostigmine may not reverse the hypoxic reflex depression.

Narcotics

Although narcotics are well known to cause respiratory depression and their effects on the response to hypercapnia has been extensively studied (see review by Keats 1985), only morphine (Weil et al 1975, Santiago et al 1979) and meperidine (Kryger et al 1976) have been studied for their effect on the hypoxic response.

Santiago et al (1979) found that after 0.2 mg/kg morphine i.m. the hypercapnic response slope was reduced by half and the hypoxic response was reduced by one-third. The CO_2 level during the hypoxic experiments was not reported, but the resting $PaCO_2$ increased from 36.8 ± 1.4 to 42.0 ± 1.2 mmHg (mean $\pm$ SE) after morphine. Weil et al (1975) described the depression of the hypoxic and hypercapnic responses 45–60 min after the administration of morphine 7.5 mg s.c. These studies illustrate the difficulties involved in comparing drug effects when alterations in the hypercapnic response are also induced. The degree of depression of the hypercapnic response was only slightly less than with thiopentone anaesthesia, as found by Knill et al (1978), and both caused similar increases in resting end-tidal CO_2. Weil, however, compared the effects of morphine with the subjects' pre-drug normocapnic hypoxic response, while Knill compared the effects of thiopentone with the subjects' pre-drug response with the CO_2 increased to match the post-drug level. With thiopentone, the hypoxic response was actually very similar to a pre-drug normocapnic response, as already noted. Morphine, however, showed a marked reduction in the hypoxic response even when compared to control runs at a lower CO_2 level. If isocapnia had been enforced between the pre- and post-drug experiments, Weil would have found an even larger depression. Thus, when the difference in controls and the interaction between hypercapnic and hypoxia are taken into account, thiopentone is probably much less depressive of hypoxic sensitivity than is morphine. Narcotics may therefore lie between thiopentone and the inhalational agents in selectively depressing the hypoxic ventilatory response.

Large doses of the opiate antagonist, naloxone (0.1 mg/kg), cause no change in either hypoxic or hypocapnic response in the absence of prior narcotic administration (Maxwell et al 1986). However, while naloxone reverses morphine's effect on the ventilatory response to hypercapnia, the ability of naloxone to reverse morphine's effect on the hypoxic ventilatory response has not been studied.

Other drugs

Although ketamine is generally regarded as having minimal or no respiratory depressant effects, the hypoxic ventilatory response has not been studied in humans. The only data available are from a study in dogs (Hirshman et al 1975b), in which hypoxic ventilatory response was decreased by a small but statistically significant amount. However, the dogs showed a decrease in the CO_2 response slope after ketamine in contrast to ketamine's lack of effect in humans. Thus species differences may prevent a direct extrapolation of this animal data to humans.

The effects of several drugs on hypoxic sensitivity are notable as much for their implications on the mechanisms of hypoxic control as for their clinical effects. Both dopamine (Welsh et al 1978, Ward & Bellville 1982) and somatostatin (Maxwell et al 1986, Filuk et al 1988) selectively depress the hypoxic response. Dopamine is a known neurotransmitter in the carotid body and may have an inhibitory role at clinically relevant (renal, or greater) doses. The role of somatostatin remains unknown. Droperidol (Ward 1984) and prochlorperazine (Maxwell et al 1986), both dopamine antagonists, increase hypoxic sensitivity. Clinical doses of droperidol will block the hypoxic depressant effects of a dopamine infusion (Ward 1984). A serotonin antagonist, methysergide, and a calcium channel blocker, verapamil (Long et al 1989), each had no effect on the hypoxic response.

Respiratory stimulants

No drug has achieved long term popularity as a non-specific respiratory stimulant. Doxapram has been advocated for use in acute and chronic respiratory failure, in post-operative respiratory depression, and in apnoea of pre-maturity, although it is not commonly used. It appears to be a non-specific respiratory stimulant which increases resting minute ventilation as well as both hypercapnic and hypoxic sensitivity by unclear mechanisms (Calverley et al 1983). It seems to have actions on the carotid bodies and its stimulating effect is blunted by halothane (Knill & Gelb 1978).

Almitrine is a piperazine derivative which is currently receiving attention as a potential therapy for a range of pulmonary diseases. It appears to exert its action on ventilation via selective stimulation of the peripheral chemo-receptors, thereby increasing resting minute ventilation and hypoxic sensitivity (Airlie et al 1989).

CONCLUSIONS

Hypoxia is quite common in the peri-operative period but the contribution of drugs used in anaesthesia to this hypoxaemia is unclear. It is not known with any certainty what role a depressed hypoxic ventilatory response may play in the development of this hypoxaemia or if the limitations of the patient's response contributes to morbidity and mortality. However, anaesthesiologists must be aware that a blunted hypoxic drive is the consequence of many drugs used during and after anaesthesia. Such a blunted drive will prevent an adequate ventilatory response and could initiate a dangerous spiral of more profound hypoxaemia.

REFERENCES

Airlie M A A, Flenley D C, Warren P M 1989 Effect of almitrine on hypoxic ventilatory drive measured by transient and progressive isocapnic hypoxia in normal man. Clin Sci 77: 431–437
Alexander C M, Gross J B 1988 Sedative doses of midazolam depress hypoxic ventilatory responses in humans. Anesth Analg 67: 377–382
Berthon-Jones M, Sullivan C E 1982 Ventilatory and arousal responses to hypoxia in sleeping humans. Am Rev Respir Dis 125: 632–639
Calverley P M A, Robson R H, Wraith P K et al 1983 The ventilatory effects of doxapram in normal man. Clin Sci 65: 65–69
Canet J, Ricos M, Vidal F 1989 Early postoperative arterial oxygen desaturation. Determining factors and response to oxygen therapy. Anesth Analg 69: 207–212
Douglas N J, White D P, Weil J V et al 1982 Hypoxic ventilatory response decreases during sleep in normal men. Am Rev Respir Dis 125: 286–289

Easton P A, Anthonisen N R 1988 Ventilatory response to sustained hypoxia after pretreatment with aminophylline. J Appl Physiol 64: 1445–1450

Easton P A, Slykerman L J, Anthonisen N R 1986 Ventilatory response to sustained hypoxia in normal adults. J Appl Physiol 61(3): 906–911

Filuk R B, Berezanski D J, Anthonisen 1988 Depression of hypoxic ventilatory response in humans by somatostatin. J Appl Physiol 65: 1050–1054

Gelb A W, Knill R L 1978 Subanesthetic halothane: Its effect on regulation of ventilation and relevance to the recovery room. Can Anaesth Soc J 25: 488–494

Gibson G E, Pulsinelli W, Blass J P, Duffy T E 1981 Brain dysfunction in mild to moderate hypoxia. Am J Med 70: 1247–1254

Gronblad M 1983 Function and structure of the carotid body. Med Biol 61: 229–248

Hanning C D 1989 Obstructive sleep apnoea. Br J Anaesth 63: 477–488

Hirshman C A, McCullough R E, Cohen P J, Weil J V 1975a Effect of pentobarbitone on hypoxic ventilatory drive in man. Br J Anaesth 47: 963–967

Hirshman C A, McCullough R E, Cohen P J, Weil J V 1975b Hypoxic ventilatory drive in dogs during thiopental, ketamine, or pentobarbital anesthesia. Anesthesiology 43: 628–634

Holtman J R, King K A 1988 Regulation of respiratory motor outflow to the larynx and diaphragm by GABA receptors. Eur J Physiol 156: 181–187

Kagawa S, Stafford M J, Waggener T B, Severinghaus J W 1982 No effect of naloxone on hypoxia-induced ventilatory depression in adults. J Appl Physiol 52: 1031–1034

Keats A S 1985 The effect of drugs on respiration in man. Ann Rev Pharmacol Toxicol 25: 41–65

Knill R L, Clement J L 1982 Variable effects of anesthetics on the ventilatory response to hypoxaemia in man. Can Anaesth Soc J 29: 93–99

Knill R L, Gelb A W 1978 Ventilatory responses to hypoxia and hypercapnia during halothane sedation and anesthesia in man. Anesthesiology 49: 244–251

Knill R L, Bright S, Manninen P 1978 Hypoxic ventilatory response during thiopentone sedation and anaesthesia in man. Can Anaesth Soc J 25: 366–372

Knill R L, Manninen P, Clement J L 1979 Ventilation and chemoreflexes during enflurane sedation and anesthesia in man. Can Anaesth Soc J 26: 353–360

Knill R L, Kieraszewicz H T, Dodgson B G, Clement J L 1983 Chemical regulation of ventilation during isoflurane sedation and anesthesia in humans. Can Anaesth Soc J 30: 607–614

Kryger M H, Yacoub O, Dosman J et al 1976 Effect of meperidine on occlusion pressure responses to hypercapnia and hypoxia with and without external inspiratory resistance. Am Rev Respir Dis 114: 333–340

Lakshminarayan S, Sahn S A, Hudson L D, Weil J V 1976 Effect of diazepam on ventilatory responses. Clin Pharm Ther 20: 178–183

Long G R, Filuk R, Balakumar M et al 1989 Ventilatory response to sustained hypoxia: effect of methysergide and verapamil. Respir Physiol 75: 173–182

Maxwell D L, Nolop K B, Hughes J M B 1986 Effects of somatostatin, naloxone and prochlorperazine on the control of ventilation in man. Clin Sci 70: 547–554

Mora C T, Torjman M, White P F 1989 Effects of diazepam and flumazenil on sedation and hypoxic ventilatory response. Anesth Analg 68: 473–478

Morris R W, Buschman A, Warren D L et al 1988 The prevalence of hypoxemia detected by pulse oximetry during recovery from anesthesia. J Clin Monitoring 4: 16–20

Neubauer J A, Melton J E, Edelman N H 1990 Modulation of respiration during brain hypoxia. J Appl Physiol 68: 441–451

Nishimura M, Suzuki A, Nishimura Y et al 1987 Effect of brain blood flow on hypoxic ventilatory response in humans. J Appl Physiol 63: 1100–1106

Nunn J F, Payne P 1962 Hypoxaemia after general anesthesia. Lancet 2: 631–632

Pavlin E G, Hornbein T F 1986 Anesthesia and the control of ventilation. In: Fishman A P, Cherniack N S, Widdicombe J G, Geiger S R (eds) The respiratory system. Bethesda, MD: Am Physiol Soc, 3, II 783–813

Raemer D B, Morris D L, Morris R et al 1987 Hypoxemia during ambulatory gynecologic surgery as evaluated by the pulse oximeter. J Clin Monitoring 3: 244–248

Rebuck A S, Davis C, Longmire D et al 1976 Arterial oxygenation and carbon dioxide tensions in the production of hypoxic electroencephalographic changes in man. Clin Sci Mol Med 50: 301–306

Santiago T V, Johnson J, Riley D J, Edelman N H 1979 Effects of morphine on ventilatory response to exercise. J Appl Physiol 47(1): 112–118

Smith D C, Crul J F 1988 Early postoperative hypoxia during transport. Br J Anaesth 61: 625–627

Taveira da Silva A M, Hartley B, Hamosh P et al 1987 Respiratory depressant effects of GABA alpha- and beta-receptor agonists in the cat. J Appl Physiol 62: 2264–2272

Tyler I L, Tantisira B, Winter P M, Motoyama E K 1985 Continuous monitoring of arterial saturation with pulse oximetry during transfer to the recovery room. Anesth Analg 64: 1108–1112

Ward D S 1984 Stimulation of hypoxic ventilatory drive by dopamine. Anesth Analg 63: 106–110

Ward D S, Bellville J W 1982 Reduction of hypoxic ventilatory drive by droperidol Anesth Analg 61: 333–337

Weil J V, McCullough R E, Kline J S, Sodal I E 1975 Diminished ventilatory response to hypoxia and hypercarbia after morphine in normal man. New Engl J Med 292: 1103–1106

Weiskopf R B, Gabel R A 1975 Depression of ventilation during hypoxia in man. J Appl Physiol 39: 911–915

Welsh M J, Heistad D D, Abboud F M 1978 Depression of ventilation by dopamine in man: Evidence for an effect on the chemoreceptor reflex. J Clin Invest 61: 708–713

Yacoub O, Doell D, Dryger M H, Anthonisen N R 1976 Depression of hypoxic ventilatory response by nitrous oxide. Anesthesiology 45: 385–389

5. Effects of general anaesthesia on the fetus during Caesarean section

P. R. Nandi   P. J. Morrison   B. M. Morgan

INTRODUCTION

The past few years have seen the development of major new diagnostic technology for examination of the fetus in utero. Ultrasonography and fetoscopy in particular can now provide detailed information about the fetal condition. This should have major implications for the obstetric anaesthetist who will increasingly have prior knowledge of the presence, and severity, of utero–placental insufficiency at Caesarean section. However, whatever the state of wellbeing of the fetus, general anaesthesia for Caesarean section remains relatively static and highly standardized. It is probably true to say that nowhere else in clinical anaesthesia is a 'standard technique' so uncritically accepted and rigidly practised as in general anaesthesia for Caesarean section. Despite the increasing popularity of conduction block, the continued use of general anaesthesia for a proportion of Caesarean sections seems inescapable, especially when there is evidence of acute fetal distress. Increased understanding of the relative contributions of different aspects of general anaesthesia to fetal status may help to reduce neonatal morbidity, especially where the fetus is compromised.

However, investigation of the effects of general anaesthesia on the fetus is difficult for a number of reasons. The fetus is relatively inaccessible in utero, and invasive studies in humans are difficult to justify on ethical grounds. The commonly used animal models may differ substantially from the situation in the pregnant woman. The difficulties are compounded by the fact that commonly used indicators of fetal distress correlate poorly with long term morbidity, even if there is evidence of severe perinatal asphyxia, and Stanley (1987) has suggested that many cases of cerebral palsy previously attributed to asphyxia are probably the consequence of other pathology unrelated to the circumstances at birth. Nevertheless, perinatal damage is not only a major, but a potentially avoidable cause of morbidity.

The anticipated fetal effects of general anaesthesia at Caesarean section may be categorized as follows:

Non-pharmacological influences on fetal oxygen delivery
1. Factors influencing uterine blood flow

    a. Reduced maternal cardiac output. (i) Posture; (ii) Controlled ventilation.

    b. Effect of catecholamine secretion.

2. Maternal arterial oxygenation/carbon dioxide tension

    a. Apnoea/hypoxia.

    b. Preoxygenation.

    c. Inspired O_2 concentration.

    d. Alveolar ventilation. (i) Hypocarbia/hypercarbia.

3. Time factors

    a. Induction–delivery and uterine incision–delivery.

Effects of drugs used in general anaesthesia

    a. Placental transfer of drugs.

    b. The fetal circulation. (i) Intravenous induction agents; (ii) Inhalational anaesthetic agents; (iii) Neuromuscular blocking agents; (iv) Opioids.

NON-PHARMACOLOGICAL INFLUENCES ON FETAL OXYGEN DELIVERY

The fetus exists in a relatively hypoxic environment, the umbilical vein Po_2 being in the order of 35 mmHg and the arrangement of the fetal circulation leads to a further decrease in arterial Po_2 from mixing of blood in the inferior vena cava and the right atrium. Fetal oxygenation is enhanced by a shift to the left of the oxyhaemoglobin dissociation curve, the fetal P50 being 19 mmHg as opposed to the maternal value of 25 mmHg. The placental blood supply arises from the uterine and ovarian arteries, the pressure being 80–90 mmHg dropping to 15 mmHg in the intervillous space. The utero–placental blood flow has been determined at 500–700 ml/min using the Fick principle, whilst the intervillous blood flow has been estimated to be in the region of 130 ml kg^{-1}/min using 133-Xenon (Jouppilla et al 1979).

    Most data on utero–placental blood flow have been derived from studies on the sheep, and some circumspection is required in extrapolating these to the human. The sheep fetus' umbilical flow is substantially greater than the human's, perhaps due to a higher temperature and lower haemoglobin concentration.

    In a series of studies on the pregnant ewe, Greiss (1966, 1967) using electromagnetic flow meters, showed the uterine vascular bed to be maximally dilated in the last half of pregnancy. Further, he showed that sympathetic nerve stimulation (Greiss & Gobble 1967) and administration of adrenaline produced reduction in blood flow due to increased vascular resistance and suggested mediation via alpha adrenergic receptors (Greiss 1963, 1964). Studies by Rosenfeld et al (1976) and Shnider et al (1979) found increased adrenaline and noradrenaline, respectively, to be associated with decreases in uterine blood flow of the order of 35–50%, whilst maternal blood pressure and cardiac output either rose or remained stable. More recently Doppler studies have been used in the pregnant woman and lend support to the animal models (Taylor et al 1985, Trudinger et al 1980).

To summarize, the evidence is that at term the uterine vascular bed is maximally vasodilated but is still responsive to the effect of catecholamines. This implies that maternal sympathetic stimulation, as well as reduced perfusion pressure, will reduce uterine blood flow.

Factors influencing uterine blood flow

Reduced maternal cardiac output

General anaesthesia may reduce maternal cardiac output; the effect this has on uterine blood flow will be determined by the relative alterations in blood pressure and uterine vascular tone.

Studies investigating maternal cardiac output at Caesarean section have been performed before delivery and depending on the measurement technique used have indicated anywhere between 50% reduction in one study to no change in another. However, these studies were performed on small numbers and the vital question of whether utero–placental flow was affected was not addressed. Other factors affecting placental blood supply are now reviewed.

Posture. The effect of posture on the haemodynamics of pregnancy has been reviewed by Bassel & Marx (1982). Early work by Lees et al (1967) focused on the problems of the supine position, the particular danger being aortocaval compression by the pregnant uterus reducing venous return and cardiac output. The mother may compensate for this by increasing peripheral vascular resistance and heart rate, but there may still be a reduction in utero–placental blood flow sufficient to result in fetal acidosis and hypoxia with lowering of one- and five-minute Apgar scores. According to Eckstein & Marx (1974), aortocaval compression may occur in up to 18% of women at term; however, Crawford et al (1972) showed it could be avoided by the use of a lateral tilt with significant improvement for the fetus at Caesarean section. Further, Buley et al (1977) showed hypotension was significantly less in the left as compared to the right lateral position. Because of the reflex cardiovascular changes, a normal brachial artery pressure does not exclude aortocaval compression.

Controlled ventilation. Intermittent positive pressure ventilation (IPPV) can compromise uterine blood flow by reducing maternal cardiac output. The mean arterial pressure in awake normal subjects is well maintained by increasing right atrial pressure due to constriction of the venous capacitance beds and with high inflation pressures arteriolar constriction may also occur.

Under anaesthesia these mechanisms are attenuated and if the circulation is already compromised by factors such as haemorrhage, dehydration and epidural or spinal blockage, then institution of IPPV can lead to a marked fall in blood pressure.

The adverse cardiovascular effects of IPPV can be minimized by reducing mean intrathoracic pressure. This may be achieved by maintaining positive pressure for only as long as necessary to effect the desired volume change, keeping minute volumes below $100-200 \, ml \, kg^{-1}/min$, and minimizing expiratory resistance and dead space.

Effect of catecholamine secretion on uterine blood flow

The effect of tracheal intubation and light anaesthesia is to produce an increase in the level of circulating maternal catecholamines and this is associated with a maternal hypertensive response and tachycardia. This has been documented in routine anaesthesia and anaesthesia for Caesarean section (Irestedt et al 1982, Jouppilla et al 1979), and has been put forward as a contributory factor by Marx et al (1984) in different fetal outcomes when general anaesthesia is compared with regional techniques.

Maternal catecholamine levels are increased significantly under general as compared to regional anaesthesia. Epidural analgesia reduced maternal catecholamine levels for both vaginal delivery and Caesarean section (Jouppilla et al 1984). Several workers have shown general anaesthesia for Caesarean section to be associated with significantly increased levels compared with epidural anaesthesia but comparable to normal vaginal delivery (Irestedt et al 1982, Jouppilla et al 1984, McCann et al 1971, Jones & Greiss 1982, Shnider et al 1983).

Raised maternal catecholamines may be a factor in producing fetal distress during labour. Adamson et al (1971) showed administration of catecholamines to cause fetal distress in the monkey when given in amounts which increased maternal blood pressure; Morishima et al (1978) showed that maternal psychological stress in the rhesus monkey could cause fetal asphyxia and Lederman et al (1981) related fetal heart rate and poor fetal outcome to increased maternal anxiety and increased catecholamine levels in the pregnant woman.

It is noteworthy that in studies of fetal, rather than maternal blood catecholamine levels, following normal vaginal delivery or Caesarean section under epidural blockade, or Caesarean section under general anaesthesia, the highest levels in the fetus were consistently associated with normal vaginal delivery and lowest with general anaesthesia. The fetal catecholamine levels did not correlate with the maternal catecholamine levels. Birth asphyxia has been shown by Lagercrantz & Bistoletti (1973) to be associated in the neonate with increased levels of adrenaline up to four-fold, and it is suggested by Eliot et al (1980) that these high levels of catecholamines at birth may be a beneficial response to asphyxia which could be reduced with general anaesthesia.

Maternal arterial oxygenation/carbon dioxide tension

The effects of anoxia on the nervous system have been described as not only stopping the machine but wrecking the machinery. Hypoxia of insufficient severity to result in fetal death may lead to either temporary or permanent neurological damage.

Apnoea/hypoxia

Pregnant women have a reduced functional residual capacity which can lead to airway closure during normal respiration, particularly when supine. Oxygen consumption is increased by 50–100 ml/min during the first stage of labour and 250 ml/min in the second stage. These changes result in increased sensitivity to periods of apnoea with hypoxia occurring more rapidly than in non-pregnant subjects.

Preoxygenation

Recent work has investigated preoxygenation by inspiring four maximal breaths of 100% oxygen within a 30-s period, compared with 5 min tidal breathing of 100% oxygen; a Pao_2 of 339 mmHg (45.2 kPa) resulted, compared with 350 mmHg (46.6 kPa). In a study by Norris & Dewan (1985) of pregnant patients the four breath technique gave a Pao_2 of 404 mmHg (53.8 kPa) compared with 385 mmHg (51.3 kPa) for the control group.

However, a more recent study by Russell et al (1987) suggests that while adequate preoxygenation using the tidal breathing technique may be achieved in only 2 min, the four-breath method is less satisfactory, and it is suggested that this is a consequence of the reduction in pregnancy of both total lung capacity and vital capacity.

Inspired oxygen concentration

Studies investigating the acid–base status, oxygenation and time to sustained respiration have generally found that fetal outcome is better if a high maternal inspired oxygen is administered prior to birth. Oxygen tension, saturation and content in both maternal and fetal blood increases significantly with increased inspired oxygen concentration. Fetal oxygen tensions were shown by Rorke et al (1968) to correlate with maternal oxygen tensions in the range 70–300 mmHg, above which the correlation ceased. Marx & Mateo (1971) found that fetal oxygenation was lowest and time to sustained respiration longest with a maternal Pao_2 less than

100 mmHg (13.3 kPa) whilst the converse was true with a maternal Pao_2 greater than 300 mmHg (40 kPa). From this they recommended an inspired oxygen concentration of at least 65% for Caesarean section. This has been corroborated by other studies (Baraka 1970, Fox et al 1969, Robertson et al 1974, James et al 1957) showing improved Apgar scores, umbilical cord blood acid–base balance and decreased time to sustained respiration with increased inspired oxygen concentrations. However, failure to adequately standardize anaesthetic technique and avoid aortocaval compression has cast doubt on the validity of the early work. In addition, the issue has been somewhat clouded by the fact that in these studies the maternal FiN_2O has been varied pari passu with the FiO_2—i.e. it is unclear whether superior neonatal condition at birth when a high maternal FiO_2 is used simply reflects a lesser fetal dose of nitrous oxide. Two recent studies have done nothing to clarify this situation, one by Lawes et al (1988) suggesting that a maternal FiO_2 of 0.3 is satisfactory, the other by Bogod et al (1988) advocating an FiO_2 of 1.0! The controversy is likely to continue until clear evidence emerges for the effect of maternal FiO_2 as a variable independent of, rather than interdependent with, maternal FiN_2O.

Alveolar ventilation

Hypocarbia. The effect of hypocarbia on the fetus has been extensively reviewed, especially as hyperventilation is usual during normal labour, and the maternal alkalosis thus produced impairs oxygen transfer by shifting the oxyhaemoglobin dissociation curve to the left. The increased maternal pH also decreases umbilical blood flow (Low et al 1970, Scott et al 1976) and increases the fetal placental vascular resistance (Crawford 1966, Motoyama et al 1966).

Early studies by Moya et al (1965) and Motoyama et al (1967) suggested that mild hyperventilation could reduce the degree of fetal acidosis and improve Apgar scores; increasing hyperventilation interfered with placental gas exchange causing fetal acidosis and increased time to sustained respiration. The critical value for the maternal carbon dioxide tension was proposed to be 17 mmHg.

Levinson et al (1974) in studying the effects of hyperventilation on pregnant ewes showed that despite an increase in maternal Pao_2 and oxygen saturation, there was an associated decline in fetal Pao_2 together with a fall of 25% in uterine blood flow. By adding CO_2 to achieve normo- or hypercapnia, the fetal Po_2 increased, although uterine blood flow remained unchanged. Their conclusion was that fetal oxygenation was impaired by the left shift in the maternal oxyhaemoglobin dissociation curve.

A study by Peng et al (1972), comparing maternal hypocapnia (mean tension 23 mmHg) with eucapnia found hypocapnia to be associated with a significant increase in fetal base deficit, lower one-minute Apgar scores and a delay in rhythmical neonatal breathing.

In marked contrast to the above studies, Baraka (1970), Crawford (1966), Low et al (1970), Scott et al (1976) and Cook (1984) found no correlation between maternal hyperventilation and fetal outcome. Much of the conflicting evidence may be the result of a lack of standardization of anaesthetic technique. Cook (1984) (in a study of 27 Crawford type 'A' infants) using lateral tilt and excluding patients with a uterine incision to delivery interval greater than 120 s, demonstrated a significant lowering of umbilical vein Po_2 with maternal end tidal Pco_2 in the range of 20–40 mmHg. However, there was no clinical difference between these (healthy) infants.

To summarize, it is suggested that maternal hyperventilation can adversely affect the fetus for the following reasons: reduction of maternal cardiac output due to mechanical ventilation and reduced carbon dioxide tension and; respiratory alkalosis which shifts the oxyhaemoglobin dissociation curve to the left and reduces umbilical and uterine blood flow by vasoconstriction.

Hypercarbia. Acute maternal hypercarbia may increase cardiac output. Early studies indicated that maternal hypercarbia dilated the placental vasculature and reduced intraplacental shunting. Motoyama et al (1967) showed that decreased maternal pH due to hypercarbia caused an increase in umbilical blood flow. Higher one-minute Apgar scores and shorter times to sustained respiration were observed with high carbon dioxide tensions, and were explained by the stimulant effect of the carbon dioxide. The increased fetal oxygen tension can be explained by a combination of the maternal oxyhaemoglobin dissociation curve being shifted to the right and increased maternal cardiac output.

Ivankovic et al (1970) studied the effect of hypercarbia in patients with normal and pathological utero–placental circulations and found that inhalation of carbon dioxide to increase the maternal $Paco_2$ above 42 mmHg during general anaesthesia for Caesarean section tended to eliminate the normally existing maternal–fetal acid–base gradient. A possible explanation is improved placental perfusion and less shunting.

The balance of available evidence would appear to suggest that some degree of maternal hypercarbia may be beneficial to the fetus.

Time factors

Induction–delivery and uterine incision–delivery interval

There are marked differences of opinion on the ideal time to deliver the fetus after induction of anaesthesia. The time intervals discussed have been categorized as the induction–delivery interval (I–D) and uterine incision to delivery interval (U–D).

It was initially thought that the I–D interval was the most important factor as regards neonatal depression. However, Crawford et al (1972) showed that the outcome was related to the supine position, with no deterioration of Apgar score related to the I–D interval when patients were anaesthetized in the lateral position. In further work, he demonstrated that if aortocaval compression and hypotension were avoided and an inspired oxygen tension of at least 65% was used, then an I–D interval of up to 30 min did not significantly affect the acid–base status of the neonate, and that the U–D interval was of greater importance, presumably because this represents the time of disruption of the fetal oxygen supply. These studies relate to apparently healthy fetuses.

EFFECTS OF DRUGS USED IN GENERAL ANAESTHESIA

Drugs administered for anaesthesia at Caesarean section may adversely affect the fetus in either of two ways. First, they may affect the fetus directly following placental transfer. Second, they may exert indirect effects via alterations in maternal physiology. In practice it may be very difficult to separate these factors in the assessment of fetal neonatal condition at Caesarean section, and their relative contribution to fetal morbidity in clinical studies can usually only be inferred and seldom, if ever, quantified. Nevertheless, the concept of direct versus indirect effects of drugs is a useful one, and will be considered in each drug subsection.

Before discussing each of the main groups of drugs individually, it is pertinent to briefly consider placental transfer of drugs in general, and also review the fetal circulation which has important implications for fetal drug levels.

Placental transfer of drugs

An in depth analysis of the factors governing placental transfer is beyond the scope of this chapter and has been well reviewed by Reynolds (1989). In the context of general anaesthesia for Caesarean section, the following points are important:

1. Essentially all drugs will cross the placenta, although the rates vary. Moreover, any drug which gains ready access to the central nervous system from the systemic circulation—a prerequisite of all general anaesthetic agents—will also readily cross the placenta by simple diffusion. The phenomenon of the awake baby delivered from an unconscious mother is not due to the presence of a 'placental barrier' to drug diffusion, but is rather a consequence of the pharmacokinetics and the arrangement of the fetal circulation.

2. Equilibrium between maternal and fetal tissues will ultimately be established for any drug administered for a long period of time to the mother. This bears little relevance to the situation in Caesarean section in which the induction–delivery time is normally much too short for equilibrium to be achieved.

3. The rate of placental transfer is the important factor in determining fetal dosage and is influenced by both placental factors and drug characteristics. Chief amongst the former is placental perfusion; the principal drug characteristics favouring rapid transfer are high lipid solubility and low ionization. kPa and protein binding influence transplacental distribution of drugs, and feto–maternal differences in pH and plasma proteins account for certain drugs, such as opioids and benzo-diazepines, achieving higher levels in the fetus than in the mother at equilibrium.

Fetal circulation

The concentration of drug delivered to fetal tissues is reduced from that in the umbilical vein by the arrangement of the fetal circulation.

Having crossed the placenta, drugs pass via the umbilical vein to the ductus venosus. A proportion of the total flow may traverse the liver parenchyma; some drug may be extracted here, although the quantitative importance of this is uncertain. The drug will then be diluted by mixing in the inferior vena cava with blood from the lower limbs, and further in the right atrium with blood from the upper body (although this is partially limited by the presence of the crista dividens which directs the major flow to the left atrium). Hence, umbilical venous drug levels are reduced both by hepatic extraction and serial dilution before reaching the aorta, and the dose received by the fetal brain and heart correspondingly reduced.

Intravenous induction agents. Drugs in this category are highly lipid soluble and therefore tend to penetrate the placenta rapidly. However, by the same token, they are also rapidly taken up by other tissues and thus share the common property of a short distribution half-life. It would be anticipated that drug levels in the fetal circulation would appear shortly after a single bolus i.v. maternal dose, rise rapidly to a peak, and thereafter, decline multiexponentially. This pattern is generally confirmed by studies. The delivery of drug to the fetus will be partly dependent on maternal blood flow to the placental site. Thus, fetal dosage may be deliberately reduced by a maternal i.v. bolus timed to coincide with uterine contraction, and it is likely that placental insufficiency of any cause will also effect a reduction in fetal dosage.

Several early studies attest to the rapid transplacental passage of thio-pentone, suggesting peak concentrations in the umbilical vein some 2–3 min after maternal administration. However, umbilical vein–maternal vein ratios have been shown by Morgan et al (1981) to correlate poorly with either total dose administered to the mother, or dose–delivery interval, and it has been suggested that maternal distribution and elimination characteristics are more important in determining fetal dosage. Moreover, neonatal and umbilical blood levels have correlated poorly with the condition of the infant at birth in a number of studies (Christensen et al

1981, Kosaka et al 1969, Finster et al 1966). In the light of this, it would appear that in normal dosage any direct deleterious effect on the neonate is slight; moreover, it has been suggested that barbiturate anaesthesia may protect the hypoxic fetus from neurological damage, although this has only been demonstrated at much higher doses than those normally employed at Caesarean section.

The case for indirectly mediated adverse effects on the fetus is, however, stronger. Thiopentone decreases cardiac output and blood pressure as a consequence of vasodilatation. Its effects are proportional to the dose and rate of injection. It would be expected to reduce uterine blood flow, and this has been shown by Volkoff et al (1965) in the pregnant ewe where a decrease of 15% was recorded and by Palahniuk & Cumming (1977) who obtained similar results (a 20% decrease). Of greater clinical relevance, are studies by Jouppilla et al (1979), who showed that induction of anaesthesia with thiopentone 4 mg/kg caused a reduction in intervillous blood flow of 35% whilst reducing maternal cardiac output by 15%. The results of these studies suggest that even a small 'sleep dose' of thiopentone might produce deterioration in the already compromised fetus.

There is evidence that thiopentone is readily taken up by the fetal liver, although the quantitative importance of a 'first pass' hepatic uptake has recently been questioned by Woods et al (1982). Saturation of this hepatic reservoir might theoretically make incremental doses post-induction likely to result in a disproportionately greater delivery of drug to the fetal brain. The fetal elimination half-life of thiopentone is much greater than that of the mother (Christensen et al 1981, Gaspari et al 1985).

Methohexitone crosses the placenta with rapidity comparable to thiopentone. Although its haemodynamic effects are similar to those of thiopentone, they are less marked and briefer, and may, according to Sliom et al (1962), result in superior fetal outcome when compared with thiopentone.

Whether drugs like ketamine and etomidate which maintain cardiac output will also maintain uterine blood flow is not certain. Ketamine produces an increase in heart rate and blood pressure with an unchanged cardiac output. In the context of pregnancy it may exert an oxytocic effect although increases above basal uterine tone were found only with a dose of 2.2 mg/kg according to Galloon (1976). This led Marx et al (1979) to conclude that a maternal dose above 100 mg could be dangerous for the fetus, particularly in the context of tonic uterine contraction, abruptio placentae and cord prolapse. As regards uterine blood flow, a study by Levinson et al (1973) in the ewe demonstrated an increase of 15% commensurate with the increase in blood pressure, whilst Eng et al (1975a) could find no change in the monkey.

In women at Caesarean section no difference was found in fetal outcome when compared with thiopentone as judged by Apgar scores and acid–base balance (Peltz & Sinclair 1973, Shulteus et al 1985). Bernstein et al (1985) however, did show a reduction in fetal Pa_{O_2} with increasing incision–delivery interval in the thiopentone group which was not present in the ketamine group. Cosmi (1977) has demonstrated, in the pregnant ewe, a variability in effect dependent on the presence of uterine contractions, such that placental perfusion was increased and fetal acid–base status preserved in the non-labouring animal while deterioration was seen in labour. Etomidate has been demonstrated to have little effect on cardiac output; however, its effects on the fetus at Caesarean section have not been widely studied. In a study by Downing et al (1979) comparing etomidate and thiopentone, the neonates in the etomidate group were rated in superior clinical condition, although the study is open to the criticism that the results for the thiopentone control group were taken from a previous study.

Propofol might be expected to approach the ideal as far as lack of direct effects on the neonate are concerned. However, hypotension may follow its use, and thus, indirectly mediated adverse effects on fetal oxygenation may prove a major drawback in obstetric practice. Recent studies by Moore et al (1989) and Valtonen et al (1989) have compared propofol with thiopentone as an induction agent in cases of uncomplicated elective Caesarean section. Neither study demonstrated clear superiority of one agent over the other; more data are needed before any conclusions can be drawn regarding the suitability of this agent for Caesarean section in cases of fetal compromise.

Benzodiazepines have not gained popularity in the UK as induction agents for Caesarean section. It is noteworthy that diazepam has been successfully used by Scher et al (1972) in this context, and in a further study by Stovner & Vangen (1974) compared favourably with thiopentone. In contrast to thiopentone, maternal and feto–placental cardiovascular dynamics appear well preserved unless large doses are used (Mofid et al 1973). Bearing this in mind, the recent availability of a specific benzodiazepine antagonist (flumazenil) should perhaps lead to a reappraisal of whether or not these drugs have a place in anaesthesia for Caesarean section. Despite the possible attainment of higher blood levels of diazepam in the fetus than the mother, the drug appears free of major hazard although Owen et al (1972) have noted an effect on early neonatal thermoregulation.

Inhalational anaesthetic agents. The low lipid solubility of nitrous oxide will result in rapid equilibration between inspired gas and maternal blood and between maternal blood and fetus. Marx et al (1971) have estimated that fetal levels of N_2O are in the order of 80% of maternal arterial levels 10–15 min after commencing a nitrous oxide anaesthetic. Thus, nitrous oxide is, for practical purposes, the only inhaled agent for which equilibration between fetus and mother is remotely likely to be approached within a plausibly short I–D interval. This in combination with the relatively high concentrations of nitrous oxide administered, raises the possibility of an effectively unique hazard of nitrous oxide, that of diffusion hypoxia in the newborn. Studies by Reid (1968), Mankowitz et al (1981) and Coleman et al (1972) have investigated this possibility with conflicting results. There is probably a slight but real risk, and although the concentration of N_2O in the neonates' end-expired gas is unlikely to be high, the already hypoxic infant may be adversely affected. In practice, the routine administration of oxygen to the neonate should adequately protect against this.

In view of the relatively rapid transplacental passage of nitrous oxide, some degree of direct neonatal depression by this agent is almost certain to occur at Caesarean section, but swift recovery is the predictable outcome of the establishment of neonatal breathing. This is the pattern typically seen in studies where maternal FiN_2O has varied, with neonatal Apgar scores being inferior at 1 min in cases of high FiO_2.

In the presence of adequate facilities for neonatal resuscitation, the use of antepartum nitrous oxide in the mother at Caesarean section appears safe in the light of current knowledge.

Much attention has been focused recently on the inhibitory effect of nitrous oxide on methionine synthase resulting in a functional hypo-vitaminosis B_{12} with neuropathy and megaloblastic anaemia. Baden et al (1984), in a study on pregnant rats, found fetal methionine synthase activity to be substantially reduced by prolonged maternal exposure to N_2O; however, a recent study by Landon & Toothill (1986) has failed to show any evidence of suppression of methionine synthase activity in human placenta post-Caesarean section and it seems likely that unless the duration of fetal N_2O exposure in Caesarean section is abnormally prolonged, this particular hazard of N_2O is negligible.

Moir (1970), in a comparison of nitrous oxide in oxygen maintenance anaesthesia with and without 0.5% halothane supplementation, showed that the infants in the halothane group had superior Apgar scores, although it should be noted that in this group the inspired O_2 concentration was greater (50% as opposed to 30%). In a later study by Latto & Waldron (1977), differing concentrations of halothane (0.65% and 0.2%) were administered to two groups of mothers undergoing Caesarean section with 50% N_2O supplementation. There was no significant difference in the condition of the neonates as assessed by Apgar scores. In general, the available evidence suggests that halothane in a concentration of 1.0 MAC or less has little or no effect on placental perfusion or fetal wellbeing, whereas higher concentrations result in deterioration (Palahniuk & Shnider 1974, Eng et al 1975b).

In a recent study by Abboud et al (1985), no adverse effect of halothane 0.25% or 0.5% on the neonate (as compared with unsupplemented O_2/N_2O maintenance) could be detected by Apgar scores, acid–base status, or early neonatal neurobehavioural scores.

It has long been recognized that halothane relaxes uterine muscle and this was initially the source of anxiety regarding the risk of increased uterine haemorrhage (Crawford 1962). Since then it has been shown that its use in low (0.5% or less) concentrations is not associated with increased blood loss. Laboratory work, however, suggests that these levels do reduce uterine contractility and therefore might be expected to increase uterine blood flow with benefit to the fetus (Shnider 1970). Unfortunately, no studies have shown any fetal benefit when compared with nitrous oxide and oxygen used alone for maintenance (in healthy full-term infants). However, it would appear to be the agent of choice for Caesarean section complicated by uterine hypertonus. Enflurane in low concentrations appears comparable to halothane in its lack of demonstrable adverse affects on the neonate, either as a supplementary agent in Caesarean section as demonstrated by Abboud et al (1985) and Coleman & Downing (1973), or when used in sub-anaesthetic concentrations as an analgesic in labour (Abboud et al 1981, Stephani et al 1982). The possibility of neonatal nephrotoxicity due to inorganic fluoride ions produced by metabolism of enflurane has been investigated by Wickstrom et al (1980) and Kristianson et al (1980), but the agent appears blameless both in the short and long term. The fluoride levels attained in the neonate are certainly well below the levels known to be nephrotoxic in adults.

Information on isoflurane, in the context of Caesarean section is somewhat limited. In a study on pregnant ewes by Palahniuk & Shnider (1974) it was associated with fetal acidosis. A reduction in fetal cardiac output occurred during a long exposure but a subsequent study by Bachman et al (1986) failed to show any detrimental effects over a 30-min exposure. Warren et al (1983) compared isoflurane, enflurane and halothane for Caesarean section and found all agents to be comparable and satisfactory. More recently, Ghaly et al (1988) found no difference in fetal Apgar scores or acid–base status following Caesarean section with isoflurane 0.75% or halothane 0.5%.

Neuromuscular blocking agents. The compounds in this group possess a mono- and bis-quaternary ammonium structure and hence share the property of being highly ionized at physiological pH. They would therefore not be expected to pass freely through lipid membranes. Evans & Waud (1973), in a study investigating fetal neuromuscular blockade in a ferret model, failed to show any depression of the fetal twitch response following doses well in excess of those required to produce complete maternal paralysis for a number of neuromuscular blockers.

Subsequent studies have by and large substantiated this impression, although some degree of placental transfer has been demonstrated for all clinically used drugs in this group.

While in most situations the fetus is not detectably affected by maternally administered neuromuscular blockers, two abnormal situations serve to demonstrate that these drugs can cross the placenta in amounts sufficient to paralyse the neonate. First, if unusually large doses of drug are administered the fetus may receive a paralysing dose despite a low umbilical vein–materal vein ratio. This has been recorded by Older & Harris (1968) in a patient with status epilepticus given a total of 245 mg of tubocurarine to control convulsions; a premature infant was born apnoeic and demonstrated to be curarized.

Second, independent reports by Baraka et al (1975) and Owens & Zeitlin (1975) have drawn attention to neonatal apnoea, or hypotonia with hypoventilation, following the administration of suxamethonium. These resulted from inherited abnormalities of plasma cholinesterase, in those cases where both mother and fetus were homozygous. In this situation, it appears that the sustained high plasma levels of the drug which follows normal clinical dosage can result in sufficient placental transfer to paralyse the fetus.

Opioids. There is a profusion of literature on the transplacental passage and neonatal effects of these drugs, particularly pethidine, when given in labour. There is no doubt that they cross the placenta rapidly, may achieve higher levels in the fetus than in the mother and may give rise to neonatal respiratory depression and take much longer to be eliminated from the neonate than the mother. The paucity of literature relating to their effects in the context of Caesarean section is perhaps surprising, and presumably reflects a reluctance to give opioids as a planned adjunct to anaesthesia for Caesarean section for fear of depression of respiration in the neonate which might result. However, Eisele et al (1982) have demonstrated that fentanyl in a dose of 1 µg/kg prior to Caesarean delivery appears to be without adverse effect on neonatal Apgar scores, acid–base status or neurobehavioural scores and recently Dann et al (1987) have used alfentanil 10 µg/kg, again with no apparent fetal detriment but with a marked reduction in the maternal pressor response to intubation and surgery.

It might be argued that a reduction in the maternal sympatho–adrenal response to tracheal intubation and surgery thus achieved might confer benefits on placental perfusion at Caesarean section and this should perhaps give grounds for the reappraisal of a potential role for potent short acting synthetic opioids in general anaesthesia for Caesarean section where the fetus is particularly at risk from placental insufficiency. Opioid-induced respiratory depression is readily reversible; hypoxic brain damage is not. It seems anomalous that while drugs known to cause neonatal depression may be administered uncritically during labour, their use in a context where possible neonatal benefit may result appears to have received so little attention.

CONCLUSIONS

Some peri-operative fetal hazards—such as aortocaval compression—are well known to anaesthetists and carefully avoided, and the avoidance measures have become incorporated into existing 'standard technique'. Expeditious delivery remains, of course, of prime importance for the acutely distressed fetus. We will concentrate on certain areas where modification of 'standard technique' may be of fetal benefit.

It is difficult to escape the conclusion that properly managed conduction block for Caesarean section has much to recommend it on theoretical grounds; a number of studies have compared regional and general anaesthesia at Caesarean section and most give support to this impression. It is interesting that in one centre it has proved possible, according to Sosis & Bodner (1983), to reduce general anaesthesia for Caesarean section to approximately 1% of all cases; however, conduction block is not an available alternative in all situations.

Several aspects of current standard technique of general anaesthesia for Caesarean section reflect a desire to keep anaesthetic dosage to a minimum so as to avoid neonatal depression—hence the eschewing of antepartum opioids as premedicants or at induction, the use of small doses of induction agent, the historical avoidance (until relatively recently) of vapour supplements to oxygen/nitrous oxide, and the attendant risk of maternal awareness at operation. An examination of the available evidence, however, suggests that direct drugging of the fetus makes an insignificant contribution to neonatal depression within the limits of judicious clinical dosage, and even when such depression does occur it is self-limiting and/or fully reversible. Moreover, the fetus most at risk is likely to receive the smallest dose of drug. In contrast, there is a real potential for imperilling the already compromised fetus by reducing utero–placental perfusion whether this is a result of reducing perfusion pressure, increasing the resistance of the utero–placental circulation, or both. While placental blood flow is well maintained under conduction block in the absence of maternal hypotension, the same does not apply under general anaesthesia if the sympatho–adrenal response gives rise to increased vascular resistance.

Arguably, the most pharmacologically rational approach to the problem of increased resistance (in the absence of conduction block) is alpha adrenergic receptor blockade. This is clearly impracticable in the context of emergency Caesarean section; first, to produce such a block while ensuring the avoidance of maternal hypotension would simply take too long, and second, the effects of alpha blockade on the fetus itself (as opposed to the placenta) might well be detrimental rather than beneficial. However, the use of potent short acting opioids at induction to obtund the sympatho–adrenal response might well preserve placental blood flow, and is, we believe, deserving of further investigation. In cases of fetal compromise, intravenous induction with thiopentone is likely to reduce placental perfusion, with further detriment to the fetus. Methohexitone may be preferable; the literature on ketamine is conflicting, and etomidate has not yet been adequately evaluated but appears deserving of further investigation. There may well be a justification for a reevaluation of benzodiazepines as induction agents, or their adjuncts, especially now that a specific benzodiazepine receptor antagonist (flumazenil) is available.

There is evidence that a high antepartum maternal inspired oxygen concentration (> 60%) improves fetal condition at delivery, although it is still unclear whether this merely reflects a concomitant lesser fetal dose of nitrous oxide. However, if an unacceptable risk of maternal awareness at operation is to be avoided at the low nitrous oxide concentrations imposed by a high maternal FIO_2, additional vapour supplementation will be required. It is clear that modest vapour supplementation will greatly reduce the 'awareness problem' while posing no added hazard to the fetus (and possibly some advantage). There can be no justification in withholding such agents in the belief that the fetus will thereby benefit.

It will be apparent to readers of this chapter that many basic questions relating to the effects on the fetus of Caesarean section remain unanswered, despite much research. One reason for this is a lack of standardization of anaesthetic techniques and patient criteria, both within and between studies. This failing has been repeatedly criticized by the late Selwyn Crawford (1988), in an editorial shortly before his death. However, the authors consider a further reason to be the paucity of data in cases of fetal distress.

The healthy fetus, like the healthy adult, has a great capacity to withstand iatrogenic insults, and it is in order to protect the minority without such capacity that the medical profession strives to improve standards of care. Superiority of one anaesthetic technique, or agent, over another is only likely to be manifest as a reduction in major morbidity when the subject is already severely compromised. The ethical problems, in cases of severe fetal distress, of using techniques which have not been tested on 'clinically acceptable ideal cases' are obvious.

Ultimately, it is to be hoped, and anticipated, that advances in the identification of the 'at risk' fetus will reduce the need for precipitous operative delivery, with the risks it imposes on both mother and neonate (Morgan et al 1990).

REFERENCES

Abboud T K, Shnider S M, Wright R G et al 1981 Enflurane analgesia in obstetrics. Anesth Analg 60: 133–137

Abboud T K, Kin S H, Henriksen E et al 1985 Comparative maternal and neonatal effects of halothane and enflurane for Caesarean section. Acta Anaesthesiol Scand 29: 663–668

Adamson K, Mueller-Heubach E, Myers R E 1971 Reproduction of fetal asphyxia in the rhesus monkey by administration of catecholamines to the mother. Am J Obstet Gynecol 109: 248–262

Bachman C R, Biehl D R, Sitar D, Cumming M, Pacci W 1986 Isoflurane potency and cardiovascular effects during short exposures in the foetal lamb. Can Anaesth Soc J 33: 41–47

Baden J M, Serra M, Mazze R I 1984 Inhibition of fetal methionine synthase by nitrous oxide. Br J Anaesth 56: 523–526

Baraka A 1970 A correlation between maternal and foetal PO_2 and PCO_2 during Caesarean section. Br J Anaesth 42: 434–437

Baraka A, Haround S, Bawssili M, Abu-Haider G, Lebanon 1975 Response of the newborn to succinycholine injection in homozygotic atypical mothers. Anaesthesia 43: 115–116

Bassel G F M, Marx G T 1982 Hazards of the supine position in pregnancy (Review). Clin Obstet Gynaecol 9: 255–271

Bernstein K et al 1985 Influence of two different anaesthetic agents on the newborn and the correlation between fetal oxygenation and I–D time in elective Caesarean section. Acta Anaesthesiol Scand 29: 157–160

Bogod D G, Rosen M, Rees G A D 1988 Maximum F_1O_2 during Caesarean section. Br J Anaesth 61: 255–262

Buley R R, Downing J W, Brock-Utne J G, Cuerden C 1977 Right versus left lateral tilt for Caesarean section. Br J Anaesth 49: 1009–1015

Christensen J H, Andreasen F, Jansen J A 1981 Pharmacokinetics of thiopental in Caesarean section. Acta Anaesthesiol Scand 21: 174–179

Coleman A J, Downing J W 1973 Enflurane anaesthesia for Caesarean section. Anaesthesia 43: 354–357

Coleman A J, Downing J W, Ripley S H, Bach P H 1972 Some implications of nitrous oxide in obstetric anaesthetic practice. S Afr J Obstet Gynaecol 31–33

Cook P T 1984 The influence on fetal outcome of maternal CO_2 tension at Caesarean section. Anaesth Intensive Care 12: 296–302

Cosmi E V 1977 Effetti della Ketamina sulla madre e sul feto studio sperimentale e clinico. Minerva Anestesiol 43: 379

Crawford J S 1962 The place of halothane in obstetrics. Br J Anaesth 34: 386–390

Crawford J S 1966 Maternal hyperventilation and the fetus. Lancet i: 430–431

Crawford J S 1988 Fetal well-being and maternal awareness (editorial). Br J Anaesth 61: 247–249

Crawford J S, Burton M, Davies P 1972 Time and lateral tilt for Caesarean section. Br J Anaesth 44: 447–484

Crawford J S, James F M, Crawley M 1976 A further study of general anaesthesia for Caesarean section. Br J Anaesth 48: 661

Dann W L, Hutchinson A, Cartwright D P 1987 Maternal and neonatal responses to alfentanil administration before induction of general anaesthesia for Caesarean section. Br J Anaesth 59: 1392–1396

Downing J W, Buley R J R, Brock-Utne J G, Houlton P C 1979 Etomidate for induction of anaesthesia at Caesarean section: Comparison with thiopentone. Br J Anaesth 51: 135–140

Eckstein K L, Marx G T 1979 Aortocaval compression and uterine displacement. Anesthesiology 40: 92–96

Eisele J H, Wright R, Rogge P 1982 Newborn and maternal fentanyl levels at Cesarean section. Anesth Analg 61: 179–180

Eliot J R, Lam R, Leake R D et al 1980 Plasma catecholamine concentrations at birth and during the first 48 hours of life. J Pediatr 96: 311–315

Eng M, Bonica J J, Akamatsu T J et al 1975a Respiratory depression in newborn monkeys at Caesarean section following ketamine anaesthesia. Br J Anaesth 47: 917–927

Eng M, Bonica J J, Akamasu T et al 1975b Maternal and fetal responses to halothane in pregnant monkeys. Acta Anaesthesiol Scand 19: 154

Evans C A, Waud D R 1973 Do maternally administered neuromuscular blocking agents interfere with fetal neuro-muscular transmission? Anesth Analg 52: 548–552

Finster M, Mar L C, Morishima H O et al 1966 Plasma thiopental concentrations in the newborn following delivery under thiopental-nitrous oxide anesthesia. Am J Obstet Gynecol 95: 621–628

Fox G S, Smith J B, Namba Y, Johnson R C 1969 Anesthesia for Cesarean section. Further studies. Am J Obstet Gynecol 133: 15–19

Galloon S 1976 Ketamine for obstetric delivery. Anesthesiology 44: 522–524

Gaspari F, Marraro G, Penna G F, Valsecchi R, Bonati M 1985 Elimination kinetics of thiopentone in mothers and their newborn infants. Eur J Clin Pharmacol 28: 321–325

Ghaley R G, Flynn R J, Moore J 1988 Isoflurane as an alternative to halothane for Caesarean section. Anaesthesia 43: 5–7

Greiss F C, 1963 The uterine vascular bed: Effect of adrenergic stimulation. Obstet Gynecol 21: 295–301

Greiss F C 1964 The uterine vascular bed: Adrenergic receptors. Obstet Gynecol 23: 209–213

Greiss F C 1966 Pressure-flow relationship in the gravid uterine vascular bed. Am J Obstet Gynecol 96: 41–47

Greiss F C 1967 A clinical concept of uterine blood flow during pregnancy. Obstet Gynecol 30: 595–603

Greiss F C, Gobble F L 1967 Effect of sympathetic nerve stimulation on the uterine vascular bed. Am J Obstet Gynecol 97: 962–967

Irestedt et al 1982 Fetal and maternal plasma catecholamine levels at elective Cesarean section under general or epidural anesthesia versus vaginal delivery. Am J Obstet Gynecol 142: 1004–1010

Ivankovic A D, Elam J, Huffman J 1970 Effect of maternal hypercarbia on the newborn infant. Am J Obstet Gynecol 107: 939–946

James L S, Weisbrodt I M, Prince C E, Holaday D A, Apgar V 1957 The acid base status of human subjects in relation to birth asphyxia and onset of respiration. J Pediatr 52: 379–394

Jones C M, Greiss F C 1982 The effect of labour on maternal and fetal catecholamines. Am J Obstet Gynecol 144: 149–153

Jouppilla P, Kiukka J, Jouppilla R, Hollmen A 1979 Effect of general anaesthesia on intervillous blood flow. Acta Anaesthesiol Scand 58: 249–253

Jouppilla R et al 1984 Maternal and umbilical cord plasma noradrenaline concentrations during labour with and without extradural analgesia and during Caesarean section. Br J Anaesth 56: 251–255

Kosaka Y, Takahashi T, Mark L C 1979 Intravenous thiobarbiturate anesthesia for Cesarean section. Anesthesiology 31: 489–506

Kristianson B, Magno R, Wickstrom I 1980 Anaesthesia for Caesarean section VI — Late effects on the infant of enflurane anesthesiology for Caesarean section. Acta Anaesthesiol Scand 24: 187–189

Lagercrantz H, Bistoletti P 1973 Catecholamine release in the newborn infant at birth. Pediatr Res 11: 889–893

Landon M J, Toothill V J 1986 Effect of nitrous oxide on placental methionine synthase activity. Br J Anaesth 58: 524–527

Latto I P, Waldron B A 1977 Anaesthesia for Caesarean section. Br J Anaesth 49: 371–378

Lawes E G, Newman B, Campbell M J, Irwin M, Dolenska S, Thomas T A 1988 Maternal inspired oxygen concentration and neonatal status for Caesarean section under general anaesthesia. Br J Anaesth 61: 250–254

Lederman K E, Lederman R P, Work B A, McCann D S 1981 Maternal psychological correlates of fetal newborn health. Am J Obstet Gynecol 139: 956–958

Lees M M, Scott D B, Kerr M G, Taylor S M 1967 The circulatory effects of recumbent postural change in late pregnancy. Clin Sci 32: 453–465

Levinson G, Shnider S M, Gildea J et al 1973 Maternal and fetal cardiovascular acid base changes during ketamine anaesthesia. Br J Anaesth 47: 917–927

Levinson G, Shnider S M, Delorimer A A, Steffonsson J L 1974 Effects of maternal hyperventilation on uterine blood flow and fetal oxygenation and acid base status. Anesthesiology 40: 340–347

Low J A, Boston R W, Cervenki F W 1970 Effect of maternal CO_2 tension on placental gas exchange. Am J Obstet Gynecol 7: 1032–1043

McCann D S, Work B, Huber M S 1971 Endogenous adrenaline and noradrenaline in last trimester pregnancy and labour. Am J Obstet Gynecol 12: 5–8

Mankowitz E, Brock-Utne J G, Downing J W 1981 Nitrous oxide elimination by the newborn. Anaesthesia 36: 1014–1016

Marx G F, Mateo C V 1971 Effects of different oxygen concentrations during general anaesthesia for elective Caesarean section. Can Anaesth Soc J 18: 587–593

Marx G F, Hwang H S, Chandra P 1979 Postpartum pressures with different doses of ketamine. Anesthesiology 50: 163–166

Marx G P, Luyky W M, Cohen S 1984 Fetal-neonatal status following Caesarean section for fetal distress. Br J Anaesth 56: 1009–1012

Mofid M, Brinkman C R III, Assali N S 1973 Effects of diazepam on uteroplacental and fetal hemodynamics and metabolism. Obstet Gynecol 41: 364–368

Moir D D 1970 Anaesthesia for Caesarean section. Br J Anaesth 42: 136–142

Moore J, Bill K M, Flynn R J, McKeating K T, Howard P J 1989 A comparison between propofol and thiopentone as induction agents for obstetric anaesthesia. Anaesthesia 44: 753–757

Morgan D J, Blackman G L, Paull J D, Wolf J 1981 Pharmacokinetics and plasma binding of thiopental: II Studies at Cesarean section. Anesthesiology 54: 474–480

Morgan B M, Magni V, Goroszenuik T 1990 Anaesthesia for emergency Caesarean section. Br J Obstet Gynaecol 97: 420–424

Morishima H O, Shnider S M, James L S 1965 The influence of maternal hyperventilation on the newborn infant. Am J Obstet Gynecol 91: 76–84

Morishima H O, Moya F, Bossers A C, Daniuel S S 1964 Adverse effects of maternal hypoxia on the new born guinea pig. Am J Obstet Gynecol 88: 524–529

Morishima H O, Pederrsen N, Finster M 1978 The influence of maternal psychological stress on the fetus. Am J Obstet Gynecol 131: 286–290

Motoyama E K, Acheson F, Rivard G, Cook C D 1966 Adverse effects of hyperventilation on the fetus. Lancet i: 286–288

Motoyama E K, Rivard G, Acheson F, Cook C D 1967 The effect of changes in maternal pH and PCO_2 and PO_2 of fetal lambs. Anesthesiology 28: 891–903

Norris M C, Dewan D M 1985 Preoxygenation for Cesarean section: A comparison of two techniques. Anesthesiology 62: 827–829

Older P O, Harris J M 1968 Placental transfer of tubocurarine. Br J Anaesth 40: 459–463

Owen J R, Irani S F, Blair A W 1972 Effect of diazepam administered to mothers during labour on temperature regulation of the neonate. Arch Dis Child 47: 107–110

Owens W D, Zeitlin G L 1975 Hypoventilation in a newborn following administration of succinycholine to the mother: A case report. Anesth Analg 54: 38–40

Palahniuk R J, Cumming M 1977 Fetal deterioration following thiopentone–nitrous oxide anaesthesia in the pregnant ewe. Can Anaesth Soc J 24: 361–370

Palahniuk R J, Shnider S M 1974 Maternal and fetal cardiovascular and acid–base changes during halothane and isoflurane anesthesia in the pregnant ewe. Anesthesiology 41: 462–472

Peltz B, Sinclair D M 1973 Induction agents for Caesarean section. A comparison of thiopentone and ketamine. Anaesthesia 28: 37–42

Peng A T C, Blancato L S, Motoyama E K 1972 Effects of maternal hypocapnia vs eucapnia on the fetus during Caesarean section. Br J Anaesth 44: 1173–1178

Reid D H S 1968 Diffusion anoxia at birth. Lancet ii: 757–758

Reynolds F 1989 Placental transfer of drugs used by anaesthetists. In: Kaufman L (ed) Anaesthesia. Review 6. Churchill Livingstone, London, pp 151–183

Robertson A, Fothergill-Hall R A, Bond R A 1974 Effects of anaesthesia with a high oxygen concentration on the acid base balance of babies delivered at Caesarean section. S Afr Med J 48: 2309–2313

Rorke N J, Davey D A, DuToit H J 1968 Fetal oxygenation during Caesarean section. Anaesthesia 23: 585–596

Rosenfeld C R, Barton M D, Meschia G 1976 Effects of epinephrine on distribution of blood flow in the pregnant ewe. Am J Obstet Gynecol 124: 156–163

Russell G N, Smith C L, Snowdon S L, Bryson T H L 1987 Pre-oxygenation and the parturient patient. Anaesthesia 42: 346–351

Scher J, Hailey D M, Beard R W 1972 The effects of diazepam on the fetus. J. Obstet Gynecol Br Comm 79: 635–638

Schulteus R R et al 1985 Haemodynamic effects of ketamine and thiopentone during anaesthetic induction for Caesarean section. Can Anaesth Soc J 32: 592–596

Scott D B, Lees M M, Davie I T, Slawson K 1976 Observations on cardiorespiratory function during Caesarean section. Br J Anaesth 41: 489–495

Shnider S M 1970 Halothane and uterine haemorrhage. (Editorial). Anesthesiology 32: 99

Shnider S M, Wright R G, Levinson G et al 1979 Uterine blood flow and plasma norepinephrine changes during maternal stress in the pregnant ewe. Anesthesiology 50: 524–527

Shnider S M, Abboua T K, Attal R et al 1983 Maternal catecholamines decrease during labour after lumbar epidural anesthesia. Am J Obstet Gynecol 147: 13–15

Sliom C M, Frankel L, Holbrook R A 1982 A comparison between methohexitone and thiopentone as induction agents for Caesarean section anaesthesia. Br J Anaesth 34: 316–326

Sosis W, Bodner A 1983 Is general anaesthesia becoming obsolete for Caesarean section? Anaesthesia 38: 702–703

Stanley F J 1987 The changing face of a cerebral palsey. Dev Med Child Neurol 29: 258–270

Stephani S J, Hughes S C, Shnider S M et al 1982 Neonatal neuro-behavioural effects of inhalation analgesia for vaginal delivery. Anesthesiology 56: 351–355

Stovner J, Vangen O 1974 Diazepam compared to thiopentone as induction agent for Caesarean sections. Acta Anaesthesiol Scand 18: 264–269

Taylor K J V, Burns P N, Wells P N T, Conway D I, Hull M G R 1985 Ultrasound Doppler flow studies of the ovarian and uterine arteries. Br J Obstet Gynaecol 92: 240–246

Trudinger B J, Giles W B, Cook C M 1980 Uterine flow velocity waveforms in pregnancy. J Ultrastruct Med 2: 10–12

Valtonen M, Kanto J, Rosenberg P 1989 Comparison of propofol and thiopentone for induction of anaesthesia for elective Caesarean section. Anaesthesia 44: 758–762

Volkoff A S, Bawded J W, Flowers C E, McGee J A 1965 The effect of anesthesia on the newborn. Am J Obstet Gynecol 93: 311–320

Warren T M, Datta S, Ostheimer G W, Naulty J S, Weiss J B, Morrison J A 1983 Comparison of the maternal and neonatal effects of halothane, enflurane and isoflurane for Cesarean delivery. Anesth Analg 62: 516–520

Wickstrom I, Kjellmer I, Kristianson B, Magno R 1980 Anaesthesia for Caesarean section VII. Early effects on neonatal renal function of enflurane anesthesiology for Caesarean section. Acta Anaesthesiol Scand 24: 190–194

Woods W A, Stanski D R, Curtis J, Rosen M, Shnider S M 1982 The role of the fetal liver in the distribution of thiopentone from mother to fetus. Anesthesiology 57: A390

6. The endocrine system

L. Kaufman

Despite the wealth of papers appearing on endocrine function during operation, there is still a lack of consensus on the desirability of inhibiting the response during elective surgery. The hormones released during surgery include corticotrophin releasing factor (CRF), ACTH, cortisol, angiotensin II, aldosterone and AVP, and in terms of quantity the amounts are far in excess of that required to produce physiological responses. However, following major trauma and multiple organ failure, suppression is probably undesirable.

Attempts to suppress the endocrine response to surgery involve the use of high dose opioids, spinal and epidural analgesia with local analgesia or opioids, and even indomethacin. Cross et al (1989) showed that hypertonic saline (1.8%) suppressed the response to surgical stimulation of ACTH, cortisol and aldosterone, but ANP altered insignificantly when compared with the control group. The rise of AVP levels was unaffected.

ALDOSTERONE AND STEROIDS

Domperidone and metoclopramide are dopamine antagonists (D_2-receptors), and metoclopramide appears to release aldosterone by direct adrenal stimulation (Stern et al 1989). Angiotensin II stimulates the release of aldosterone and may have a central influence on cardiovascular and body fluid homeostasis (Harding et al 1989). Metoclopramide increases serum aldosterone levels significantly and this effect is reduced in the presence of neostigmine, suggesting that acetylcholine is involved (Sommers et al 1989). Dopamine improves oxygen supply to tissues more than it increases oxygen consumption (Ruttimann et al 1989).

The place of corticosteroids in homeostasis has been reviewed by Dallman et al (1989), noting that under both normal and conditions of stress, corticosteroids provide adequate stores of energy by their ability to mobilize and convert them to glucose. In animals who are deficient of steroids, cortisone stimulates food intake and this is seen in patients with Addison's disease whose appetite improves with therapy. They exert the anti-insulin effects peripherally. Animals readily respond to haemorrhage and hypotension provided that they are well nourished, but this is reduced when the animals are starved for 24 h. Dallman et al (1989) suggest that glucocorticoids exert a 'low profile' action and it is the peptides and neurotransmitters which act rapidly in the cell membrane, an effect which is enhanced by steroids.

It has always been assumed that the conversion of cortisol to cortisone took place in the liver, under the influence of 11β-hydroxysteroid dehydrogenase. However, Whitworth et al (1989) found that the kidney is a major site where cortisol is converted to cortisone, and it is also responsible for cortisone formation. This study may elucidate the mechanism of hypertension and the relationship to the renin–angiotensin–aldosterone system.

Helfer & Rose (1989) have reiterated the complications of steroid therapy of which hypothalamic–pituitary–adrenal suppression is of paramount importance. This can be detected by an injection of cosyntropin (250 µg), estimating the serum cortisol and aldosterone responses in 30 min to 1 h. Normal aldosterone response and reduced cortisol response indicate secondary adrenal insufficiency while if both hormones are subnormal, it indicates primary adrenal insufficiency (normal peak cortisol level should be > 550 nmol/l). They listed other complications including those affecting the CNS (psychiatric disturbances); ophthalmological (glaucoma and cataract); cardiovascular (hypertension, sodium and water retention, oedema, hypokalaemic alkalosis); gastrointestinal (peptic ulcer, haemorrhage, pancreatitis); musculoskeletal (necrosis of bone, osteoporosis, myopathy); fibre tissues (impaired healing); immunological (decreased immune response, infection); metabolic (hyperglycaemia, hyperlipidaemia); and endocrine (growth failure, secondary amenorrhoea, suppression of hypothalamic–pituitary–adrenal axis. A rectal suppository of 200 mg hydrocortisone produced adequate levels of cortisol and may be of value in the self-treatment of preventing Addisonian crises (Newrick et al 1990).

In the absence of stress, suppression of corticosteroids in the adrenal either via surgical removal or pharmacological means required 18–21 h for the brain–pituitary axis to respond by increasing secretion of ACTH (Jacobson et al 1989). However, in the presence of surgical stimulation, cortisone significantly attenuates the ACTH response to surgical stimulation, this effect being accentuated by fentanyl. There appears to be two distinct responses: fast feedback in the presence of stress and delayed feedback (Raff et al 1988). Kong et al (1989) has described physiological models for assessing the suppressive effects of methylprednisolone on serum cortisol.

CORTICOTROPHIN RELEASING FACTOR (CRF)

The physiology of CRF has been reviewed by Linton & Lowry (1989): it is a peptide of 41 amino acids and is involved in the release of ACTH and beta-endorphin from the pituitary; the highest concentration is in the hypothalamus although it can be detected in the cerebral cortex and in some of the nuclei. Its role in the stress response has still to be defined, but it is one of the most potent factors in the release of ACTH as well as AVP. CRF causes a rapid rise in plasma ACTH within 2 min, peaking at 10–15 min and falling rapidly at 90 min. There then follows a rise to a second major peak at 2–3 h and this lasts for several hours. Plasma cortisol follows a similar pattern. Although AVP has little effect on ACTH release, it augments the action of CRF. Insulin-induced hypoglycaemia results in a greater release of ACTH and cortisol than can be achieved by simultaneous administration of CRF and AVP. It is also worthy of note that during operation the levels of cortisol and ACTH peak at about 90 min following stimulation, and the early rise seen following CRF administration does not occur or measurements are too infrequent to detect this change (Loveland & Kaufman, unpublished data). The measurements of CRF in stress situations do not necessarily reflect hypothalamic activity because of the release of CRF from extrahypothalamic sites.

CRF levels are high in the third trimester of pregnancy, increase during labour and then fall dramatically, returning to normal within 24 h following delivery.

CRF also stimulates respiration, an effect which is not mediated by ACTH or cortisol (Huber et al 1989). Centrally, catecholamines have little direct effect on ACTH secretion, but the increased CRF secretion affects ACTH and cortisol. The stimulated responses involving alpha-1-mediated and alpha-2-receptors are probably inhibited. Evidence for beta-receptor activities is controversial (Plotsky et al 1989).

Mu- and kappa-opioid receptors are involved in the apparent stimulating and depressing action of endogenous opioids which affect the release of CRF in response to stress. Mu-receptors are stimulants while delta- and kappa-agonists have a depressing action, although delta-receptors are probably less involved (Cover & Buckingham 1989). Mu-receptor stimulation increases the autonomic outflow resulting in vasodilatation (Marson et al 1989). Interleukin-1 also stimulates the hypothalamic pituitary system, possibly by CRF stimulation (Berkenbosch et al 1989).

ACTH

Pro-opiomelanocortin (POMC) is the precursor of ACTH, melanocyte-stimulating hormone (MSH), endorphins and lipotrophins. Animal experiments indicate that ACTH can cause an increase in blood pressure and heart rate as well as a loss of sodium. Gamma-MSH has activity which is 100 times more than ACTH on the cardiovascular system and 1000 times more effective as a natriuretic hormone. It may play a part in endotoxic shock or haemorrhage (Gruber & Callahan 1989).

ATRIAL NATRIURETIC HORMONE (ANF, ANP)

Atrial natriuretic hormone promotes diuresis with the loss of sodium and inhibits the renin–angiotensin–aldosterone system. The major stimulus causing release of ANP is atrial distension, and elevated levels are seen in congestive cardiac failure and supraventricular tachycardia. The release is specific, transient and less effective in response to further atrial stretching. This may be due to depletion of stores or adaptation (Ferrari & Agnoletti 1989). Atrial contraction also affects the release while hyperosmotic saline increases not only AVP levels but also that of ANP. Other factors affecting the release are opioids, anaesthesia and beta-agonists. Although it is synthesized in the atria, it also appears to have a central action decreasing mean arterial pressure, possibly via centrally acting opioids (Levin et al 1989). ANP may also be synthesized in the lungs and may have a role in the prevention of pulmonary oedema (Gutkowska et al 1989). As it is a vasodilator, it may well be that it is a natural antagonist to angiotensin II and AVP, and a disturbance in the balance between these hormones and their vascular receptors may cause hypertension (Schiffrin 1989).

Obata et al (1989) found that there was an increase in ANP during cardiac pacing, even though there was no increase in the atrial pressure. During cardiac surgery, cross clamping of the aorta and vena cavae did not lead to a significant decrease in plasma ANP (Asari et al 1989), but following the termination of bypass there was a marked diuresis and sodium loss associated with an increase in ANP, presumably due to atrial distension but the ADH levels were normal (Schaff et al 1989, also see Ardaillou & Dussaule 1990).

The action of clonidine, a centrally acting agonist of alpha-2 sympathetic receptors, may be in part due to ANP which, however, does not potentiate the effects of dihydralazine (Wehling et al 1989).

In young subjects adrenaline increased the plasma ANP, an effect which was absent in the elderly. The significance of this has still to be determined as it is not known if adrenaline in fact has a place in the physiological regulation of ANP secretion (Morrow et al 1989).

In acute renal failure, plasma levels of ANP and cGMP increased but returned to normal during recovery. These increases are related to changes in blood volume during acute renal failure, and it may be an attempt of adaptation in controlling renal failure (Kanfer et al 1989).

In normal patients, intravenous infusion of saline results in an increase in ANP and suppression of plasma renin activity and plasma aldosterone, but in patients with hepatic cirrhosis, plasma aldosterone and plasma renin activity remained normal. There may be other factors which promote the 'resistance' of renal function to ANP (Tesar et al 1989). ANP interacts with angiotensin II in the glomerulus which leads to diuresis and loss of sodium; it also inhibits the angiotensin II-induced tubular sodium reabsorption (Rakugi et al 1989). It is a potent inhibitor of angiotensin II, reducing the secretion of aldosterone (Metzler & Ramsay 1989); even in small doses there was a marked suppression of aldosterone (Shenker 1989). Groban et al (1989) demonstrated that high levels of plasma ANP did not affect renal hormonal function, presumably due to the fact that ANP led to a reduction in cardiac preload which activated sympathetic activity. The results of infusions of hypertonic saline are contradictory, and Burrell & Baylis (1990) have drawn attention to the fact that the release of ANP is influenced by posture and not hyperosmolality—in response to hypertonic saline, ANP rises in the supine position but not in the sitting position.

Urinary prostaglandins increased under the influence of ANP, presumably as a result of increased prostaglandin synthesis. This may affect the diuretic effect but not the natriuretic action (Benzoni et al 1989). Sympathetic activity may play a part in the release of ANP which does not occur in diabetics with autonomic dysfunction, and it may in fact be a useful test to detect the decrease in autonomic activity (Donckier et al 1989). ANP enhances the hypoglycaemic action of insulin, possibly by affecting insulin breakdown in the liver (Jungmann et al 1989). There are high levels of ANP in patients with aldosterone-secreting adenoma (Nakada et al 1989).

ENDOCRINE RESPONSE TO SURGERY

The intrapleural instillation of local anaesthetics has been advocated for the relief of post-operative pain as well as inhibiting the metabolic response to surgery. Scott et al (1989) have shown that both intrapleural and thoracic epidural bupivacaine had little effect on plasma glucose or cortisol levels following cholcystectomy. FEV_1, FVC and peak expiratory flow rate were still reduced in both groups. Although analgesia was satisfactory, afferent blockades were ineffectual in blocking the respiratory effects and endocrine response.

The hormonal and haemodynamic effects of intravenous indomethacin have been assessed by Manner et al (1989); it had little effect on limiting the actions of 5% hypertonic saline on plasma renin activity, aldosterone and AVP. Although indomethacin appears to augment the efficacy of analgesic agents, it has little effect on blood glucose, serum cortisol and C-reactive protein following hysterectomy (Engel et al 1989).

In portal hypertension, prostacyclin (PGI_2) is involved in the vascular responses in the splanchnic area to noradrenaline (Sitzmann et al 1989). Psychological stress results in increased levels of ACTH and beta-endorphins (Mutti et al 1989) and decreased renal blood flow (Tidgren & Hjemdahl 1989). Adrenaline does not affect renal blood flow directly but enhances renin release.

Re-exposure to trauma may affect pain sensitivity, resulting in what is termed stress-induced analgesia. Animal experiments indicate that previous exposure to stress results in higher plasma cortisol levels following further exposure (Caggiula et al 1989). Reduction in pain intensity following exposure to trauma has also been demonstrated in Vietnam veterans (van der Kolk et al 1989). This may imply that there is a centrally mediated opioid response and that post-traumatic stress disorder might respond to tricyclic antidepressants and monoamine oxidase inhibitors (Davidson & Nemeroff 1989, Pitman et al 1989).

Hyperthermia increases plasma beta-endorphins and ACTH but not plasma enkephalin. This indicates that possibly plasma methionin–enkephalin are derived from other sources such as the adrenal medulla (Vescovi et al 1990). In response to stress, insulin levels rise significantly but blood sugar is also influenced by the release of steroids (Alvarez et al 1989). The effects of stress on immunity are not mediated entirely by glucocorticoids and catecholamines, endogenous opioids and growth hormone are also involved (Dantzer & Kelley 1989).

Patients with advanced carcinoma have an increased rate of glucose production in the liver (gluconeogenesis), despite normal levels of insulin, cortisol and growth hormone. There is also an increase in protein turnover and fat mobilization (Douglas & Shaw 1990). This may be due to tumour necrosis factor (cachectin) which is also raised in chronic heart failure and which is associated with a marked increase in renin–angiotensin activity (Levine et al 1990).

In malnourished patients, increasing glucose intake promotes nitrogen balance, especially with a high nitrogen intake. High nitrogen intake increases plasma insulin and glucagon and reduces glycerol, fatty acids and 3-hydroxybutyrate concentrations. Glucagon concentrations were decreased by adding glucose in those with a high nitrogen intake. The alteration of nitrogen balance was entirely due to a decrease in urea excretion (Forse et al 1990).

In surgical patients following major abdominal surgery, bradykinin improved the rate of nitrogen retention and this was probably due to its aerobic effects on stimulation of protein synthesis (Hartl et al 1990). In sepsis, there is a reduction in hepatic gluconeogenesis (Ardawi et al 1989).

Temperature may have an effect on the outcome of metabolism during surgery (Carli et al 1989). Carli maintained that normothermia during hip surgery appeared to decrease but not entirely eliminate the protein breakdown and nitrogen loss following operation. Some patients may be abnormally sensitive to low environmental temperature and have an abnormally low core temperature (Allen et al 1989). During total hip replacement, there is an increase in platelet activation and this is unaffected by high doses of corticosteroids (Hogevold et al 1990).

During prostatic surgery under epidural analgesia, there were no significant changes in blood glucose or cortisol except when there was a significant increase in blood loss of more than 800 ml. When there was an absorption of more than 300 ml of irrigating solution, hyponatraemia readily developed (Hahn 1989). The absorption of irrigating fluids results in transurethral resection syndrome (TURS), with not only hyponatraemia but also hypo-proteinaemia leading to cerebral and pulmonary oedema. Stewart & Barlow (1989) suggested that the syndrome may also be due to a rise in plasma ammonia resulting from the metabolism of glycine contained in the irrigating solutions. The absorption of glycine leads to increasing concentrations of non-essential amino acids and stimulates the release of AVP, resulting in antidiuresis (Hahn & Rundgren 1989).

Epidural analgesia whether with general anaesthesia or not, suppresses the immune response to surgical stimulation as reflected by leucocyte and leucocyte migration. The stress-free anaesthesia is not necessarily advantageous in patients who are undergoing inguinal herniorrhaphy which is only likely to evoke limited endocrine response to surgical stimulation (Edwards et al 1990).

During cardiac surgery, somatostatin augments the inhibiting action on the endocrine response of sufentanil except the release of catecholamines which also proved refractory to ganglion blocking agents such as tri-metaphan (Desborough et al 1990).

Laryngoscopy results in circulatory responses and these can be prevented by an infusion of fentanyl. Esmolol, a cardioselective adrenergic receptor-blocking agent with a short half-life of 9 min, has a less depressant effect on diastolic pressure (Ebert et al 1989).

ARGININE VASOPRESSIN (AVP)

Insulin-induced hypoglycaemia leads to a maximum increase of cortisol levels at 90 min while those of ACTH, AVP and CRF peak at 45 min. AVP and CRF are the mediators of ACTH release following hypoglycaemia (Ellis et al 1990). AVP appears to interact with CRF to promote tumour growth and ACTH release in Cushing's disease (Wittert et al 1990).

AVP also influences sympathetic nerve activity, but the central site is still unknown and is unlikely to be in the tractus solitarius (Suzuki et al 1989). There is a link between angiotensin II and AVP involving prostacyclin, but other receptors besides V_1 or V_2 may be implicated (Vallotton et al 1989). AVP interacts centrally to limit reflex increase in sympathetic outflow (DiCarlo et al 1989).

Sodium loading increases blood pressure associated with increased sympathetic activity, and AVP appears to be involved via central AVP receptors (Gavras & Gavras 1989). In the foetus, hypoxaemia results in hypertension, bradycardia and redistribution of cardiac output, and these effects appear to be mediated by AVP (Perez et al 1989). However, in animal experiments, AVP lowers cardiac output by coronary vasoconstriction. It also causes a marked increase in mesenteric blood flow due to vasoconstriction, in a manner similar to that of alpha-adrenergic receptors (Veelken et al 1989). A decrease in central venous pressure does not stimulate AVP secretion, nor does the hypotension produced by nitroprusside (Goldsmith 1989). Low-pressure baroreceptors have little effect on the regulation of AVP release but high pressure baroreflexes are more important (Norsk 1989).

Although AVP increases systemic vascular resistance, it has little effect on the pulmonary vasculature (Wallace et al 1989). Hyperosmolar saline increases AVP secretion and this is augmented in the presence of cortisol (Bennett & Rose 1989). GABA activity reduces AVP responses to hypovolaemic and hyperosmotic stimuli (Chiodera et al 1989a). Alpha-2 adrenergic activity, however, does not affect the regulation of AVP in CSF or plasma (Peskind et al 1989). Centrally administered hypertonic saline increases blood pressure and AVP release but not methionine–enkephalin, and this effect can be abolished by V_1-antagonists (Ota et al 1990).

Intrathecally, AVP increases blood pressure and heart rate by increasing the sympathetic outflow rather than by direct effect on the blood vessels (Riphagen & Pittman 1989).

It has been assumed that changes in atrial pressure prompt a fall in plasma AVP leading to diuresis. Bennett & Linden (1989) postulated that AVP is not directly involved in this response but only acts as a trigger to another diuretic agent.

Metoclopramide stimulates the release of AVP, but the mechanism of this has only recently been ascertained. Coiro et al (1989) showed that this response is not influenced by serotonin (5-HT1- or 5-HT2-receptors) but is cholinergic. The release of AVP is mediated by muscarinic receptors (M1, M2) at the M1-receptors within the blood–brain barrier or at M2-receptors, either inside or outside the barrier.

Asthma

The possibility that AVP might be involved in asthma has been examined, but Knox et al (1989) were unable to demonstrate any effect on bronchial reactivity, even in asthmatic patients.

Endotoxic shock

Endotoxaemia involves the stimulation of alpha-1 adrenergic receptors as well as those for vasopressin, with resultant effects on lipid metabolism (Spitzer & Rodriguez de Turco 1989). AVP in high doses is antinociceptive, without involving the opioid pathways (Hart & Oluyomi 1990). In burns, AVP has a deleterious action by increasing the renal arterial pressure initially followed by a large fall. On ECG there was elevated ST segment, T-wave inversion followed by ventricular fibrillation. AVP also raises the levels of beta-endorphin which may be the mediating agent for the adverse response (Sun et al 1989).

The administration of V_1AVP antagonist does not attenuate the cardiovascular responses or mortality associated with endotoxaemia (Egan et al 1989).

Brain death

A novel use for AVP is the maintenance of blood pressure following brain death. The use of adrenaline to maintain blood pressure results in myocardial damage whereas the combination of a small dose of adrenaline with AVP can maintain circulation without myocardial damage, allowing the heart to be possibly of use for cardiac transplantation (Kinoshita et al 1990).

In addition to the antidiuretic and cardiovascular effects of AVP, there are effects on clotting and memory. This has been confirmed by Koob et al (1989) who suggests that AVP derived from pituitary is effective in enhancing memory, either through processing information in the limbic system or through increased performance. However, the use of the synthetic AVP, desmopressin, has little effect in cardiac surgery (Hackmann et al 1989).

AVP and ANP

It is speculative to conclude that AVP and ANP have opposing actions on urinary output. Following a water load AVP levels fall and there is also an increase in urinary output. However, studies by Hellebrekers et al (1989) failed to demonstrate a concomitant rise in ANP. Similarly, ANP had little effect on blood pressure compared with that of AVP (Szczepanska-Sadowska 1989). Osmoreceptors within the blood brain barrier are involved in AVP release as well as changes in blood pressure, but are without effect on ANP (Iitake et al 1989). AVP rises in response to haemorrhage and any changes in ANP were related to the reduction in atrial pressure associated with haemorrhage, and there was no correlation between the release of AVP and ANP (Courneya et al 1989). In hypoxic animals, AVP lowers the pulmonary arterial pressure due to the release of ANP (Jin et al 1989).

Syndrome of inappropriate antidiuretic hormone (SIADH)

SIADH is a condition with excess AVP secretion causing water retention; in this syndrome there is a rapid elimination of a large amount of sodium loading despite the presence of hyponatraemia. This has led to suggestions that ANP might be a causative factor but this has not been substantiated by Gross et al (1989). On the other hand, Weinand et al (1989) demonstrated that there was a reciprocal relationship between AVP and ANP in some patients and not in others, and judging by the response, SIADH must include at least three subtypes depending on the response. Hyponatraemia and non-osmolar AVP release occurs in patients with AIDS, with the high levels of AVP being related to mortality rate (Vitting et al 1990). Post-operative diabetes insipidus occurs in patients who have undergone transsphenoidal surgery, however, there is a release of an antagonist later leading to normal AVP activity (Seckl et al 1990).

OXYTOCIN (OT)

Although OT andAVP are synthesized in the neurons of the hypothalamus, only AVP concentrations appear to rise significantly following surgical stimulation. Ether and stress increase OT concentrations in animals within minutes (Hashimoto et al 1989). Callahan et al (1989) found that the paraventricular nuclei were involved in the cardiovascular responses to stress, and the mediator may be oxytocin.

In foetal and neonatal sheep, OT increases glucagon and insulin release, an effect not seen with AVP (Wallin et al 1989). Futhermore, in insulin dependent diabetics, oxytocin increases plasma glucagon and adrenaline under normal conditions and also during insulin-induced hypoglycaemia, while at the same time reducing the plasma cortisol levels. It may have a place in the recovery from hypoglycaemia (Paolisso et al 1989). Hypoglycaemia produces a rise in OT which is inhibited by somatostatin and naloxone-sensitive endogenous opioids (Chiodera et al 1989b). OT has little effect on the release of growth hormone, TSH and prolactin but inhibits the increase in plasma ACTH in response to CRF (Page et al 1990).

AVP is known to rise dramatically during surgical stimulation, not only during the initial incision but also during closure of the perineum and suturing of the skin. No such effect can be demonstrated with OT in man. Haemorrhage increases AVP levels but Loveland et al (1990) have demonstrated that this also applies to OT. It may well be that OT is only released in response to profound haemorrhage to augment the vasoconstrictor action of AVP.

Antagonists of AVP and OT

Detailed studies have indicated that there are OT receptors and AVP receptors which were initially divided into V_1 and V_2; there are other subdivisions of these receptors including V_{1a} receptors in the hepatocytes and V_{1b} receptors in the pituitary. The receptors in other sites are less clearly distinguished. The V_2 receptors are in the renal tubular cells and in addition to the antidiuretic effects may also affect the peripheral vasculature. OT and AVP can interact at each other's receptor sites. OT can combine and activate V_{1a} and V_2 receptors while AVP can activate OT-like receptors. This has made designing antagonists particularly difficult but four types of antagonists can be recognized: OT, V_{1a}, V_{1b}, and V_2.

Oxytocin (OT) antagonists can block V_{1a} receptors and also may be of value in premature labour;

V_{1a} antagonists selectively block the vascular effects of AVP but also the effects of OT as well as AVP releasing action on ACTH;

V_{1b} antagonists block the ACTH-releasing effects of AVP, and also the V_{1a} antagonists;

V_2 and V_{1a} antagonists block both the vascular and the antidiuretic action of AVP as well as oxytocin;

V_2 antagonists selectively block the antidiuretic actions of AVP.

Clinically there is little use yet for these antagonists except possibly in the care of SIADH or to antagonize the vasopressor actions of AVP (Manning & Sawyer 1989).

REFERENCES

Allen J, Boyd K, Hawkins S A, Hadden D R 1989 Poikilothermia in a 68-year-old female. A risk factor for accidental hypothermia, or hyperthermia. Q J Med 70: 103–112

Alvarez M A, Portilla L, Gonzalez R, Ezcurra E 1989 Insulin response to a short stress period. Psychoneuroendocrinology 14: 241–244

Ardaillou E, Dussaule J C 1990 Atrial natriuretic factor—Role in the physiopathology of cardiac and renal diseases. La Presse Medicale 19: 76–82

Ardawi M S M, Ashy A A, Jamal Y S, Khoja S M 1989 Metabolic control of hepatic gluconeogenesis in response to sepsis. J Lab Clin Med 114: 579–586

Asari H, Kondo H, Ishihara A, Ando K, Marumo F 1989 Extracorporeal circulation influence on plasma atrial natriuretic peptide concentration in cardiac surgery patients. Chest 96: 757–760

Bennett K L, Linden R J 1989 Effect of the cessation of an infusion of vasopressin in acutely hypophysectomized anaesthetized dogs. Q J Exp Physiol 74: 841–849

Bennett T L, Rose J C 1989 Effect of cortisol on vasopressin response to hypertonic saline in fetal sheep. Am J Physiol 257: R861–R865

Benzoni D, Geoffroy J, Waeber B, Brunner H R, Biollaz J, Sassard J 1989 Atrial natriuretic peptide and urinary prostaglandins in man. Br J Clin Pharmacol 28: 397–402

Berkenbosch F, de Goeij D E C, Rey A D, Besedovsky H O 1989 Neuroendocrine, sympathetic and metabolic responses induced by interleukin-1. Neuroendocrinology 50: 570–576

Burrell L M, Baylis P H 1990 Release of atrial natriuretic peptide during hypertonic saline infusion: the importance of posture. Clin Endocrinol 32: 491–496

Caggiula A R, Antelman S M, Aul E, Knopf S, Edwards D J 1989 Prior stress attenuates the analgesic response but sensitizes the corticosterone and cortical dopamine responses to stress 10 days later. Psychopharmacology 99: 233–237

Callahan M F, Kirby R F, Cunningham J T et al 1989 Central oxytocin systems may mediate a cardiovascular response to acute stress in rats. Am J Physiol 256: H1369–H1377

Carli F, Emery P W, Freemantle C A J 1989 Effect of perioperative normothermia on postoperative protein metabolism in elderly patients undergoing hip arthroplasty. Br J Anaesth 63: 276–282

Chiodera P, Gnudi A, Volpi R et al 1989a Effect of the GABAergic agent sodium valproate on the arginine vasopressin responses to hypertonic stimulation and upright posture in man. Clin Endocrinol 30: 389–399

Chiodera P, Gnudi A, Bianconi L et al 1989b Naloxone abolishes the inhibiting effect of somatostatin on the release of oxytocin evoked by insulin-induced hypoglycemia in humans. Metab Clin Exp 38: 709–711

Coiro V, Capretti L, Speroni G et al 1989 Muscarinic cholinergic, but not serotoninergic mediation of arginine vasopressin response to metoclopramide in man. Clin Endocrinol 31: 491–498

Courneya C A, Wilson N, Ledsome J R 1989 Plasma vasopressin and atrial natriuretic factor during haemorrhage: influence of cardiac and aortic receptors. Clin Exp Pharmacol Physiol 16: 651–658

Cover P O, Buckingham J C 1989 Effects of selective opioid-receptor blockade on the hypothalamo–pituitary–adrenocortical responses to surgical trauma in the rat. J Endocrinol 121: 213–220

Cross J S, Gruber D P, Gann D S, Singh A K, Moran J M, Burchard K W 1989 Hypertonic saline attenuates the hormonal response to injury. Ann Surg 209: 684–692

Dallman M F, Darlington D N, Suemaru S, Cascio C S, Levin N 1989 Corticosteroids in homeostasis. Acta Physiol Scand 583: 27–34

Dantzer R, Kelley K W 1989 Stress and immunity: an integrated view of relationships between the brain and the immune system. Life Sci 44: 1995–2008

Davidson J R T, Nemeroff C B 1989 Pharmacotherapy in posttraumatic stress disorder: historical and clinical considerations and future directions. Psychopharmacol Bull 25: 422–425

Desborough J P, Hall G M, Hart G R, Burrin J M, Bloom S R 1990 Hormonal responses to cardiac surgery: effects of sufentanil, somatostatin and ganglion block. Br J Anaesth 64: 688–695

DiCarlo S E, Stahl L K, Hasser E M, Bishop V S 1989 The role of vasopressin in the pressor response to bilateral carotid occlusion. J Auton Nerv Syst 27: 1–10

Donckier J E, De Coster P M, Buysschaert M et al 1989 Exercise and posture-related changes of atrial natriuretic factor and cardiac function in diabetes. Diabetes Care 12: 475–480

Douglas R G, Shaw J H F 1990 Metabolic effects of cancer. Br J Surg 77: 246–254

Ebert J P, Pearson J D, Gelman S, Harris C, Bradley E L 1989 Circulatory responses to laryngoscopy: the comparative effects of placebo, fentanyl and esmolol. Can J Anaesth 36: 301–306

Edwards A E, Smith C J, Gower D E et al 1990 Anaesthesia, trauma, stress and leucocyte migration: influence of general anaesthesia and surgery. Eur J Anaesthesiol 7: 185–196

Egan J W, Jugus M, Kinter L B, Lee K, Smith E F III 1989 Effect of a selective V_1 vasopressin receptor antagonist on the sequelae of endotoxemia in the conscious rat. Circ Shock 29: 155–166

Ellis M J, Schmidli R S, Donald R A, Livesey J H, Espiner E A 1990 Plasma corticotrophin-releasing factor and vasopressin responses to hypoglycaemia in normal man. Clin Endocrinol 32: 93–100

Engel C, Kristensen S S, Axel C, Lund B, Nielsen J B 1989 Indomethacin and the stress response to hysterectomy. Acta Anaesthesiol Scand 33: 540–544

Ferrari R, Agnoletti G 1989 Atrial natriuretic peptide: its mechanism of release from the atrium. Int J Cardiol 24: 137–149

Forse R A, Elwyn D H, Askanazi J, Iles M, Schwarz Y, Kinney J M 1990 Effects of glucose on nitrogen balance during high nitrogen intake in malnourished patients. Clin Sci 78: 273–281

Gavras H, Gavras I 1989 Salt-induced hypertension: the interactive role of vasopressin and of the sympathetic nervous system. J Hypertens 7: 601–606

Goldsmith S R 1989 The effect of moderate hypotension on vasopressin levels in normal humans. Am J Med Sci 298: 295–298

Groban L, Ebert T J, Kreis D U, Skelton M M, van Wynsberghe D M, Cowley A W Jr. 1989 Hemodynamic, renal, and hormonal responses to incremental ANF infusions in humans. Am J Physiol 256: F780–F786

Gross P, Lang R, Ketteler M et al 1989 Natriuretic factors and lithium clearance in patients with the syndrome of inappropriate antidiuretic hormone (SIADH). Eur J Clin Invest 19: 11–19

Gruber K A, Callahan M F 1989 ACTH-(4-10) through gamma-MSH: evidence for a new class of central autonomic nervous system-regulating peptides. Am J Physiol 257: R681–R694

Gutkowska J, Nemer M, Sole M J, Drouin J, Sirois P 1989 Lung is an important source of atrial natriuretic factor in experimental cardiomyopathy. J Clin Invest 83: 1500–1504

Hackmann T, Gascoyne R D, Naiman S C et al 1989 A trial of desmopressin (1-desamino-8-d-arginine vasopressin) to reduce blood loss in uncomplicated cardiac surgery. N Engl J Med 321: 1437–1443

Hahn R G 1989 Influence of the fluid balance on the cortisol and glucose responses to transurethral prostatic surgery. Acta Anaesthesiol Scand 33: 638–641

Hahn R G, Rundgren M 1989 Vasopressin and amino acid concentrations in serum following absorption of irrigating fluid containing glycine and ethanol. Br J Anaesth 63: 337–339

Harding J W, Jensen L L, Quirk W S, Dewey A L, Wright J W 1989 Brain angiotensin: critical role in the ongoing regulation of body fluid homeostasis and cardiovascular function. Peptides 10: 261–264

Hart S L, Oluyomi A O 1990 Vasopressin and stress-induced antinociception in the mouse. Br J Pharmacol 99: 243–246

Hartl W H, Jaunch K-W, Herndon D N, Cohnert T U, Wolfe R R, Schildberg F W 1990 Effect of low-dose bradykinin on glucose metabolism and nitrogen balance in surgical patients. Lancet 335: 69–71

Hashimoto K, Murakami K, Takao T, Makino S, Sugawara M, Ota Z 1989 Effect of acute ether or restraint stress on plasma corticotropin-releasing hormone, vasopressin and oxytocin levels in the rat. Acta Med Okayama 43: 161–167

Helfer E L, Rose L I 1989 Corticosteroids and adrenal suppression characterising and avoiding the problem. Drugs 38: 838–845

Hellebrekers L J, Biewenga W J, Mol J A 1989 Effect of arginine vasopressin on urine formation and plasma atrial natriuretic peptide level in conscious dogs. Eur J Pharmacol 164: 55–62

Hogevold H E, Mundal H H, Norman N, Reikeras O 1990 Platelet release reaction and plasma catecholamines during total hip replacement. No effects of high doses of corticosteroids. Thromb Res 57: 21–29

Huber I, Krause U, Nink M, Lehnert H, Beyer J 1989 Dexamethasone does not suppress the respiratory analeptic effect of corticotropin-releasing hormone. J Clin Endocrinol Metab 69: 440–442

Iitake K, Kimura T, Ota K et al 1989 Responses of vasopressin, atrial natriuretic peptide, and blood pressure to central osmotic stimulation. Am J Physiol 257: E611–E616

Jacobson L, Akana S F, Cascio C S, Scribner K, Shinsako J, Dallman M F 1989 The adrenocortical system responds slowly to removal of corticosterone in the absence of concurrent stress. Endocrinology 124: 2144–2152

Jin H, Chen Y-F, Yang R-H, McKenna T M, Jackson R M, Oparil S 1989 Vasopressin lowers pulmonary artery pressure in hypoxic rats by releasing atrial natriuretic peptide. Am J Med Sci 298: 227–236

Jungmann E, Konzok C, Holl E, Fassbinder W, Schoffling K 1989 Effect of human atrial natriuretic peptide on blood glucose concentrations and hormone stimulation during insulin-induced hypoglycaemia in healthy man. Eur J Clin Pharmacol 36: 593–597

Kanfer A, Dussaule J-C, Czekalski S, Rondeau E, Sraer J-D, Ardaillou R 1989 Physiological significance of increased levels of endogenous atrial natriuretic factor in human acute renal failure. Clin Nephrol 32: 51–56

Kinoshita Y, Okamoto K, Yahata K et al 1990 Clinical and pathological changes of the heart in brain death maintained with vasopressin and epinephrine. Pathol Res Pract 186: 173–179

Knox A J, Britton J R, Tattersfield A E 1989 Effect of vasopressin on bronchial reactivity to histamine. Clin Sci 77: 467–471

Kong A-N, Ludwig E A, Slaughter R L et al 1989 Pharmacokinetics and pharmacodynamic modeling of direct suppression effects of methylprednisolone on serum cortisol and blood histamine in human subjects. Clin Pharmacol Ther 46: 616–628

Koob G F, Lebrum C, Bluthe R-M, Dantzer R, Le Moal M 1989 Role of neuropeptides in learning versus performance: focus on vasopressin. Brain Res Bull 23: 359–364

Levin E R, Mills S, Weber M A 1989 Central nervous system mediated vasodepressor action of atrial natriuretic factor. Life Sci 44: 1617–1624

Levine B, Kalman J, Mayer L, Fillit H M, Packer M 1990 Elevated circulating levels of tumor necrosis factor in severe chronic heart failure. N Engl J Med 323: 236–241

Linton E A, Lowry P J 1989 Corticotrophin releasing factor in man and its measurement: a review. Clin Endocrinol 31: 225–249

Loveland R C, Kaufman L, Robinson I C A F 1990 Arginine vasopressin and oxytocin during major colorectal surgery (in press)

Manner T, Kanto J, Ruskoaho H et al 1989 Hormonal, haemodynamic, and subjective effects of intravenously infused indomethacin: no change in the physiological response to hypertonic saline challenge. Pharmacol Toxicol 65: 231–235

Manning M, Sawyer W H 1989 Discovery, development, and some uses of vasopressin and oxytocin antagonists. J Lab Clin Med 114: 617–632

Marson L, Kiritsy-Roy J A, van Loon G R 1989 Mu-opioid peptide modulation of cardiovascular and sympathoadrenal responses to stress. Am J Physiol 257: R901–R908

Metzler C H, Ramsay D J 1989 Physiological doses of atrial peptide inhibit angiotensin II-stimulated aldosterone secretion. Am J Physiol 256: R1155–1159

Morrow L A, Morganroth G S, Hill T J et al 1989 Atrial natriuretic factor in the elderly: diminished response to epinephrine. Am J Physiol 257: E866–E870

Mutti A, Ferroni C, Vescovi P P et al 1989 Endocrine effects of psychological stress associated with neurobehavioral performance testing. Life Sci 44: 1831–1836

Nakada T, Furuta H, Katayama T, Sumiya H, Shimazaki J 1989 The effect of adrenal surgery on plasma atrial natriuretic factor and sodium escape phenomenon in patients with primary aldosteronism. J Urol 142: 13–18

Newrick P G, Braatvedt G, Hancock J, Corrall R J M 1990 Self-management of adrenal insufficiency by rectal hydrocortisone. Lancet 335: 212–213

Norsk P 1989 Influence of low- and high-pressure baroreflexes on vasopressin release in humans. Acta Endocrinol 121 (suppl 1): 10–27

Obata K, Yasue H, Okumura K et al 1989 Increased secretion of atrial natriuretic polypeptide in response to cardiac pacing. Jpn Circ J 53: 1055–1060

Ota K, Kimura T, Matsui K et al 1990 Effects of central osmotic stimulation on vasopressin and enkephalin release into the blood and cerebrospinal fluid and blood pressure. Acta Endocrinol 122: 62–70

Page S R, Ang V T Y, Jackson R, White A, Nussey S S, Jenkins J S 1990 The effect of oxytocin infusion on adenohypophyseal function in man. Clin Endocrinol 32: 307–313

Paolisso G, Sgambato S, Giugliano D et al 1989 Effects of oxytocin delivery on counter-regulatory hormone response in insulin-dependent (type 1) diabetic subjects. Horm Res 31: 250–255

Perez R, Espinoza M, Riquelme R, Parer J T, Llanos A J 1989 Arginine vasopressin mediates cardiovascular responses to hypoxemia in fetal sheep. Am J Physiol 256: R1011–R1018

Peskind E R, Veith R C, Dorsa D M, Gumbrecht G, Raskind M A 1989 Yohimbine increases cerebrospinal fluid and plasma norepinephrine but not arginine vasopressin in humans. Neuroendocrinology 50: 286–291

Pitman R K, Orr S P, Steketee G S 1989 Psychophysiological investigations of posttraumatic stress disorder imagery. Psychopharmacol Bull 25: 426–431

Plotsky P M, Cunningham E T Jr, Widmaier E P 1989 Catecholaminergic modulation of corticotropin-releasing factor and adrenocorticotropin secretion. Endocr Rev 10: 437–458

Raff H, Flemma R J, Findling J W with the technical assistance of Nelson D K 1988 Fast cortisol-induced inhibition of the adrenocorticotropin response to surgery in humans. J Clin Endocrinol Metab 67: 1146–1148

Rakugi H, Ogihara T, Nakamaru M et al 1989 Renal interaction of atrial natriuretic peptide with angiotensin II: glomerular and tubular effects. Clin Exp Pharmacol Physiol 16: 97–107

Riphagen C L, Pittman Q J 1989 Mechanisms underlying the cardiovascular responses to intrathecal vasopressin administration in rats. Can J Physiol Pharmacol 67: 269–275

Ruttimann Y, Chiolero R, Jequier E, Breitenstein E, Schutz Y 1989 Effects of dopamine on total oxygen consumption and oxygen delivery in healthy men. Am J Physiol 257: E541–E546

Schaff H V, Mashburn J P, McCarthy P M, Torres E J, Burnett J C 1989 Natriuresis during and early after cardiopulmonary bypass: relationship to atrial natriuretic factor, aldosterone, and antidiuretic hormone. J Thorac Cardiovasc Surg 98: 979–986

Schiffrin E L 1989 Vascular receptors for angiotensin, vasopressin, and atrial natriuretic peptide in experimental hypertension. Can J Physiol Pharmacol 67: 1118–1123

Scott N B, Mogensen T, Bigler D, Kehlet H 1989 Comparison of the effects of continuous intrapleural vs epidural administration of 0.5% bupivacaine on pain, metabolic response and pulmonary function following cholecystectomy. Acta Anaesthesiol Scand 33: 535–539

Seckl J R, Dunger D B, Bevan J S et al 1990 Vasopressin antagonist in early postoperative diabetes insipidus. Lancet 355: 1353–1356

Shenker Y 1989 Atrial natriuretic hormone and aldosterone regulation in salt-depleted state. Am J Physiol 257: E583–E587

Sitzmann J V, Li S-S, Lin P-W 1989 Prostacyclin mediates splanchnic vascular response to norepinephrine in portal hypertension. J Surg Res 47: 208–211

Sommers De K, Meyer E C, van Wyk M 1989 Effect of neostigmine on metoclopramide-induced aldosterone secretion in man. Eur J Clin Pharmacol 36: 411–413

Spitzer J A, Rodriguez de Turco E B 1989 Modification of adrenergic and vasopressin receptor-linked lipid metabolism during endotoxemia. In: Roth B L et al (eds) Molecular and Cellular Mechanisms of Septic Shock. Alan R Liss Inc. New York; pp 77–99

Stern N, Eggena P, Chandler W, Tuck M L 1989 Effects of central and peripheral dopamine antagonism on aldosterone secretion: evidence for adrenal mechanism. Am J Physiol 257: E588–E594

Stewart P A H, Barlow I M 1989 Metabolic effects of prostatectomy. J R Soc Med 82: 725–728

Sun K, Lin B C, Zhang C, Wang C H, Zhu H N 1989 Possible involvement of beta-endorphin in the deteriorating effect of arginine vasopressin on burn shock in rats. Circ Shock 29: 167–174

Suzuki S, Takeshita A, Imaizumi T et al 1989 Central nervous system mechanisms involved in inhibition of renal sympathetic nerve activity induced by arginine vasopressin. Circ Res 65: 1390–1399

Szczepanska-Sadowska E 1989 Interaction of vasopressin and of the atrial natriuretic peptide in blood pressure control. Acta Physiol Scand 136 (suppl 583): 79–87

Tesar V, Horky K, Petryl J et al 1989 Atrial natriuretic factor in liver cirrhosis—the influence of volume expansion. Horm Metab Res 21: 519–522

Tidgren B, Hjemdahl P 1989 Renal responses to mental stress and epinephrine in humans. Am J Physiol 257: F682–F689

Vallotton M B, Gerber-Wicht C, Dolci W, Wuthrich R P 1989 Interaction of vasopressin and angiotensin II in stimulation of prostacyclin synthesis in vascular smooth muscle cells. Am J Physiol 257: E617–E624

van der Kolk B A, Greenberg M S, Orr S P, Pitman R K 1989 Endogenous opioids, stress induced analgesia, and posttraumatic stress disorder. Psychopharmacol Bull 25: 417–421

Veelken R, Danckwart L, Rohmeiss P, Unger T 1989 Effects of intravenous AVP on cardiac output, mesenteric hemodynamics, and splanchnic nerve activity. Am J Physiol 257: H658–H664

Vescovi P P, Gerra G, Pioli G, Pedrazzoni M, Maninetti L, Passeri M 1990 Circulating opioid peptides during thermal stress. Horm Metab Res 22: 44–46

Vitting K E, Gardenswartz M H, Zabetakis P M et al 1990 Frequency of hyponatremia and nonosmolar vasopressin release in the acquired immunodeficiency syndrome. JAMA 263: 973–978

Wallace A W, Tunin C M, Shoukas A A 1989 Effects of vasopressin on pulmonary and systemic vascular mechanics. Am J Physiol 257: H1228–H1234

Wallin L A, Fawcett C P, Rosenfeld CR 1989 Oxytocin stimulates glucagon and insulin secretion in fetal and neonatal sheep. Endocrinology 125: 2289–2296

Weinand M E, O'Boynick P L, Goetz K L 1989 A study of serum antidiuretic hormone and atrial natriuretic peptide levels in a series of patients with intracranial disease and hyponatremia. Neurosurgery 25: 781–785

Wehling M, Muller T, Heim J M et al 1989 Effects of clonidine and dihydralazine on atrial natriuretic factor and cGMP in humans. J Appl Physiol 67: 938–944

Whitworth J A, Stewart P M, Burt D, Atherden S M, Edwards C R W 1989 The kidney is the major site of cortisone production in man. Clin Endocrinol 31: 355–361

Wittert G A, Crock P A, Donald R A et al 1990 Arginine vasopressin in Cushing's disease. Lancet 335: 991–994

7. Sweating and thermoregulation in anaesthesia: a review of the physiology and pharmacology and their relationship to anaesthesia

C. S. Martin   A. J. Asbury

Autonomic nervous system activity is important clinically because it is used, with other signs, to give some estimate of the depth of anaesthesia. Furthermore, autonomic activity, of which sweating is one component, has to be considered in judging responses under anaesthesia and in intensive care to challenges such as pain and fluid loading or loss. Finally, there are many drugs and disease states which affect sweating, and their effects need to be considered when assessing a patient.

A DESCRIPTION OF THE SWEAT GLANDS

The sweat glands were divided into eccrine and apocrine glands by Schiefferdecker in 1917 (Weiner & Hellman 1960). The apocrine glands are of little significance in man. The eccrine glands consist of a single coiled unbranched tubule leading to the secretory coil of the gland which lies between 2–5 mm below the epidermis (Sato & Sato 1983). The total number of sweat glands in the adult is between 2–4 million and they are distributed throughout the skin but are absent from the lips, nail bed, glans penis and eardrum. They are most densely distributed on the plantar and palmar areas and on the forehead. The density ranges from $60/cm^2$ on the thigh to $350/cm^2$ on the forehead and $620/cm^2$ on the sole of the foot (Sato 1977). The number of active sweat glands is variable and dependent on acclimatization (Peter & Wyndham 1966). The density of eccrine glands decreases as the body surface area increases from infancy (Thomson 1954).

The secretory coil gives rise to precursor sweat by active chloride secretion driven by Na/K ATPase in the particular cell membrane (Quinton & Tormey 1976, Bijman & Quinton 1987). The precursor sweat is similar to plasma in osmolarity and in sodium, chloride and bicarbonate concentration. The content of the final sweat appearing at the orifice of the gland suggests that sweat undergoes several modifications in the sweat duct. Active reabsorption of sodium and chloride in the distal part of the gland can produce hypotonic sweat. The observation that sweat pH is proportional to the rate of sweating suggests that sodium/proton exchange may occur. Potassium is secreted into the sweat but the mechanism is unclear (Bijman 1987). The ability to produce hypotonic sweat is unique to primates and possibly most highly developed in man (Quinton 1983). This ability conserves extracellular solutes and the circulating volume by mobilizing water from the intracellular compartment.

COMPOSITION OF SWEAT

Sweat is a hypotonic liquid which is very different from both intracellular and extracellular fluid. The composition is influenced by the rate of sweating because the reabsorptive capacity is a function of flow. The sodium concentration is normally 10–20 mmol/l at relatively low sweat rates but can be near 100 mmol/l near the maximum sweat rate (Bijman 1987). Potassium concentration is normally greater than in the extracellular fluid at 6–7 mmol/l (Sato et al 1989a). The pH is also rate dependent, from 5.0 at low rates, to 7.0 at high rates (Sato 1977). Other constituents are chloride, lactate, ammonia, bicarbonate, glucose, urea, calcium, magnesium, phosphate, mucopolysaccharides, prostaglandins, amino acids and proteins including immunoglobulins (Page & Remington 1967) and enzymes (Quinton 1983).

Drugs appearing in sweat include carbamazepine, phenobarbitone, phenytoin, alcohol, griseofulvin and ketoconazole (Sato et al 1989a).

Acclimatization to heat enables a subject to secrete a more hypotonic sweat thus preserving the extracellular fluid volume more efficiently. Salt deprivation increases the reabsorption of sodium, partly due to increased aldosterone secretion (Sigal & Dobson 1968). The glands increase their ability to reabsorb sodium in these circumstances by hypertrophy and lengthening of the duct (Sato & Sato 1983).

Sweat induced by thermal exposure has been shown to have lower sodium and chloride concentrations than sweat induced by running exercise. There was a similar rise in serum aldosterone during thermal exposure and running exercise. These aldosterone responses cannot account for the differences in composition; other factors must be involved (Fukomoto et al 1988).

INNERVATION OF SWEAT GLANDS

The eccrine sweat glands are innervated principally by post-ganglionic fibres of the sympathetic nervous system and are probably unique in that the transmitter is acetylcholine (Dale & Feldburg 1934) thus explaining the similarity in response to those glands which are under parasympathetic control. Acetylcholine is released from the nerve endings by the arrival of a nerve impulse and it combines with the receptor to stimulate sweating by a mechanism involving calcium influx, potassium release and other molecular changes (Sato et al 1989a). The quantity of acetylcholine released is proportional to the number of nerve impulses arriving at the junction. Acetylcholine is removed from the nerve ending mainly by acetylcholinesterase. The eccrine glands also receive some adrenergic innervation (Uno 1977) although noradrenaline is less effective than acetylcholine as a stimulant of sweat secretion (Sato 1977). Vasoactive intestinal polypeptide has also been observed in human eccrine glands and has been shown to be capable of stimulating sweat secretion by a mechanism mediated by cAMP (Sato & Sato 1987).

SWEATING AND THERMOREGULATION

Evaporation of the sweat from the skin is the main mechanism of heat loss when the body temperature starts to rise, although evaporation also occurs from the respiratory tract. The latent heat of vaporization of water is 0.58 kcal/g. In addition to sweating, water is lost from the skin by simple diffusion which accounts for 600–800 ml/24 h and is largely independent of environmental factors.

Sweating is stimulated when body temperature rises to a threshold where thermosensitive neurones in the preoptic anterior hypothalamus detect changes in internal temperature and initiate appropriate thermoregulatory responses to maintain constant internal temperature (Nakayama 1985). A rise in the mean skin temperature will also stimulate sweating through the hypothalamus, but increases in core temperature are the major determinants. Thermosensitive neurones have also been identified in the spinal cord, lower brain stem and are probably widely distributed throughout the body core (Hammel 1988). Thermosensitive neurones in the spinal cord are responsible for initiating the shivering associated with extradural anaesthesia (Walmsley et al 1986). The injection of cold bupivacaine into the extradural space was associated with shivering in 47% of patients. Those patients who were shivering most violently were given a dose of bupivacaine warmed to 41°C, which abolished the shivering in 50% of cases. Cessation of shivering corresponded with the periods in which the extradural temperature increased. In addition to skin temperature, the response of the hypothalamus is inversely related to body fluid osmolality (Quinton 1987).

The maximum rate of thermal sweat secretion in one hour may be as high as 1.7 l but this cannot be sustained and the maximum in a 24-h period is about 12 l. The efficiency of sweating as a mechanism of heat loss is hindered by humidity, absence of wind and clothing. In such circumstances a greater volume of sweat is required to achieve the same amount of cooling and sweat may be wiped away without dissipating any heat.

Temperature regulation has physiological priority over the maintenance of salt and water balance; sweating will continue in the face of severe dehydration and salt loss until circulatory failure occurs (Guyton 1986).

NORMAL PATTERNS OF SWEATING

Differences can be detected in the distribution of sweating provoked by thermal or emotional stimuli (Chalmers & Keele 1952). Thermal sweating is most profuse on the forehead, neck, chest and dorsum of the hand and is less marked on the palms and soles.

In contrast, sweating provoked by anxiety or emotion occurs mainly on the palms and soles but often involves the axillae in addition and may become generalized in severe cases. Both types of sweating are under the control of the central nervous system. Thermal sweating is controlled by the hypothalamus but emotional sweating is controlled by other centres, which may be situated in the cerebral cortex.

DETECTION AND MEASUREMENT OF SWEATING

There is a variety of methods available for the detection of sweating. The most basic is simple clinical observation which is subject to observer variability. Colorimetric indicators include sodium chinazerin 2, 6 disulphide, alcoholic cobalt chloride, phenolphthalein or bromophenol blue in silicone. These indicators tend to be toxic, irritant or staining. The iodine-starch method is more satisfactory. The iodinated starch is sprayed onto the skin and sweat droplets are visualized as discrete purple dots. This method is sensitive, can be used over a large part of the body surface and sweating can be assessed repeatedly on the same skin area when elicited by different stimuli (Sato et al 1988). These methods are qualitative.

Quantitative recordings of sweat rate can be obtained from small areas of skin using galvanic methods. A plexiglass sweat capsule is attached to the skin and the local sweat rate can be monitored continuously using resistance hygrometry. This technique measures sweating by detecting the fall in electrical resistance of the skin which occurs as sweat is secreted into the ducts (Kenney et al 1986, Bullard 1962). An optical method involving the absorption of infra-red radiation and a photographic method have also been used. The variety of recording methods indicates the difficulty in setting up a reliable system (Millington & Williamson 1983). The Servo Med evaporimeter has been used clinically in anaesthesia to record palmar sweat production as a measure of the sympathetic response to stress (Maryniak & Bishop 1987a, b).

INFLUENCE OF DRUGS ON THE SWEAT GLANDS

Parasympathomimetic agents

The parasympathomimetic agents which influence sweating are primarily of experimental interest. Acetylcholine produces sweating in a muscarinic fashion, working directly on the glands, whereas nicotine acts at a site on the axon remote from the neuroeffector junction (Randall & Kimura 1954).

Drugs such as physostigmine and neostigmine which inhibit cholinesterase also have a sudorific action. Beta-adrenergic agonists and theophylline also stimulate sweating by a mechanism involving cAMP production (Sato & Sato 1981).

Anticholinergic agents

Atropine and hyoscine act both on the central nervous system and peripherally on smooth muscle and secretory glands innervated by post-ganglionic cholinergic nerves. Glycopyrrolate on the other hand, does not cross the blood–brain barrier and is therefore only available to act peripherally. All the muscarinic effects of acetylcholine can be attenuated by the action of these anticholinergic agents. The site of action of atropine appears to be on the effector cell where the transmitter is prevented from stimulating the receptor. Atropine has no effect on the release of acetylcholine from the nerve ending.

The systemic administration of atropine has been found to reduce general body sweating by 40–50% (Craig 1952) but the dose required would cause severe cardiovascular reactions to occur before a concentration sufficient to produce anhidrosis is reached.

Beta-adrenergic blocking agents

It may be deduced that any effect of beta blocking agents occurs at the sympathetic ganglia because sweating is under cholinergic control. Beta-blockers are the agents of choice in the treatment of anxiety associated with physical symptoms such as tremor and palpitations besides sweating, although patients with predominantly psychic symptoms may deteriorate (Rogers & Spector 1983).

Atenolol, metoprolol and propranolol have been shown to increase sweating during exercise (Gordon et al 1955, Wilcox et al 1984).

Beta-blockade attenuates the autonomic responses to hypoglycaemia, and it has been shown in both normal subjects (Deacon 1977, Schluter & Kerp 1983) and those with diabetes mellitus (Strom 1978) that palpitations and tremors do not occur. However, sweating was markedly increased and in diabetics had become the most prominent symptom of hypoglycaemia.

Hyperhidrosis can be a feature of sudden withdrawal of beta-blockade (O'Brien 1975). However, beta-blockade is not recommended for the treatment of hyperhidrosis because of the cardiovascular side effects.

Adrenal corticoid agents

During acclimatization to heat it has been noted that as the sodium chloride content of sweat falls, there is an increase in the secretion of adrenocortical hormones (Conn et al 1946). Administration of deoxycorticosterone acetate causes similar change in sweat composition. The sodium chloride content of sweat in Addisonian patients is more than the expected figure (Conn 1949). Conversely, salt levels are low in Cushingoid subjects. Spironolactone increases salt concentration.

Diuretics

Frusemide and bumetanide both inhibit the secretion of sweat (Quinton 1987).

SWEATING AND ANAESTHESIA

Sweating is often observed in the clinical practice of anaesthesia, and would normally be considered an indication of inadequate anaesthesia, but obviously it would be considered in the light of other signs. While sweating as a sign in anaesthesia is highly subjective, it is still important because when muscle relaxants are used, it is one of the few signs left to guide the anaesthetist. The causes of sweating in anaesthesia are said to be pyrexia, hypercapnia, light anaesthesia, shock, anxiety and high nervous tone (Atkinson et al 1987).

The effects of anaesthetics on sweating have been studied in the cat, using the hairless skin of the paw (Janig & Rath 1980). Reflex sweating was induced by nociceptive and vibrational stimuli, which have separate spinal pathways. Ketamine was found to enhance the sweating induced by vibrational stimulation but to inhibit the sweating induced by noxious stimulation of the skin. In contrast, methohexitone was found to inhibit reflexes to vibrational stimuli but enhanced response to noxious stimuli. The differing actions of these two drugs probably reflect their actions on different pathways at spinal cord level or higher. Halothane and althesin were both found to depress both types of reflexes. These results show that the effects of anaesthetics on sweating depend on the type of reflex tested and also the agent used. In further studies in chronic spinal cats, these authors showed that ketamine and methohexitone act on supraspinal brain structures and not at all (or only to a minor degree) at the spinal cord level.

Layman (1984) has shown that sweating can occur during surgery independent of the depth of anaesthesia as assessed by a cerebral function monitor (CFM). In this study factors inducing or masking sweating were avoided. No sweating was observed in patients undergoing abdominal or thoracic surgery at the time of skin incision or suturing. However, sweating that was clinically demonstrable occurred with regularity at times of bowel handling and pleural retraction. There were no associated changes in cortical activity, blood pressure or heart rate. The sweating was therefore assumed to indicate a subcortical autonomic reflex and it was obtunded by an althesin/opiate/relaxant anaesthetic.

The production of palmar sweat is part of the sympathetic response to stress which can be measured using an evaporimeter. Maryniak & Bishop (1987a) have evaluated the production of palmar sweat and its correlation with heart rate during anaesthesia for cystoscopy. The correlation was positive and it was concluded that the measurement of palmar sweat production may be a useful, sensitive and non-invasive method of assessing the degree of sympathetic activity during anaesthesia and surgery.

In a further investigation (Maryniak & Bishop 1987b) the same authors studied palmar sweat and heart rate changes during an attempt to attenuate the response to laryngoscopy and intubation by pretreatment with alfentanil 30 μg/kg. It was found that this pretreatment attenuated the tachycardia associated with intubation, but palmar sweat production increased after induction and the increase was sustained during intubation. This suggested that heart rate may not be as good a measure of stress as has been previously assumed and that pharmacological damping of the cardio-vascular system may not necessarily indicate an ablation of the stress response to laryngeal stimulation.

Anhidrosis can be used as an indicator of sympathetic blockade. Other indicators which have been used include increase in pulse amplitude and increase in skin temperature. However these latter two changes merely signify degrees of sympathetic blockade but do not show complete sympathetic blockade unless accompanied by the absence of sweating (Benzen et al 1985).

It is beneficial to have a reliable sign of complete sympathetic blockade in the treatment of patients with chronic pain associated with sympathetic imbalance. In such patients, an attempted therapeutic blockade may fail for one of two reasons which can be distinguished by anhidrosis. The first reason is that the block is incomplete and the second is that the aetiology of the pain is multifactorial (for example, combined sympathetic dystrophy and somatic sensory pain) and sweating will be abolished.

Reduction in plantar sweating has been used in the comparison of neurolytic and surgical lumbar sympathectomy and was found to be reduced in both groups of patients (Walsh et al 1984).

The effect of post-ganglionic sympathetic blockade with intravenous guanethidine in palmar sweating has been studied (Glynn et al 1981). No significant changes occurred in palmar sweating before or after treatment despite a significant decrease in reported pain. However, the site of action of guanethidine is the post-ganglionic sympathetic nervous system where it displaces noradrenaline from the presynaptic vesicles and prevents its re-uptake as well as blocking its release in response to nerve stimulation. As palmar sweating is mediated by acetylcholine the absence of any change in sweating was not unexpected.

The topical application of a eutectic mixture of 5% lignocaine and 5% prilocaine has been found to inhibit sweating in patients with axillary hyperhidrosis. There was a marked decrease in efficacy after a period of several weeks, the reason for which is uncertain (Juhlin et al 1979).

The measurement of depth of anaesthesia assumes considerable importance in modern clinical anaesthesia which involves the widespread use of neuromuscular blocking drugs. The need to prevent awareness must be balanced against the administration of an overdose to a patient with its implications both intra-operatively and in the recovery phase. At the moment there is no practical means of objective measurement of the depth of anaesthesia and so the anaesthetist must base an indirect judgement on the clinical information which is available. This includes the readily measured cardiovascular variables of pulse rate and rhythm and blood pressure as well as subjective signs which include lacrimation, pupillary dilatation and skin pallor in addition to sweating.

Sweating in anaesthesia is influenced by a wide range of factors including drugs, surgery and thermal balance, and these should be taken into account before any significance is attached to the presence or absence of sweating as a clinical sign.

ABNORMAL PATTERNS OF SWEATING

Heat stroke

The characteristic features of heat stroke or heat exhaustion are hyperpyrexia, salt loss and dehydration. It may be preceded by the sudden cessation of sweating. The typical cause is strenuous activity during hot weather with prolonged profuse sweating accompanied by inadequate water and salt intake causing both hypovolaemia and hypernatraemia, both of which elevate the hypothalamic threshold temperature for sweating (Fortney et al 1981). In addition, hypovolaemia may reduce cutaneous blood flow. These factors may lead to a rise in body temperature to 41° or even higher and can be accompanied by convulsions. Increasing body temperature stimulates metabolism and additional heat production. Circulatory failure supervenes with impaired skin blood flow and exacerbating the inability to dissipate heat, finally producing heat stroke, thus exacerbating the problems.

Sweat gland fatigue

Prolonged exposure to heat may result in an increase in the sodium chloride content of sweat in association with a fall in the volume of sweat produced. Prickly heat is an unrelated condition affecting persons moving from a temperate to a tropical climate (Ryan 1987).

Fever

Fever is defined as a raised core temperature and results from disturbance in the function of the thermoregulating centre in the hypothalamus

(Ganong 1987). It is one manifestation of the acute phase response usually initiated by pyrogenic stimuli including micro-organisms or their products, inflammatory processes or tissue injury. Toxins from bacteria such as endotoxin act on macrocytes, macrophages and Kupffer cells to produce interleukin-1, which together with other pyrogens can act on the central nervous system to produce an upward shift in body temperature. During the onset of fever the activities of the thermoregulatory functions are consistent with those of a hypothermic state. Heat production is maintained by metabolic production and possibly shivering and heat loss is minimized by cutaneous vasoconstriction. For every 1°C rise in body temperature, metabolic rate and oxygen consumption increase by 13% (Baracas et al 1987). However, in septic patients the increase in heat production does not necessarily correlate with fever, although the changes in metabolism do parallel the severity of infection. The sweat glands are inactive at this stage. During the phase of defervescence when the temperature falls, marked sweating occurs and heat loss is greater than heat production.

Antipyretic drugs such as aspirin probably function by acting on the hypothalamus to reset the thermostat and bring down body temperature by cutaneous vasodilation and sweating (Guyton 1986). Naproxen has been shown to abolish the rise in temperature induced by endotoxin. However, it has no effect on the rise in metabolic heat production (Baracas et al 1987).

Hyperhidrosis

Systemic hyperhidrosis is most commonly due to autonomic dysfunction or a thermoregulating disorder. Hyperhidrosis occurs in thyrotoxicosis, diabetes mellitus, congestive heart failure, the menopause and with phaeochromocytoma (Sato et al 1989b). Sweating associated with the last condition may be obtunded by the local injection of an anticholinergic agent (Prout & Wardell 1969) indicating that the mechanism is not one of direct stimulation by circulating catecholamines. It is possible that sweating in phaeochromocytoma is the result of inappropriate thermo-genesis induced by catecholamines, accompanied by cutaneous vasoconstriction.

Sweating also occurs in hypovolaemic shock and in hypoglycaemia, but both the reasons and the mechanisms are poorly understood.

Anhidrosis

Anhidrosis is defined as a relative or absolute deficiency of sweat production in the presence of an appropriate stimulus, whether physiological or pharmacological. Lesions of the preoptic anterior region of the hypothalamus including haemorrhage, trauma and tumours result in anhidrosis (Quinton 1987). Spinal cord transection causes sudden anhi-drosis below the level of the interruption so that patients with high cervical trauma are at risk from heat stroke (Pledger 1962). More distal lesions permit a compensatory increase proximal to the transection (Huckaba et al 1976).

Some patients with spinal injuries, however, experience episodes of profuse sweating which develop months after the injury affecting the skin area outside the denervated sensory or autonomic dermatomes. This hyperhidrosis may be associated with autonomic hyperreflexia (Jane et al 1982), orthostatic hypotension (Khurana 1987) or post-traumatic syringomyelia (Stanworth 1982).

Damage to a peripheral nerve produces an area of anhidrosis which matches the area of paraesthesia.

The autonomic neuropathy of diabetes mellitus also causes anhidrosis which most often affects the extremities and lower body. Burns and scars destroy the sweat glands which are unable to regenerate. This may account for the difficulties which some subjects exhibit in responding to heat stress (Roskind et al 1978) after a major burn. Some compensation is achieved by the remaining glands which can increase their output (McGibbon et al 1973). Total body radiation abolishes sweating for some six months.

Abnormalities in the composition of sweat

The most significant abnormality in the composition of sweat is an increased sodium and chloride concentration. This predisposes the patient to heat stroke because sweating occurs at the expense of the extracellular fluid volume rather than the intracellular volume. This increase in salt concentration occurs in Addison's disease, in chronic pancreatitis and in cystic fibrosis. Sodium and chloride concentrations are greater than 60 mmol/l in fibrocystic disease and the potassium concentration is also greater than normal. Diagnostic sweat tests are carried out on patients suspected of having the disease in which sweating is elicited by pilocarpine iontophoresis.

ANAESTHESIA AND THERMOREGULATION

Anaesthesia influences thermal balance by diminishing autonomic and behavioural responses to thermal stresses imposed on the body. An anaesthetized patient cannot make changes to retain or generate heat like a conscious patient.

Peri-operative hypothermia may occur in association with major operations, reduced metabolic rate, in cool theatres, at extremes of age or when patients are deliberately cooled. The only thermoregulatory responses available during anaesthesia are vasoconstriction and non-shivering thermogenesis.

The effects of different anaesthetic techniques on thermoregulation have been studied, and epidural and high dose fentanyl (50 µg/kg) were associated with a greater fall in core temperature compared with halothane 0.5% or low dose fentanyl (10 µg/kg). When however, total body heat was calculated the intergroup differences disappeared, suggesting that redistribution of heat was occurring, an effect possibly related to depth of anaesthesia. Interestingly in the recovery period the patients who had received epidural anaesthesia were slower to rewarm despite a higher incidence of shivering (Holdcroft et al 1979).

The effect of halothane 1%, enflurane 1% and 2% and isoflurane 1% and 2%, were studied during and after surgery (Ramachandra 1989). More body heat was lost in the halothane group compared with the enflurane group. Halothane caused a greater decrease in mean skin temperature and this accounted for the greater loss of body heat. Core temperature decrease was greatest in the halothane, enflurane 2% and the isoflurane 2% groups. The patients in these groups took significantly longer to return to preoperative values, a fact which has significant implications for patients with poor cardiorespiratory reserve as rewarming can increase oxygen demand by 400–500% (Bay et al 1968).

Similar studies in volunteers produced conflicting results (Stevens et al 1971, Calverley et al 1978). Enflurane and isoflurane produced an increase in skin temperature at higher concentration. However, surgical stimulation, neuromuscular blockade and exposure of the peritoneal or other body cavity are all important factors in surgical patients.

Another study found no difference between ether, halothane and methoxyflurane (Morris 1971), although halothane in nitrous oxide produced a significantly greater decrease in core temperature than ketamine (Engelman & Lockhart 1972). A comparison of heat loss during anaesthesia for pelvic surgery showed little difference between halothane 0.5%, halothane 1% and low dose fentanyl. Those patients who received halothane 1% reduced their heat loss in the third hour of anaesthesia (Holdcroft & Hall 1978).

A further study found no difference in rectal temperature change during N_2O/fentanyl or O_2/halothane anaesthesia for eye surgery. In both groups the temperature fell 0.6°C and a thermal steady state was reached after 2 h of anaesthesia resulting from passive interaction with the environment (Sessler et al 1987a).

A subsequent study found that in patients undergoing general anaesthesia thermal steady state develops passively in warm patients, but in patients who become sufficiently hypothermic profound vasoconstriction develops with a ten-fold reduction in cutaneous blood flow. However, the cold patients did not increase their oxygen consumption suggesting that non-shivering thermogenesis did not occur (Sessler et al 1987b). The same authors also showed that active thermoregulation occurs during halothane anaesthesia, but that it does not occur until core temperature is about 2.5°C below normal. In these cases thermoregulation was achieved by cutaneous vasoconstriction. A thermal steady state developed after about 2 h when the temperature stopped decreasing, heat loss to the environment then being equal to metabolic heat production (Sessler et al 1988a).

During recovery from isoflurane anaesthesia electromyographic patterns were found to differ from those of normal thermogenic shivering. It was suggested that shivering during recovery from anaesthesia was due to spinal reflex hyperactivity resulting from inhibition of descending cortical control by residual anaesthetic, rather than a thermoregulatory mechanism (Sessler et al 1988b).

The concept of depression of the thermoregulatory threshold and explanation of post-anaesthetic shivering were challenged in an editorial by Hammel (1988), who identified three stages of temperature regulation during and after the administration of anaesthesia. Initially thermoregulation is inactivated by anaesthetic action on the preoptic and hypothalamic nuclei. In the second stage, when the anaesthetic is being eliminated, the patient is hypersensitive to cooling of the preoptic anterior hypothalamic nuclei and the temperature threshold of these nuclei is raised due to hypothermia of the body core. In the third stage, when the body core is hyperthermic, the thermal sensitivity of these nuclei is again diminished to below normal.

In the paper which reported active thermoregulation during halothane anaesthesia (Sessler et al 1988a) halothane did in fact eliminate temperature regulation in the first 2 h of anaesthesia. During this time heat was transferred from the core to the periphery, but the resulting core hypothermia did not elicit any thermoregulatory response. In a normal unanaesthetized subject, this degree of hypothermia would increase the hypothalamic temperature threshold for both cutaneous vasoconstriction and shivering to a high temperature; vasoconstriction and shivering would also be maximum. The fact that some vasoconstriction developed in the third hour of surgery suggests that some degree of temperature regulation occurred in these patients. Despite the hypothalamic threshold for vasoconstriction and shivering being well above the actual hypothalamic temperature, there was some vasoconstriction but no shivering in these patients. This indicates that the preoptic and hypothalamic nuclei remained largely dysfunctional.

The study on post-anaesthetic shivering was also open to further interpretation (Hammel 1988). The suggestion that descending cortical control is inhibited is retained, but added to this is the restoration of thermoregulation by preoptic and hypothalamic nuclei as sufficient isoflurane is removed in the initial post-anaesthetic stage. The hypothalamic nuclei then become hypersensitive to changes in local temperature thus eliciting a strong shivering response, even though the responding muscles receive less than normal inhibition from the motor cortex. According to this, the shivering response to a given change of hypothalamic temperature is variable, so the amount of shivering cannot be expected to correlate with core temperature.

Opioids and thermoregulation

Morphine has long been known to produce changes in body temperature. However, the effects are species specific and also dependent on dose, route of administration, ambient temperature, circadian rhythms and age. The endogenous opioid system is also thought to play a role in thermoregulation.

Some species exhibit a hypothermic response to morphine (dog, rabbit and bird) while others develop excitation and hyperthermia (cat, cattle and horse). However, in rats, mice and primates there is a dose-dependent dual response with low dose hyperthermia and high dose hypothermia. Naloxone blocks and antagonizes the effects of morphine on body temperature, suggesting that the effects are mediated through opioid receptors.

The mechanisms of these changes are not fully understood. Hypothermia induced by morphine has been shown to be associated with decreased oxygen consumption and metabolic heat production, although the hyper-thermic response in the rat has been shown to be due to peripheral vasoconstriction (Adler et al 1988).

Epidural sufentanil has been shown to influence body temperature in man (Johnson et al 1989). Following Caesarean section under epidural lignocaine anaesthesia, a patient was shivering despite the use of warming blankets and warmed intravenous fluids. Sufentanil 100 μg was ad-ministered by the epidural route to provide post-operative analgesia, following which the shivering stopped and the patient's temperature fell from 35°C to 33°C. She later developed nausea and vomiting which resolved after naloxone 0.1 mg. This also caused the shivering to restart and the temperature to increase towards normal.

Further study of epidural sufentanil following Caesarean section showed a dose-dependent reduction in core temperature in doses up to 100 μg (Sevarino et al 1989). This occurred without shivering suggesting a direct action on spinal cord receptors altering the hypothalamic set-point and thus influencing temperature. These patients had a high level of sympathetic blockade at the time of administration of sufentanil, hence vasoconstriction was largely lost as a means of thermoregulation.

The interaction of morphine with opioid receptors is influenced by temperature (Puig 1987). The potency of morphine increased five-fold as temperature increased from 30°C to 37°C in the guinea pig ileum preparation. This could be related to a change in the dissociation constant of morphine for the mu receptor. In the same study, the affinity of the opioid receptors for naloxone was not affected by temperature. However, in clinical practice the effects of temperature on dose requirements of drugs are the result of changes in both pharmacokinetic and pharmacodynamic variables. That is, temperature may change the distribution, bio-transformation or excretion of drugs, or the interaction with the ultimate site of action. The question of opioid requirements during hypothermia and hyperthermia has not been addressed in the anaesthetic literature (Adler et al 1988).

Changes in body temperature can affect the requirements for other drugs during anaesthesia. The MAC of the volatile agents increases with hyperthermia (Steffey & Eger 1974) and decreases with hypothermia (Vitez et al 1974, Eger & Johnson 1987). Similarly, hypothermia has the net effect of reducing the requirement for the non-depolarizing muscle relaxants pancuronium and tubocurarine (Miller et al 1978), although the concentration of tubocurarine needed to produce neuromuscular blockade during hypothermia was greater than normal, both in vitro (Holmes et al 1976) and in vivo (Ham et al 1978). However, hypothermia decreased serum clearance and elimination of tubocurarine and the net effect was prolongation of the neuromuscular blockade.

The influence of temperature on the action of atracurium has been shown to affect the train-of-four response to neuromuscular stimulation (Thornberry & Mazumdar 1988). When one arm was wrapped in cotton wool to maintain temperature, and the other was exposed to the ambient conditions, it was found that a difference developed between the arms in the train-of-four response. This difference was directly proportional to the difference in temperature between the two arms. Neuromuscular transmission was suppressed in the cooler arm when the temperature fell below 32°C.

Post-operative rewarming

Patients lose heat during surgery and are frequently hypothermic on arrival in the recovery room. This may represent a significant clinical risk, particularly to the patient with poor cardiorespiratory reserve, as oxygen demand may increase by 400% (Bay et al 1968). Patients over the age of 60 years and those receiving subarachnoid or extradural anaesthesia rewarm more slowly in the first post-operative hour than their younger counterparts and those receiving general anaesthesia (Carli et al 1986). There was no correlation with body fat or duration of surgery in this study.

Sequential changes in body temperature have been measured after major elective surgery. Core temperature increased immediately after surgery and showed a biphasic response with peaks of 37.5°C 14 h after surgery and 37.4°C 32 h after surgery. Resting energy expenditure also increased after surgery, to reach a peak 30% greater than the pre-operative control value after 16 h (Carli & Aber 1987).

MEASUREMENT OF TEMPERATURE

Monitoring of body temperature is indicated for surgery associated with the administration of large volumes of blood and intravenous fluids, where the patient is to be deliberately cooled, for hypothermic patients and for malignant hyperthermia subjects or suspects. It is also advisable for pyrexial patients, for patients undergoing combined regional and general anaesthesia and for the elderly (Holloway 1988).

Various sites have been used to measure core temperature. These include the nasopharynx, oesophagus, rectum, tympanic membrane, bladder and axilla. The oesophageal temperature probe requires accurate placement distal to the bifurcation of the trachea to avoid fluctuations associated with movement of respiratory gases (Siegel & Gravenstein 1989). This may be achieved with the aid of the oesophageal stethoscope to place the sensor at the point where heart sounds are maximal (Cork et al 1983). However, another study showed that the sensor may be proximal to the tracheal bifurcation even with this technique. The distribution of temperature along the oesophagus was found to be non-uniform, the lowest quarter being the warmest (Kaufman 1987).

Rectal temperature is less precise than bladder temperature (Cork et al 1983), and changes in rectal temperature lag behind changes at other core sites (Bone & Feneck 1988). Nasopharyngeal and tympanic membrane temperatures serve as estimates of brain temperature, although the nasopharynx is an air-filled cavity and the result may be unreliable (Cohen & Hercus 1959). Positioning of the tympanic membrane sensor has resulted in perforation of the tympanic membrane (Wallace et al 1974).

Monitoring of bladder temperature with the aid of a thermistor tipped urinary catheter has been used successfully, both intra- and post-operatively (Cork et al 1983, Bone & Feneck 1988, Editorial 1988). The axilla has also been used to measure core temperature non-invasively, but is less accurate than other sites (Cork et al 1983).

The temperature of the great toe correlates poorly with core temperature, although this correlation improves greatly after 2 h of anaesthesia (Cork et al 1983). Mean skin temperature (MST) can be calculated from measurements from four sites: lower leg, thigh, chest wall and upper arm:

$$\text{MST} = 0.3 \, (\text{chest wall} + \text{upper arm}) + 0.6 \, (\text{leg} + \text{thigh})$$

(Ramanathan 1964).

This has been shown to correlate well with a 15 site formula (Holdcroft & Hall 1978). Mean body temperature (MBT) can be calculated from the MST and core temperature:

$$\text{MBT} = (0.66 \times \text{core temperature}) + (0.33 \times \text{MST})$$

and from this total body heat (TBH) can be calculated:

$$\text{TBH} = \text{MBT} \times \text{specific heat} \times \text{mass} \; (\text{Colin et al 1971}).$$

PREVENTING HEAT LOSS

As described previously, anaesthetized patients tend to cool. The thermo-neutral temperature for the unclothed adult is 29°C, but at this temperature operating theatre personnel suffer discomfort. Simple measures can be undertaken to minimize heat loss. These include maintaining the ambient temperature over 20°C and ambient humidity over 50%, preventing draughts, preventing skin contact with cold surfaces and preventing exposure of the patient with drapes, blankets and head coverings (Holloway 1988). Surgical measures include covering exposed bowel and using warm fluids for washing out body cavities.

Anaesthetic steps to reduce heat loss include warming intravenous fluids, employing low fresh gas flows in circle systems and heat and moisture exchangers (HME).

As blood is stored at 4°C, warming is necessary. The more efficient warmers pass blood over a dry heating element and are capable of providing flows of 150 ml/min at 32°C. The water bath type of heater is less efficient (Russell 1974). Crystalloids and colloids may also be passed through these warmers or alternatively placed in a warming cabinet before use.

Anaesthetic gases are cold and dry. High fresh gas flows and high minute volumes increase the rate of heat loss. The use of a circle with low flow conserves heat and moisture. Heat and moisture exchangers (HME, condenser humidifiers or artificial noses) also conserve heat and reduce water loss by up to 50% (Haslam & Niesen 1986, Shanks et al 1988). A comparison of HME found humidities ranging from 18–32 mg/l at 27–30°C, both inversely proportional to fresh gas flow (Turtle et al 1987). The disadvantages of resistance and dead space make them unsuitable for paediatric anaesthesia. The Pall Ultipor has the advantage of being the most efficient antibacterial device (Shelley et al 1986).

Heated water bath humidifiers are more commonly used in paediatric practice and in intensive therapy. They are cumbersome, and require sterile water and protection against overheating (Stone et al 1981). A two-stage heater/humidifier employing a heated wire in the inspiratory limb of a circle system reduced both heat loss and duration of stay in the recovery room (Conahan et al 1987). In a similar study using HME, it was found that these humidifiers did not preserve body temperature and the duration of stay in the recovery room was not reduced (Goldberg et al 1988).

Mattresses through which warm water can circulate can be used, but the heating is peripheral. They can also be used in malignant hyperthermia suspects, to be switched on to aid cooling if required (Holloway 1988). Radiant heat has been shown to be more effective than a warm water blanket in stopping post-anaesthetic shivering. In this study, the radiant heat abolished shivering in hypothermic patients before the core temperature had returned to normal. Certain regions, particularly the head, neck and chest, have great sensitivity to warmth and a powerful input to the hypothalamus and hence overall control of body temperature (Sharkey et al 1987).

In anaesthetized children, it is possible to increase the ambient temperature by creating a microclimate around the patient using a device consisting of a fan heater and wide bore hose. The patient is covered by a large plastic drape under which warm air is directed from the fan (Nightingale & Meakin 1986).

REFERENCES

Adler M W, Geller E B, Rosow C E, Cochin J 1988 The opioid system and temperature regulation. Annu Rev Pharmacol Toxicol 28: 429–449

Atkinson R S, Rushman G B, Alfred Lee J 1987 Accidents, complications and sequelae. In: A synopsis of anaesthesia. IOP Publishing Ltd, Bristol: 321

Baracas V E, Whitmore W T, Gale R 1987 The metabolic cost of fever. Can J Physiol Pharmacol 65: 1248–1254

Bay J, Nunn J F, Prys-Roberts C 1968 Factors influencing arterial pO_2 during recovery from anaesthesia. Br J Anaesth 40: 398–406

Benzen H T, Cheng S C, Avrom M J, Molloy R E 1985 Sign of complete sympathetic blockade. Sweat test or sympathogalvanic response? Anaesth Analg 64: 415–419

Bijman J 1987 Transport processes in the eccrine sweat gland. Kidney Int 32 (Suppl 21): S109–112

Bijman J, Quinton P M 1987 Lactate and bicarbonate uptake in the sweat duct of cystic fibrosis and normal subjects. Pediatr Res 21: 79–82

Bone M E, Feneck R O 1988 Bladder temperature as a measure of body temperature during cardiopulmonary bypass. Anaesthesia 43: 181–185

Bullard R 1962 Continuous recording of sweating rate by resistance hygrometry. J Appl Physiol 17: 735–737

Calverley R K, Ty Smith N, Prys-Roberts C, Eger E I, Jones C W 1978 Cardiovascular effects of enflurane anesthesia during controlled ventilation in man. Anesth Analg 57: 619–628

Carli F, Aber V R 1987 Thermogenesis after major elective surgical procedures. Br J Surg 74: 1041–1045

Carli F, Gabrielczyk M, Clark M M, Aber V R 1986 An investigation of factors affecting the postoperative rewarming of adult patients. Anaesthesia 41: 363–369

Chalmers T M, Keele C A 1952 The nervous and chemical control of sweating. Br J Dermatol 64: 43–54

Cohen D, Hercus V 1959 Controlled hypothermia in infants and children. Br Med J 1: 1435–1439

Colin J, Timbal J, Houdas Y, Boutelier C, Guieu J D 1971 Computation of mean body temperature from rectal and skin temperature. J Appl Physiol 31: 484–489

Conahan T J, Williams G D, Apfelbaum J L, Lecky J H 1987 Airway heating reduces recovery time (cost) in outpatients. Anesthesiology 67: 128–130

Conn J W 1949 The mechanism of acclimatisation to heat. Arch Int Med 83: 416–428

Conn J W, Johnston M W, Louis L H 1946 Relations between salt intake and sweat salt concentration under conditions of hard work in humid heat. Fed Proc 5: 230

Cork R C, Vaughan R W, Humphrey L S 1983 Precision and accuracy of intra-operative temperature monitoring. Anesth Analg 62: 211–214

Craig P N 1952 Effects of atropine, work and heat on heart rate and sweat production in man. J Appl Physiol 4: 826–833

Dale H H, Feldberg W 1934 The chemical transmission of secretory impulses to the sweat glands of the cat. J Physiol 82: 121–128

Deacon S P 1977 Effect of atenolol and other beta blockers on insulin induced hypoglycaemia. Proc R Soc Med 70 (Suppl 5): 50–56

Editorial 1988 Where to measure body temperature? Lancet 1: 1318

Eger E I, Johnson B H 1987 MAC of I-653 in rats, including a test of the effect of body temperature and anesthetic duration. Anesth Analg 66: 974–976

Engelman D R, Lockhart C H 1972 Comparisons between temperature effects of ketamine and halothane anesthetics in children. Anesth Analg 51: 98–107

Fortney S M, Nadel E R, Wegner C B, Bove J R 1981 Effect of blood volume on sweating rate and body fluids in exercising humans. J Appl Physiol 51: 1594–1600

Fukomoto T, Tanaka T, Fujioka H, Yoshihara S, Ochi T, Kuroiwa A 1988 Differences in the composition of sweat induced by thermal exposure and by running exercise. Clin Cardiol 11: 707–709

Ganong W F 1987 Thermoregulation. In: Review of medical physiology 12th edn. Lange Medical Publications, California, p 203

Glynn C T, Basedow R W, Walsh J A 1981 Pain relief following post ganglionic sympathetic blockade with IV guanethidine. Br J Anaesth 53: 1297–1302

Goldberg M E, Jan R, Gregg C E, Berko R, Marr A T, Larijani G E 1988 The heat and moisture exchanger does not preserve body temperature or reduce recovery time in outpatients undergoing surgery and anesthesia. Anesthesiology 68: 122–123

Gordon N F, Kruger P E, Van Rensberg J P, Vander Linde A, Kielblock A J, Gilliers J F 1955 Effect of beta-adrenoceptor blockade on thermoregulation during prolonged exercise. J Appl Physiol 58: 899–906

Guyton A C 1986 Sweating and its regulation by the autonomic nervous system. In: Dreibelbis D (ed) Textbook of medical physiology 7th edn. W B Saunders, Philadelphia, pp 852–858

Ham J, Miller R D, Bevet L Z, Matteo R S, Roderick L L 1978 Pharmacokinetics and pharmacodynamics of d-tubocurarine during hypothermia in the cat. Anesthesiology 49: 324

Hammel H T 1988 Anesthetics and body temperature regulation. Anesthesiology 68: 833–835

Haslam K R, Niesen C H 1986 Do passive heat and moisture exchangers keep the patient warm? Anesthesiology 64: 379–381

Holdcroft A, Hall G M 1978 Heat loss during anaesthesia. Br J Anaesth 50: 157–164

Holdcroft A, Hall G M, Cooper G M 1979 Redistribution of body heat during anaesthesia. Anaesthesia 34: 758–764

Holloway A M 1988 Monitoring and controlling temperature. Anaesth Intensive Care 16: 44–47

Holmes P B E, Jenden D J, Taylor D B 1976 The analysis of the mode of action of curare on neuromuscular transmission; the effect of temperature change. J Pharmacol Exp Ther 103: 382

Huckaba C E, Frewin D B, Dourney J A, Tarn H S, Dorling R C, Cheh H Y 1976 Sweating responses of normal, paraplegic and anhidrotic subjects. Arch Phys and Med Rehabil 57: 268–274

Jane M J, Freehafer A A, Hazel C, Lindan R, Joiner E 1982 Autonomic dysreflexia. A cause of morbidity and mortality in orthopedic patients with spinal cord injury. Clin Orthop 169: 151–154

Janig W, Rath B 1980 Effects of anaesthetics on reflexes elicited in the sudomotor system by stimulation of Pacinian corpuscles and of cutaneous nociceptors. J Auton Nerv Syst 2: 1–14

Johnson M D, Sevarino F B, Lema M J 1989 Cessation of shivering and hypothermia associated with epidural sufentanil. Anesth Analg 68: 70–71

Juhlin L, Evers H, Brobery F 1979 Inhibition of hyperhidrosis by topical application of a local anaesthetic composition. Acta Derm Venereol 59: 556–559

Kaufman R D 1987 Relationship between oesophageal temperature gradient and heart and lung sounds heard by oesophageal stethoscope. Anesth Analg 66: 1046–1048

Kenney M J, Owen M D, Wall P T, Gisolfi C V 1986 Characterisation and quantification of sweating in a systemic hyperhidrotic patient. Clin Exp Dermatol 11: 543–552

Khurana R K 1987 Orthostatic hypotension-induced autonomic dysreflexia. Neurology 37: 1221–1224

Layman P R 1984 Sweating during anaesthesia. Anaesthesia 39: 846

McGibbon B, van Beaumont W, Strand J, Paletta F X 1973 Thermal regulations in patients after the healing of large deep burns. Plast Reconstr Surg 52: 164–170

Maryniak J K, Bishop V A 1987a Cardiovascular and palmar sweat changes in patients undergoing cystoscopy. Br J Anaesth 59: 654

Maryniak J K, Bishop V A 1987b Palmar sweat and heart rate changes during stress response attenuation with alfentanil. Br J Anaesth 59: 133–134

Miller R D, Agoston S, Van der Pol F, Booij L H, Crul J F, Ham J 1978 Hypothermia and the pharmacokinetics and pharmacodynamics of pancuronium in the cat. J Pharmacol Exp Ther 207: 532

Millington P R, Williamson R 1983 Sweat glands. In: Harrison R J, McMinn R M H (eds)

Biological structure and function 9—skin. Cambridge University Press, Cambridge, pp 42–47

Morris R H 1971 Operating room temperature and the anaesthetised paralysed patient. Arch Surg 102: 95–97

Nakayama T 1985 Thermosensitive neurones in the brain. Jpn J Physiol 5: 375–389

Nightingale P, Meakin G 1986 A new method for maintaining body temperature in children. Anesthesiology 65: 447–448

O'Brien E T 1975 Beta-blockade withdrawal. Lancet 2: 819

Page C O Jnr, Remington J S 1967 Immunologic studies in normal human sweat. J Lab Clin Med 69: 634–650

Peter J, Wyndham C H 1966 Activity of the human eccrine sweat gland during exercise in a hot humid environment before and after acclimatisation. J Physiol 187: 583–594

Pledger H G 1962 Disorders of temperature regulation in acute traumatic tetraplegia. J Bone Jt Surg 44B: 110–113

Prout B J, Wardell W M 1969 Sweating and peripheral blood flow in patients with phaeochromocytoma. Clin Sci 36: 109–117

Puig M M, Warner W, Tang C K, Laorden M L, Turndorf H 1987 Effects of temperature on the interaction of morphine with opioid receptors. Br J Anaesth 59: 1459–1464

Quinton P M 1983 Sweating and its disorders. Annu Rev Med 34: 429–452

Quinton P M 1987 Physiology of sweat secretion. Kidney Int 32 (Suppl 21): S102–S108

Quinton P M, Tormey J M 1976 Localisation of Na/K ATPase sites in the secretory and reabsorptive epithelia of perfused eccrine sweat glands; a question to the role of the enzyme in secretion. J Membr Biol 29: 383–399

Ramachandra V, Moore C, Kaur N, Carli F 1989 Effect of halothane, enflurane and isoflurane on body temperature during and after surgery. Br J Anaesth 62: 409–414

Ramanathan N L 1964 A new weighting system for mean skin temperature of the human body. J Appl Physiol 19: 531–533

Randall W C, Kimura K R 1954 The pharmacology of sweating. Pharmacol Rev 7: 365–397

Rogers H, Spector R 1983 How drugs relieve symptoms of anxiety (propranolol, oxprenolol, acebutolol). Monthly Index of Medical Specialities Magazine: 47–52

Roskind J L, Petrofsky J, Lind A R, Paletta F X 1978 Quantitation of thermoregulatory impairment in patients with healed burns. Ann Plast Surg 1: 172–176

Russel W J 1974 A review of blood warmers for massive transfusion. Anaesth Intensive Care 2: 109–130

Ryan T J 1987 Diseases of the skin. In: Weatherall D J, Ledingham J G G, Warrell D A (eds) Oxford textbook of medicine 2nd edn. Oxford Medical Publications, Oxford, pp 20–56

Sato K 1977 The physiology, pharmacology and biochemistry of the eccrine sweat gland. Rev Physiol Biochem Pharmacol 79: 51–131

Sato K, Sato F 1981 Cyclic AMP accumulation in the beta adrenergic mechanism of eccrine sweat secretion. Eur J Physiol 390: 41–53

Sato K, Sato F 1983 Individual variations in structure and function of the human eccrine sweat gland. Am J Physiol 245: R203–R208

Sato K, Sato F 1987 Effect of VIP on sweat secretion and cAMP accumulation in isolated simian eccrine glands. Am J Physiol 253: R935–R941

Sato K, Kang W H, Saga K, Sato K T 1989a Biology of sweat glands and their disorders. I. Normal sweat gland function. J Am Acad Dermatol 20: 537–563

Sato K, Kang W H, Saga K, Sato K T 1989b Biology of sweat glands and their disorders. II. Disorders of sweat gland function. J Am Acad Dermatol 20: 713–726

Sato K T, Richardson A, Timm D E, Sato K 1988 One step starch iodine method for direct visualisation of sweating. Am J Med Sci 295: 528–531

Schluter K J, Kerp L 1983 Beta adrenoceptor blocking agents induce different counter-regulatory responses to insulin (propranolol, metoprolol, pindolol). J Pharmacol 4 (Suppl 2): 49–60

Sessler D I, Rubinstein D H, Eger E I 1987a Core temperature changes during N_2O/fentanyl and halothane/O_2 anesthesia. Anesthesiology 67: 137–139

Sessler D I, Olofsson C I, Rubinstein C H 1987b Active thermoregulation during isoflurane anesthesia. Anesthesiology 67: A405

Sessler D I, Olofsson C I, Rubinstein E H, Beebe J J 1988a The thermoregulatory threshold in humans during halothane anesthesia. Anesthesiology 68: 836–842

Sessler D I, Israel D, Pozos R S, Rubinstein E H 1988b Spontaneous post-anesthetic tremor does not resemble thermoregulatory shivering. Anesthesiology 68: 843–850

Sevarino F B, Johnson M D, Lema M J, Datta S, Ostheimer G W, Naulty J S 1989 The effect of epidural sufentanil on shivering and body temperature in the parturient. Anesth Analg 698: 530–533

Shanks C A, Ronai A K, Schafer M F 1988 The effects of airway heat conservation and skin surface insulation on thermal balance during spinal surgery. Anesthesiology 69: 956–958

Sharky A, Lipton J M, Murphy M T, Giesecke A H 1987 Inhibition of post-anaesthetic shivering with radiant heat. Anesthesiology 66: 249–252

Shelley M, Bethune D W, Latimer R D 1986 A comparison of five heat and moisture exchangers. Anaesthesia 41: 527–532

Siegel M N, Gravenstein N 1989 More on thermoregulatory thresholds with halothane. Anesthesiology 70: 370–371

Sigal C B, Dobson R L 1968 The effect of salt intake on sweat gland function. J Invest Dermatol 50: 541–545

Stanworth P A 1982 The significance of hyperhidrosis in patients with post-traumatic syringomyelia. Paraplegia 2: 282–287

Steffey E P, Eger E I 1974 Hyperthermia and halothane MAC in the dog. Anesthesiology 41: 392

Stevens W C, Cromwell T H, Halsey M J, Eger E I, Shakespeare T F, Bahlman S H 1971 The cardiovascular effect of a new inhalation anaesthetic, Forane, in human volunteers at constant arterial carbon dioxide tension. Anesthesiology 35: 8–16

Stone D R, Downs J B, Paul W 1981 Adult body temperature and heated humidification of anesthetic gases during general anesthesia. Anesth Analg 60: 736–741

Strom L 1978 Propranolol in insulin dependent diabetes. N Engl J Med 299: 487

Thomson M L 1954 A comparison between the number and distribution of functioning eccrine sweat glands in Europeans and Africans. J Physiol 123: 225–233

Thornberry E A, Mazumdar B 1988 The effect of changes in arm temperature on neuro-muscular blockade in the presence of atracurium blockade. Anaesthesia 43: 447–449

Turtle M J, Ilsley A H, Rutten A J, Runciman W B 1987 An evaluation of six disposable heat and moisture exchangers. Anaesth Intensive Care 15: 317–322

Uno H 1977 Sympathetic innervation of the sweat glands and piloarrector muscles of macaques and human beings. J Invest Dermatol 69: 112–120

Vitez T S, White P F, Eger E I 1974 Effects of hypothermia on halothane MAC and isoflurane MAC in the rat. Anesthesiology 41: 80

Wallace C T, Marks W E, Atkins W Y, Mahaffey J E 1974 Perforation of the tympanic membrane, a complication of tympanic thermometry during anesthesia. Anesthesiology 41: 290–291

Walmsley A J, Giesecke A H, Lipton J M 1986 Contribution of extradural temperature to shivering during extradural anaesthesia. Br J Anaesth 58: 1130–1134

Walsh J A, Glynn C J, Cousins M J, Basedow R W 1984 Bloodflow, sympathetic activity and pain relief following lumbar sympathetic blockade or surgical sympathectomy. Anaesth Intensive Care 13: 18–24

Weiner J S, Hellman K 1960 The sweat glands. Biol Rev 35: 141–186

Wilcox R G, Bennett T, MacDonald I A, Herbert M, Skene A M 1984 The effects of acute or chronic ingestion of propranolol or metoprolol on the physiological responses to prolonged submaximal exercise in hypertensive men. Br J Clin Pharmacol 17: 273–281

8. Anaesthesia for renal transplantation

S. Cottam   J. Eason

Renal dialysis and transplantation have transformed the outlook for patients with end-stage renal disease (ESRD). The last decade has seen further improvements, most notably the widespread use of continuous ambulatory peritoneal dialysis (CAPD) and a marked broadening of the indications for renal transplantation. The old and very young, diabetics and patients with spina bifida or spinal cord injury may now be considered for transplant (Editorial 1990). Currently, approximately 80% of first cadaveric kidney transplants will function for at least one year and perioperative mortality has declined from 16 to under 1% (Heino et al 1986). The operation has to some extent become a victim of its own success. There are now 3600 patients awaiting a transplant in the UK but the total number of procedures performed (1575 in 1988) is limited by the availability of donor organs. Unless it becomes ethically acceptable to electively ventilate

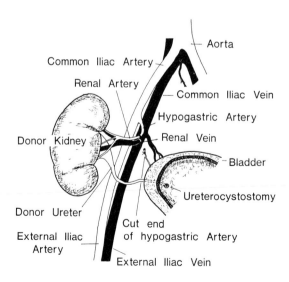

Fig. 8.1   The surgical field.

159

victims of cerebral catastrophe specifically in order to provide organs for transplantation, demand will inevitably outstrip supply.

The student will be saddened and the surgeon surprised to hear that the successful anaesthetic management of patients undergoing renal transplantation presupposes a knowledge of the aetiology, pathophysiology, clinical manifestations (vi) and medical management of patients in ESRF (Innes & Catto 1989), together with a detailed appreciation of the pharmacological consequences of renal dysfunction (vi). In addition, some understanding of surgical technique (see Fig. 8.1) and transplant immunology is required. Considerations of space forbid discussion of these topics, which have been reviewed in detail elsewhere (Graybar & Bready 1987, Sear & Holland 1989).

CANDIDATES FOR TRANSPLANTATION

Patients with progressive ESRF may be managed conservatively until an organ becomes available, or they may have been maintained on haemodialysis (HD) or CAPD. The underlying causes of their condition are numerous (Table 8.1) and only a few of these (such as rapidly progressive glomerulonephritis with high titres of anti-basement membrane antibody,

Table 8.1 Causes of end-stage renal failure

Cause		Comments
Chronic Glomerulo-nephritis*		Do not transplant rapidly progressive glomerulonephritis
Interstitial nephritis*	Drugs, Exogenous toxins, Endogenous toxins	Congenital metabolic defects may require combined hepatic and renal transplantation
Metabolic nephropathy	Diabetic*, Amyloid, Hypercalcaemic	
Vascular nephropathy	Hypertensive*, Renal artery stenosis	
Polycystic disease*		Combined hepatic and renal transplant in some cases
Collagen vascular disease		Do not transplant in the acute phase of the disease e.g. SLE
Chronic obstruction ±pyelonephritis		Congenital metabolic defects may require combined hepatic and renal transplantation
Malignancy	Myeloma, Lymphoma, Carcinoma with obstruction	Unsuitable for transplantation
Infection	Tuberculosis, Bacterial endocarditis, Tropical disease	Do not transplant HIV positive patients and those with uncontrolled infection
Unresolved acute renal failure		
Congenital renal tubular acidosis		

*Common indication for transplantation

acute systemic lupus erythematosus or Wegener's granulomatosis, sepsis and malignancy) are considered to be contraindications to transplantation.

PROBLEMS ASSOCIATED WITH RENAL TRANSPLANTATION

Cardiovascular

Hypertension is almost universal in these patients and may be essential or secondary to salt and water retention, or drug treatment; the majority of cases will require antihypertensive medication although dialysis may suffice to control secondary hypertension. Left ventricular failure often supervenes despite such treatment, exacerbated by the increased cardiac output necessitated by shunts through arterio-venous (AV) fistulae and the universal anaemia which accompanies ESRF. Cardiomyopathy and pericardial effusion, associated with uraemia and dialysis, may compound cardiac compromise. More than 50% of patients in renal failure will suffer from accelerated atherosclerosis, resulting in ischaemic heart disease and peripheral vascular disease (Morgan & Lumley 1975), although many cases will be asymptomatic. Abnormalities in cardiac conduction, due to coronary artery disease, hyperkalaemia or other electrolyte imbalances, or calcification of the conducting system are an ever present risk. Autonomic neuropathy, manifesting as postural hypotension and failure to respond normally to acute changes in blood volume is not uncommon (Thomas & Pollard 1989).

Pulmonary

Fluid overload may result in pulmonary congestion in periods between dialysis. Haemodialysis may produce acute hypocapnia or hypoxia. In addition, dialysis membranes may activate complement, resulting in leucocyte sequestration in the pulmonary microcirculation. These effects are usually mild and self-limiting although the occasional patient may develop a picture identical to adult respiratory distress syndrome. CAPD causes diaphragmatic splinting, resulting in atelectasis and an increased intrapulmonary shunt. Pulmonary infection is common.

Haematological

Patients in ESRF are invariably anaemic, their haemoglobin concentration being between 3 and 9 g/dl with a normochromic, normocytic picture. The aetiology of the anaemia is complex (Dodds & Nicholls 1983), perhaps the most important factor being decreased renal production of erythropoietin (EPO). Other factors include: marrow depression resulting from chronic uraemia and osteitis fibrosa cystica (OFC), aggravated by deficiency of haematinics such as iron, folic acid, and vitamins B12 and B6; increased red cell fragility and haemolysis; and increased losses from blood sampling and haemodialysis (the vampire effect) or from chronic gastric ulceration. Aluminium toxicity, which inhibits EPO is largely a thing of the past (Rosenlof et al 1990).

This anaemia causes a 50% reduction in oxygen carrying capacity for which most patients compensate by increasing cardiac output. Tissue oxygen delivery is enhanced by metabolic acidosis and an increased concentration of 2, 3–diphosphoglycerate. Transfusion is controversial. A beneficial effect of pre-transplant transfusion, first described in 1972 (Opelz et al 1973), has been confirmed by several hundred subsequent publications. However, with the introduction of cyclosporin in the 1980s, the advantage of transfusion seems to have disappeared (Opelz 1987), possibly because its immunosuppressant actions were similar to those of cyclosporin (Groth 1987). Disadvantages of transfusing these patients include the risk of inducing broadly reactive anti-HLA cytotoxic antibodies (particularly in patients who have had previous transplants). Patients so sensitized become virtually untransplantable. The risk can be reduced by transfusion with HLA matched donors (Scornik et al 1989). Transfusion will confer no long term benefit due to the increased red cell destruction, and with multiple transfusions the risks of blood-borne infection increase as do complications such as iron overload and bone marrow depression.

A possible solution to the problem of the transplant candidate whose haemoglobin is 4 g/dl or less may be the use of human recombinant erythropoietin (r-HuEPO). This potentially abolishes the need for transfusion, enhances wellbeing, increases exercise capacity and improves haemostatic function in uraemia (Macdougall et al 1990). Potential problems may stem from an elevation in the haematocrit, and an increase in the incidence of thrombosis (particularly of AV fistulae) has been reported. The cost of treatment is around £5000 per year.

The haemostatic defect of ESRF is partially corrected by dialysis and by restoring the haematocrit towards 30%. In untreated renal failure, bleeding is a common cause of death, and can still be a fatal complication for uraemic patients requiring major surgery. The precise mechanism of the bleeding tendency remains obscure. The most consistent finding in patients with a bleeding tendency seems to be a prolongation of the skin bleeding time (BT) (Remuzzi 1988). This points to a defect in primary haemostasis, i.e. the process of forming a platelet plug at the site of vessel injury. The BT may be prolonged by a low platelet count, although thrombocytopenia severe enough to cause bleeding is rare in renal failure. This suggests a defect in platelet release of ADP and serotonin, substances normally stored in platelet dense bodies whose number is decreased in uraemia.

The fact that platelet function can be improved by dialysis implies a dialysable factor, possibly urea, guanidosuccinic acid, various phenols or hypermagnesaemia. There is some evidence of increased production of (non-dialysable) prostacyclin by vessel walls in uraemic patients, which may explain persisting poor platelet adhesion in patients on regular dialysis. Changes in the coagulation cascade are variable, the most consistent findings being an increase in factor VIII and fibrinogen concentrations, and a decrease in antithrombin III. Paradoxically, there may exist a prothrombotic state despite a prolonged BT. This may provide some explanation of the accelerated atherosclerosis found in patients in renal failure. The clinical implications of these findings are: the skin BT is the best test to identify patients at risk from excessive haemorrhage; dialysis, a haematocrit approaching 30% and the avoidance of antiplatelet drugs such as aspirin provide the best prophylaxis against haemorrhage. In the face of abnormal haemorrhage, preliminary evidence suggests that desmopressin acetate (DDAVP) 0.3 µg/kg will reduce BT for about four hours. DDAVP causes the release of von Willebrand factor from the vascular endothelium, which enhances platelet adhesion via specific glyco-protein receptors. Cryoprecipitate has also been reported to correct the bleeding tendency in uraemic patients.

The incidence of haematological and other malignancies is increased in patients on long term immunosuppressant treatment.

Nervous system

A peripheral neuropathy is common in patients in ESRF. This starts as a predominantly sensory loss (most marked in the lower limbs) but motor involvement may develop. This may be reversed by successful transplantation, although below knee neuropathy rarely recovers. Autonomic neuropathy is common, especially amongst diabetics and may present serious problems in the peri-operative period.

Most patients presenting for renal transplantation are well motivated and co-operative. A proportion of patients however are highly anxious or dependent, especially those with longstanding disease who may have spent significant periods of their lives in hospital or on dialysis.

Mental changes have been associated with chronic dialysis. A mild uraemic encephalopathy may indicate inadequate dialysis, and post-dialysis disequilibrium syndrome is well described, resulting from sudden reduction of extracellular volume and cerebral oedema. In the past a characteristic toxic encephalopathy with anaemia and bone disease was associated with the use of oral aluminium hydroxide (as a dietary phosphate binder) and traces of the metal in dialysis fluids. Untreated renal failure ultimately leads to myopathy, myoclonus, grand mal fits and terminal uraemic coma.

Gastrointestinal

A high proportion of patients suffer from gastrointestinal inflammation and bleeding. This group of patients have increased gastric acid secretion and delayed gastric emptying (which may double whilst a patient is undergoing haemodialysis). A proportion will have deranged liver function attributable to the high incidence of transfusion-related hepatitis (Frey et al 1989). Gastrointestinal symptoms are common in untreated uraemia and include anorexia, nausea, vomiting and intractable hiccoughs. The risk of aspiration is considerable.

Endocrine

Deteriorating renal function leads to phosphate retention, which reduces serum calcium levels. Together with decreased absorption of dietary calcium (due to the inability of the failing kidney to hydroxylate vitamin D) this causes parathyroid overactivity in an attempt to maintain normal serum calcium levels. Parathormone induces bone decalcification, EPO antagonism, increased absorption of aluminium from the gut and ectopic calcification of soft tissues such as the eye, skin, heart and lungs. Further calcium losses produce secondary hyperparathyroidism and OFC. Corticosteroid therapy may add osteoporosis to the osteomalacia and OFC. Reduced plasma insulin clearance leads to carbohydrate intolerance and levels of somatostatin, calcitonin, glucagon, vasopressin, growth hormone, vasoactive intestinal polypeptide and renin (on occasion) are elevated (Innes & Catto 1989).

Acid–base and electrolyte balance

Progressive renal disease is associated with a chronic metabolic acidosis due to failure of hydrogen ion excretion and increased urinary bicarbonate loss despite secondary hyperventilation. Hyponatraemia (< 130 mmol/l) occurs due to water retention and loss of renal concentrating ability. It also reduces the MAC for inhalational agents. Hyperkalaemia is a serious abnormality in the later stages of ESRF and may be relatively asymptomatic. Hypermagnesaemia is a problem in patients with gastrointestinal disease (who may ingest large amounts of proprietary antacids) and especially when coupled with hypocalcaemia, potentiates neuromuscular blocking drugs.

Hypernatraemia (> 150 mmol/l), hypokalaemia and hypomagnesaemia may also occur in patients whose kidneys can no longer control their plasma chemistry.

DRUGS AND RENAL FAILURE

This complex subject has been well reviewed elsewhere (Nancarrow & Mather 1983, Bennett et al 1983) and can only be briefly considered here (see Table 8.2).

Table 8.2 Anaesthetic drugs in renal failure

Drug	Elimination half-life in ESRF	Comments
Thiopentone	Small decrease	Same dose, decrease rate of administration
Methohexitone	? Small decrease	Same dose, decrease rate of administration
Diazepam	Halved	Same dose, decrease rate of administration
Midazolam	Unchanged	Same dose, decrease rate of administration
Ketamine	?	Contraindicated due to CVS effects
Propofol	$\sim 40\%$ increase	Same dose, decrease rate of administration
Fentanyl	$\sim 25\%$ increase	Use with care
Alfentanil	$\sim 15\%$ increase	Use with care
Phenoperidine	50% increase	Use with care
Pethidine	Unchanged	Norpethidine accumulation
Buprenorphine	Unchanged	1500% increase in active metabolites
Morphine	Unchanged	Morphine-6-glucuronide accumulation
Suxamethonium	Probably increased	Hyperkalaemic risk
Gallamine	Vast increase	Contraindicated
Tubocurarine	85% increase	Use a nerve stimulator
Pancuronium	100% increase	Avoid, or use a nerve stimulator
Vecuronium	30–40% increase	Use a nerve stimulator
Atracurium	Unchanged	Relaxant of choice?
Neostigmine	150% increase	Expect a prolonged action
Edrophonium	50% increase	Expect a prolonged action
Lignocaine	? Small increase	Action shortened, toxicity increased, decrease dose
Bupivacaine	? Small increase	Action shortened, toxicity increased, decrease dose

Pharmacokinetics

Uraemia and its accompanying acidosis and hypoalbuminaemia decrease the total amount of protein binding of drugs such as thiopentone. This increases the percentage of free, unbound drug available to act on its target organ. However, more free drug, together with a hyperdynamic circulation, means a greater initial volume of distribution and more rapid redistribution and elimination. It is widely stated that these antagonistic effects largely cancel one another out in the case of the short acting barbiturates, the benzodiazepines, and etomidate. Consequently, the total dosage remains unaltered, although the rate of administration should be slower than usual.

Basic drugs are less affected by hypoalbuminaemia, although those that bind to acute phase proteins such as alpha-1-acid glycoprotein, which is increased in uraemia, may show reduced levels of unbound free drug. Lignocaine and bupivacaine are two such drugs; this increased glyco-protein binding, together with more rapid systemic absorption due to a high cardiac output, may explain Bromage's observation of a decreased duration of action of local anaesthetics in patients with chronic renal failure.

Metabolism

Uraemia has little effect on the principal hepatic drug breakdown systems

Table 8.3 Drugs actively secreted by the kidney

Atropine, neostigmine
Paracetamol, indomethacin, aspirin
Penicillins, cephalosporins, sulphonamides
Isoprenaline
Morphine, pethidine (insignificant amounts)
Procaine (also hydrolysed by plasmacholinesterase)

(oxidation, demethylation and glucuronide formation) although minor effects attributable to reduced levels of pseudocholinesterase (and consequently ester hydrolysis) have been reported. Although urea (probably) and cyclosporin A (definitely) inhibit cytochrome P450 the overall effects of ESRF on hepatic drug metabolism are slight, in the absence of coexisting hepatic disease.

Elimination

Lipid soluble drugs are metabolized to water soluble compounds which are eliminated either in bile or by the kidney. Water soluble compounds which are excreted by passive filtration at the glomerulus will accumulate in renal failure. So too will compounds which are eliminated by active tubular secretion (see Table 8.3). The activity and toxicity of drug metabolites clearly must also be considered, although there is a dearth of published information.

The muscle relaxants vary considerably in the extent to which they are renally eliminated. Widely quoted figures for the percentage renal excretion of the more commonly used drugs are: gallamine $> 90\%$, alcuronium $60-90\%$, pancuronium 60%, d-tubocurarine $25-60\%$ (biliary excretion is increased in renal failure), vecuronium and atracurium $< 25\%$.

The extent of drug elimination via dialysis membranes is largely determined by the size and pKa of the molecule in question and the blood flow through the dialysing system. Nevertheless, drug levels should be assayed wherever possible and in the case of uncommonly used drugs, appropriate pharmacological literature should be consulted.

Toxicity

Nephrotoxic agents such as tetracycline obviously should be avoided in patients with compromised renal function. When their use is unavoidable, as with cyclosporin A or aminoglycoside antibiotics, careful monitoring of levels is mandatory. Although the inhalational agents are principally eliminated via the lungs, metabolism of the halogenated agents cannot be ignored. Methoxyflurane is deservedly obsolete largely because its extensive metabolism generated toxic levels of free fluoride ions; prolonged administration of enflurane, although it rarely generates enough free fluoride to exceed the toxic threshold of 50 μmol/l identified by Cousins et al (1974), is generally felt to be unwise. Halothane is extensively metabolized but generates little fluoride, isoflurane in clinically realistic amounts is also reasonably safe in this regard (Kong et al 1990).

PRE-OPERATIVE PREPARATION

The surgical techniques of vascular anastomosis upon which renal transplantation surgery are based were worked out at the turn of the century by Ullman, Decastello, Carrel and Jaboulay. The first human cadaveric transplant was performed by Voronoy in 1933 but it was not until the mid 1950s that anything other than transient success was achieved (Graybar & Bready 1987, Graybar & Tarpey 1987). The pioneer surgeons and anaesthetists had to cope with the whole horrendous gamut of complications described above but there is no longer any justification for heroic procedures in ill-prepared patients. Organ preservation techniques (Farman 1989) have advanced to a point where it is no longer admissible to plead extreme urgency; anaesthetists should not allow themselves to be pressurized into abetting the implantation of a superannuated organ into a grossly metabolically deranged patient.

All patients must be assessed pre-operatively. Patients are naturally anxious and a pre-operative visit by the anaesthetist will hopefully provide reassurance. It is advisable to discuss the possibility of post-operative ventilation in the high risk patient. While assessing the patient specific attention must be paid to the following.

Fluid and electrolyte status

Patients who have not been recently dialysed and all those who significantly exceed their 'dry weight', or whose serum sodium or potassium, or pre-operative chest X-ray are seriously abnormal, must undergo haemodialysis or haemofiltration pre-operatively.

Hypertension

All transplant candidates should undergo cardiological assessment pre-operatively. Hypertension must be controlled and antihypertensive medication continued up to the time of surgery.

Arterio-venous fistulae

The site of any AV fistulae must be noted and suitable intra-operative protection provided. Puncture of limb veins and arteries is to be avoided.

Gastric emptying

All patients in ESRF are at increased risk of aspiration and the routine use of metoclopramide and ranitidine is advised.

Diabetes

Insulin dependent diabetics should receive a continuous dextrose and insulin infusion with frequent monitoring of blood sugar. This may also be appropriate, but is not mandatory, in non-insulin dependent diabetics.

DONOR MANAGEMENT

Management of the cadaveric donor centres on maintenance of arterial blood pressure and urine output until the moment of organ harvesting. Details may be found in Graybar & Bready (1987).

MANAGEMENT OF THE RECIPIENT

Choice of anaesthetic technique

Initial reports of anaesthesia for renal transplantation concentrated almost exclusively on the use of regional anaesthesia (Vandam et al 1962). Techniques using continuous or single shot spinal, and lumbar or sacral epidural anaesthesia are well described (Linke & Merin 1976). When patients were poorly prepared and fluid overloaded, regional anaesthesia with sympathetic blockade was an attractive proposition. Recent reviews on anaesthesia for renal transplantation do not emphasize regional anaesthesia, although the technique still has its adherents. Linke & Merin (1976) report 64 cases who were managed successfully using a single high dose spinal technique, although 'some form of supplementation was always necessary'. Increased clearance of local anaesthetic may necessitate larger than normal dosage in patients with renal failure, although there is evidence of enhanced sensitivity to the toxic effects of local anaesthetics in the presence of a metabolic acidosis. The objections to regional anaesthesia based on the risks of epidural haematoma are not supported by any reports in the literature. The use of regional anaesthesia in patients with autonomic neuropathy is definitely unwise. It is generally agreed that vasopressors are to be avoided, in view of the risk of cardiac arrhythmias, hypertension and renal ischaemia.

Technical improvements have led to a widespread preference for general anaesthesia in renal transplantation, not least because a difficult procedure is not made easier by an anxious, talking or (worst of all) coughing subject.

Premedication

It is our practice to omit anticholinergic or opiate premedication in view of

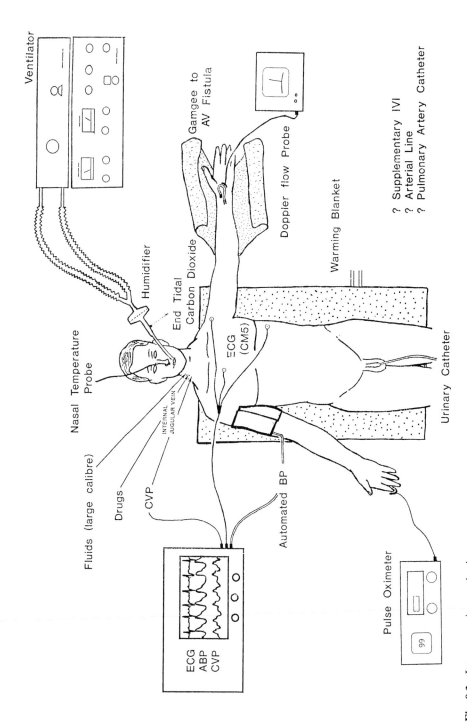

Fig. 8.2   Intra-operative monitoring.

delayed gastric emptying. Atropine and glycopyrrolate, unlike hyoscine, are eliminated renally (20–50% of the total dose); if a vagolytic drug is specifically indicated we would recommend a small dose of intravenous glycopyrrolate given at induction when its effects can be monitored. Phenothiazine drugs have undesirable dopamine antagonist properties and their alpha blocking effects may complicate induction of anaesthesia in a hypovolaemic, recently dialysed patient and act synergistically with beta blockers. If anxiolysis is required a short acting benzodiazepine such as temazepam can be given along with oral ranitidine and metoclopramide. All intramuscular injections are undesirable.

Monitoring

This should be commenced prior to induction of anaesthesia (see Fig. 8.2).

Arterial cannulation

This has been routinely employed in Brussels since 1974 (Carlier et al 1986). In the UK the practice is less widespread (Sear & Holland 1989), in the possibly erroneous belief that arterial cannulation permanently damages vessels which may be required for the fashioning of AV fistulae. In many cases previous shunts will have reduced the number of sites available for cannulation. Advances in non-invasive monitoring have weakened the arguments in favour of routine invasive monitoring. The new generation of non-invasive, continuous blood pressure monitors, in combination with pulse oximetry and capnography are adequate for the majority of patients.

Central venous access

There is no clinical or non-invasive substitute for measurement of central venous pressure (CVP) in the peri-operative period. Patients will require reliable central venous access for several days. Forearm veins are best avoided, in case they are required for a shunt. It is our practice to use a triple lumen catheter inserted under strict asepsis either pre-operatively, or after induction of anaesthesia. The Seldinger technique may be safer than traditional catheter-over-needle methods. Our preferred approach is via the internal jugular vein, although a subclavian approach may be necessary if the patient has had tunnelled indwelling haemodialysis catheters inserted via the external or internal jugular veins. The use of a catheter with one large lumen which can be used for rapid transfusion, and two small lumina for pressure monitoring and drug infusion is advantageous.

Pulmonary artery catheters

There is good evidence that optimal hydration at the time of release of the vascular clamps improves the early function of the graft. Although immediate function is not essential for ultimate success, it is a powerful psychological boost to both patient and physician and makes post-operative fluid and drug administration easier. Rejection can be diagnosed at an earlier stage. A retrospective study by Carlier et al (1986) revealed a reduction in acute tubular necrosis in patients whose mean pulmonary artery pressure was greater than 20 mmHg at the time of unclamping. Interestingly, the CVP was also significantly higher at the time of unclamping although the differences measured were smaller. Post-operatively there was no difference in the incidence of pulmonary complications in patients monitored with pulmonary artery catheters when compared with a group monitored with CVP alone. The mechanism by which maximum hydration improves immediate graft function appears to involve the release of atrial natriuretic peptide (ANP). This was studied by Gianello et al (1989) in dogs; these investigators suggest that maximal hydration could be replaced by normohydration and concomitant infusion of ANP. More recent studies by Carlier et al (1989) have indicated that the change in filling pressures correlates with ANP levels rather than absolute pressure values. In rats, storage granules for ANP appear predominantly in the right atrium.

Arterio-venous fistulae

The patient must be adequately protected intra-operatively. Limbs should be well padded, and if an AV fistula is present, intravenous lines and the blood pressure cuff should be sited elsewhere. A doppler probe positioned over the fistula is a useful guide to its continued patency. A haemodialysis catheter, if present should also be protected and the temptation to use it for transfusion and drug infusions resisted.

Induction and intubation

Induction of anaesthesia is potentially hazardous in renal patients so pre-induction monitoring is mandatory. Monitoring consists of ECG (CM5 lead), non-invasive blood pressure and pulse oximetry (see Fig. 8.2). Intubation is performed after preoxygenation and a rapid sequence induction with cricoid pressure. Hypertension and tachyarrhythmias during intubation are common. It is our practice to use fentanyl together with the short-acting beta-blocker esmolol in this group of patients in an attempt to attenuate pressor responses. The induction agent of choice is still thiopentone although etomidate is useful in the high risk patient. We have used propofol, whose disposition is unaltered in chronic renal failure (Morcos & Payne 1985), in fitter patients. The need for suxamethonium can be a problem; the only absolute contraindications are hyperkalaemia of greater than 5.0 mmol/l or extensive neuropathy. Decreased levels of pseudo-cholinesterase during chronic HD are not a practical problem. With the

advent of the newer competitive neuromuscular blocking drugs, atracurium has emerged as the drug of choice (Orko et al 1987), although
concern has been expressed over its histamine-releasing properties and
potential accumulation of its renally excreted metabolite laudanosine. If
histamine release gives rise to concern then vecuronium is a practical
alternative. Vecuronium does accumulate in patients with renal failure if
given by infusion, although its elimination is largely hepatic. Both drugs
can cause hypotension and bradycardia. New relaxants such as mivacurium
and doxacurium (Cashman et al 1990) await further evaluation before their
use can be recommended. We avoid infusions of muscle relaxants during
renal transplant surgery. The inclusion is extraperitoneal so full muscle
relaxation is seldom required; patients can often be managed with a single
dose of relaxant at the beginning of the procedure. If the patient is
especially muscular or obese then repeated doses can be given and monitored with a nerve stimulator. The general aim is to avoid high plasma
concentrations of relaxant at the end of the procedure.

Maintenance of anaesthesia

All anaesthetic techniques reduce renal blood flow. There is no ideal
technique, although hyperventilation, hypercapnia and high
concentrations of inhalational agents seem unwise. The elimination of
awareness and ventilation to normocapnia with maintenance of
oxygenation and cardiac output are obviously of paramount importance.
Neuroleptic techniques have their advocates but in practice most anaesthetists use a combination of isoflurane and fentanyl.

Volatile anaesthetics

Inhalational agents decrease the incidence of awareness, help reduce hypertension and are not renally excreted. Among their disadvantages are the
potential for organ toxicity, myocardial depression, coronary artery steal,
sensitization of the myocardium to the effects of catecholamines both endogenous and exogenous, and pollution. Of the published studies comparing
halothane, enflurane and isoflurane with repect to post-operative graft
function, no agent seems to have a clear advantage (Mazze et al 1984,
Cronelly et al 1984). The choice of agent would seem to depend more on
individual patient characteristics plus the anaesthetist's experience and
preference. Medicolegal considerations and the fear of liver damage have
reduced the use of halothane. Enflurane has theoretical disadvantages with
respect to free fluoride production and myocardial depression. Wickstrom
(1981) has reported ten patients undergoing renal transplantation in whom,
after an average of 2.4 MAC hours of enflurane, mean values of 21 µmol/l
of fluoride were found. Fluoride levels exceeded 40 µmol/l in one patient.
Isoflurane is recommended for its limited metabolism, which reduces its

potential for organ damage. A low blood-gas solubility facilitates rapid changes in anaesthetic depth, and arrhythmias are rare. Some may wish to avoid it in the patient with coronary artery disease.

Nitrous oxide

Whilst acknowledging its potential for hypoxia, gas embolism, myocardial depression, methionine synthetase inhibition and vomiting, we still find the use of 50–70% nitrous oxide useful.

Narcotic analgesics

Most narcotic analgesics are metabolized by the liver, with the possible exception of phenoperidine of which 50% is excreted unchanged in the urine. Fentanyl may be the drug of choice on account of its relatively unchanged pharmacokinetics in renal failure; Gulden et al (1984) have reported some prolongation of the elimination half-life in juvenile onset diabetics undergoing renal transplantation, but a bolus dose of $25\,\mu g/kg$ and an operative time of four hours make this study difficult to interpret. The pharmacokinetics of alfentanil again appear relatively unaltered although studies have been confined to single bolus doses of the drug and have produced conflicting results (Koehntop et al 1990). Potential problems with the commonly used opiates centre on the excretion of their water soluble metabolites. Morphine-6-glucuronide accumulates in renal failure (Osbourne et al 1986), which may explain reports of prolonged effects in the absence of high levels of morphine itself in renal failure (Casthely & Villanueva 1983). Pethidine is best avoided because its renally excreted metabolite norpethidine is potentially convulsant. Overall, whatever opiate is used, infusions are hazardous and it is our practice to give small regular doses, with an awareness of the potential for accumulation of the drug or its metabolites.

Non-anaesthetic drug administration

This differs widely from unit to unit. In general terms the following categories of drugs will be used.

Prophylactic antibiotics

These are administered intravenously at induction of anaesthesia. The possible interactions of antibiotics with anaesthetic and other drugs must be constantly borne in mind, for example the aminoglycoside antibiotics potentiate competitive neuromuscular blocking agents, and probably enhance frusemide nephrotoxicity.

Immunosuppressant drugs

Immunosuppression begins pre-operatively; most centres use triple therapy with prednisolone, azathioprine and cyclosporin. Potential problems exist with pre-operative oral cyclosporin, because its foul taste necessitates its administration in large (200 ml) volumes—chocolate milk is popular. Intravenous cyclosporin must be diluted in 5% dextrose or 0.9% saline and infused over 2–6 h. The preparation is dissolved in polyethoxy-lated castor oil which has been associated with anaphylactoid reactions. Side effects of cyclosporin are usually related to chronic administration and may be seen in patients presenting for re-transplantation; these include hypertension, fluid retention and convulsions, especially in children. Azathioprine may be given by slow intravenous injection (to avoid hypo-tension), prior to surgery. It is reported to antagonize the action of competitive neuromuscular blockers such as d-tubocurarine (although data on atracurium are lacking). Finally, methylprednisolone, often given at induction of anaesthesia, has been associated with cardiac arrest, arrhythmias, and circulatory collapse. It is wise to administer the drug at a rate not exceeding 500 mg in 10 min.

Intra-operative hypertension

This is mainly a problem on intubation and on revascularization of the graft. Glyceryl trinitrate, trimetaphan, or lipid soluble beta-blockers such as propranolol or metoprolol are the saftest agents to use; sodium nitro-prusside can be used provided the increased risk of cyanide and particulary thiocyanate toxicity in ESRF is borne in mind. Inadvertent inclusion of the adrenal gland in the donor organ is a rare cause of hypertension (Freilich et al 1984).

Intra-operative hypotension

This usually reflects hypovolaemia. If a vasopressor must be used a selective beta$_1$-agonist such as dobutamine or dopexamine is preferable. Occasionally, surgical manipulation or the presence of a large polycystic liver or kidney may lead to caval compression.

Fluid and diuretic therapy

This should represent a balance between the patient's cardiac status and the need to elevate cardiac filling pressures prior to revascularization of the graft. The relative proportions of crystalloid and colloid will depend on pre-operative haematocrit and electrolytes, and ongoing losses. In a patient with known poor left ventricular function a pulmonary artery catheter will be necessary to guide adequate volume replacement. High volume crystalloid loading has been advocated by Carlier et al (1982). We prefer to use smaller volumes of colloid aiming to increase the CVP to 10 cm prior to unclamping. Hartmann's solution is undesirable due to its potassium and lactate content.

Diabetic patients receive a maintenance infusion of 10% dextrose and insulin. We use a low dose $(1-3 \mu g \, kg^{-1}/min)$ infusion of dopamine throughout surgery in an attempt to improve renal perfusion; (the use of the combined dopaminergic and beta$_1$-agonist dopexamine is an attractive alternative) this is continued into the post-operative period. Diuretic therapy is also frequently employed at unclamping. Frusemide in doses of 0.5 mg/kg in the live related graft to 3 mg/kg in the cadaveric graft, may be given (remembering possible interactions with aminoglycosides and cyclosporin). Mannitol is given immediately prior to clamp release in some centres, although this will cause problems if the donor graft fails to function and mannitol is not eliminated. It also tends to increase the serum potassium concentration.

THE POST-OPERATIVE PERIOD

Recovery from anaesthesia

In some centres patients are electively ventilated for 2–3 h before weaning (Carlier et al 1986). We do not have the facilities to do this routinely although a unit where selected patients can be ventilated post-operatively must be available. At the end of the procedure any residual neuromuscular blockade is reversed with conventional doses of neostigmine with glycopyrrolate.

If patients fail to recover rapidly from anaesthesia, it is best to continue ventilation. Possible drug interactions can be discussed at leisure.

Early post-operative care

Post-operatively, patients are nursed in a high dependency area, where intra-operative monitoring can be continued. A chest X-ray is indicated to confirm the placement of CVP lines and to exclude pulmonary oedema. Post-operative analgesia will consist of regular small doses of a suitable opiate supplemented by wound infiltration or regional nerve block. Bupivacaine is probably the agent of choice, but for reasons already discussed it is wise to reduce the dose by 25% to a maximum of 1.5 mg/kg. Low dose dopamine is continued for 24 h and the urine output replaced with a combination of 5% dextrose and 0.9% saline in equal proportion. Central venous pressure is maintained with suitable colloidal solutions.

Post-operative complications

Complications include those of the patient's pre-existing condition, of the anaesthetic and surgical procedures, and of the immunosuppressant drugs given peri-operatively. Grafted kidneys may not function immediately—this usually reflects a degree of acute tubular necrosis in the graft which should recover—although acute rejection associated with preformed cytotoxic antibodies may also occur. Primary graft failure may also be attributed to mechanical problems with vascular or ureteric anastomoses. Initially functioning grafts may undergo chronic rejection or may fail due to recurrence of primary pathology. Immunosuppressant drug treatment produces widespread effects, amongst which opportunist infection, cyclosporin toxicity, and the development of malignancy merit a mention. It has been claimed that excellent results can be obtained by changing from cyclosporin to prednisolone and azathioprine at three months post-transplantation (Hall et al 1988).

Outcome

Transplant recipients are in no doubt of the enormous benefits of renal transplantation. Better than 80% one-year and 60% five-year organ survival is now the rule. The causes of death in transplanted patients are, in order of frequency, sepsis, cardiovascular disease, suicide, and gastrointestinal perforation. For all the ethical, logistical and technical problems of renal transplantation, it is nevertheless a privilege to participate in an endeavour which is consistently rewarding, often challenging and rarely dull.

General surgical procedures in renal transplant patients

The success of renal transplant surgery has ensured that increasing numbers of patients with renal transplants will present for further elective or emergency surgical procedures (Castaneda & Garvin 1986). Whatever the procedure, early communication with the renal physician concerned with the patients management is obviously vital. The majority of elective procedures are well tolerated; renal handling of drugs becomes less of a problem although renal function is rarely normal. The patient's immunosuppressive regime must be continued throughout the perioperative period and should never be altered without consultation with a renal physician.

REFERENCES

Bennett W M, Aronoff G R, Morrison G et al 1983 Drug prescribing in renal failure: dosing guidelines for adults. Am J Kidney Dis 3: 155–193
Carlier M, Squifflet J-P, Pirson Y 1982 Maximal hydration during anaesthesia increases

pulmonary artery pressures and improves early function of human renal transplants. Transplantation 34: 201–204

Carlier M, Squifflet J-P, Pirson Y et al 1986 Anesthetic protocol in human renal transplantation: twenty-two years of experience. Acta Anaesthesiol Belg 37: 89–94

Carlier M, Gianello P, Squifflet J-P et al 1989 Correlation between atrial natriuretic peptide levels and cardiac filling pressures in renal transplant recipients. Transplantation 48: 700–701

Cashman J N, Luke J J, Jones R M 1990 Neuromuscular block with doxacurium (B W A938U) in patients with normal or absent renal function. Br J Anaesth 64: 186–192

Castaneda M A, Garvin P J 1986 General surgical procedures in renal allograft recipients. Am J Surg 152: 717–721

Casthely P A, Villanueva R 1983 Level of consciousness after cadaveric kidney transplant under halothane anaesthesia. Can Anaesth Soc J 30: 587–592

Cousins M J, Mazze R I, Losek J C et al 1974 The aetiology of methoxyflurane nephrotoxicity. J Pharmacol Exp Ther 190: 530–541

Cronelly R, Salvatierra O, Feduska N J 1984 Renal allograft function following halothane, enflurane or isoflurane anesthesia. Anesth Analg 63 (Abstract): 202

Dodds A, Nicholls M, 1983 Haematological aspects of renal disease. Anaesth Intensive Care 11: 361–368

Editorial 1990 Organ donors in the UK—getting the numbers right. Lancet 335: 80–82

Farman J V 1989 Transplantation surgery. In: Nimmo W S, Smith G (eds) Anaesthesia. Blackwell Scientific Publications, London, pp 817–829

Freilich J D, Waterman P M, Rosthental J M 1984 Acute haemodynamic changes during renal transplantation. Anesth Analg 63: 158–160

Frey F J, Schaad H J, Renner E L et al 1989 Impaired liver function in stable renal allograft patients. Hepatology 9: 606–613

Gianello P, Squifflet J-P, Carlier M et al 1989 Evidence that atrial natriuretic peptide is the humoral factor by which volume loading or mannitol infusion produces an improved renal function after acute ischaemia. Transplantation 48: 9–14

Graybar G B, Bready L L 1987 Anaesthesia for renal transplantation. Martinus Nijhoff, Boston

Graybar G B, Tarpey M 1987 Kidney transplantation. In: Gelman S (ed) Anesthesia for organ transplantation. W B Saunders, Philadelphia

Groth C G 1987 There is no need to give blood transfusions for renal transplantation in the cyclosporine era. Transplant Proc 19: 153–154

Gulden D, Koehntop D, Rodman J et al 1984 Fentanyl pharmacokinetics during renal transplantation. Anesthesiology 61: (3A) abstract A243

Hall B M, Tiller D J, Hardie I et al 1988 Comparison of three immunosuppressive regimens in cadaver renal transplantation: long-term cyclosporine, short term cyclosporine therapy followed by azathioprine and prednisolone without cyclosporine. N Engl J Med 318: 1499–1506

Heino A, Orko R, Rosenberg P H 1986 Anaesthesiological complications in renal transplantation: a retrospective study of 500 transplantations. Acta Anaesthesiol Scand 30: 574–580

Innes A, Catto G R D 1989 Renal failure. In: Nimmo W S, Smith G (eds) Anaesthesia. Blackwell Scientific Publications, London, pp 1341–1362

Koehntop D E, Noormohamed S E, Fletcher C V 1990 Pharmacokinetics of alfentanil during renal transplantation in diabetic and non-diabetic patients. Anesth Analg 70: S212

Kong K L, Tyler J E, Willats S M, Prys-Roberts C 1990 Isoflurane sedation for patients undergoing mechanical ventilation: metabolism to inorganic fluoride and renal effects. Br J Anaesth 64: 159–162

Linke C L, Merin R G 1976 A regional anesthetic approach for renal transplantation. Anesth Analg 55: 69–73

Macdougall I C, Hutton R D, Cavill I et al 1990 Treating renal anaemia with recombinant human erythropoietin: practical guidelines and a clinical algorithm. Br Med J 300: 655–659

Mazze R I, Sievenpiper T S, Stevenson J 1984 Renal effects of enflurane and halothane in patients with abnormal renal function. Anesthesiology 60: 161–163

Morcos W E, Payne J P 1985 The induction of anaesthesia with propofol (Diprivan) compared in normal and renal failure. Postgrad Med J 61 (3): 62–63

Morgan M, Lumley J 1975 Anaesthetic considerations in chronic renal failure. Anaesth Intensive Care 3: 218–226

Nancarrow C, Mather L E 1983 Pharmacokinetics in renal failure. Anaesth Intensive Care
    11: 350–360
Opelz G 1987 Improved kidney graft survival in nontransfused recipients. Transplant Proc
    19: 149–152
Opelz G, Sengar D P S, Mickey M R et al 1973 Effect of blood transfusions on subsequent
    kidney transplants. Transplant Proc 5: 253–259
Orko R, Heino A, Bjorksten F et al 1987 Comparison of atracurium and vecuronium in
    anaesthesia for renal transplantation. Acta Anaesthesiol Scand 31: 450–453
Osbourne R J, Joel S P, Slevin M L 1986 Morphine intoxication in renal failure: the role of
    morphine-6-glucuronide. Br Med J 292: 1548–1549
Remuzzi G 1988 Bleeding in renal failure. Lancet 1: 1205–1208
Rosenlof K, Fyhrquist F, Tenhunen R 1990 Erythropoietin, aluminium and anaemia in
    patients on haemodialysis. Lancet 1: 247–249
Scornik J C, Salomon D R, Howard R J et al 1989 Prevention of transfusion-induced broad
    sensitisation in renal transplant candidates. Transplantation 47: 617–620
Sear J W, Holland D E 1989 Anaesthesia for patients with renal dysfunction. In: Nimmo W
    S, Smith G (eds) Anaesthesia. Blackwell Scientific Publications, London, pp 912–932
Thomas A N, Pollard B J 1989 Renal transplantation and diabetic autonomic neuropathy.
    Can J Anaesth 36: 590–592
Vandam L D, Harrison J H, Murray J E et al 1962 Anaesthetic aspects of renal homotrans-
    plantation in man. Anesthesiology 23: 783–792
Wickstrom I 1981 Enflurane anesthesia in living related donor renal transplantation. Acta
    Anaesthesiol Scand 25: 263–269

9. Halothane and the implications of hepatitis

J. M. Neuberger

INTRODUCTION

Liver damage following anaesthesia and surgery occurs relatively frequently. For example, in patients following major surgery, mild jaundice is found in approximately 17% of cases and marked jaundice in 4% (Evans et al 1974). After open heart surgery jaundice is even more common, occurring in about 25% of patients (Chu et al 1984). In most instances liver damage is usually mild and of little clinical significance. However hepatitis, which may occur either as a consequence of exacerbation of pre-existing liver disease or as a result of surgical or anaesthetic factors inducing new liver disease, may rarely be severe or even fatal.

CAUSES OF POST-OPERATIVE LIVER DYSFUNCTION

The major causes of post-operative liver injury are listed in Table 9.1. In many instances the cause of the liver injury can be deduced from the clinical history or by simple investigations. Of those syndromes which present with a clinical picture of hepatitis, the important diagnoses to consider are: viral hepatitis, ischaemia, sepsis, exacerbation of pre-existing liver disease, cholangitis and drug-induced hepatitis.

The diagnosis of viral hepatitis is usually made serologically. Hepatitis A virus is readily diagnosed by the detection of IgM antibodies to the hepatitis A virus; IgG antibodies will persist for many years after the initial

Table 9.1 Major causes of post-operative hepatitis

Hypoxia
Hypotension/circulatory failure
Drugs (including halothane)
Viral infection
Sepsis
Cholecystitis
Pre-existing liver disease
   (exacerbated by anaesthesia/surgery)
Pancreatitis

179

infection. An acute episode of hepatitis B viral infection is confirmed by demonstration of the presence of IgM antibodies to the core antigen (IgM anti-HBc). The presence of HBsAg (the Australia antigen) does not differentiate acute from chronic viral infection.

It has been clear for some years that there are other hepatitis viruses which are defined loosely as the non-A, non-B viruses. Of these, two have more recently been defined: hepatitis C virus (HCV), which has many similarities with flavi viruses, is spread parenterally. A number of antibody assays are currently being marketed. Although the initial results of sero- logical testing were considered highly promising, it is now becoming recognized that there exists an increasing number of false positive results and more specific tests are being developed. It must be remembered that the hepatitis C virus is currently detectable only by the presence of antibody and it may be several months after the initial infection that these antibodies are detectable in the serum. The hepatitis E virus, which is spread in outbreaks, has no serological marker. There are a number of other viruses which may rarely cause hepatitis, including Echo, coxsackie, herpes, Epstein-Barr and adenoviruses.

Ischaemic hepatitis may occur as a result of intra-operative hypotension. In this instance the cause is usually readily identified and is associated with damage to other organs. The diagnosis can be confirmed histologically. Anaesthesia, whether general, epidural or spinal, may cause a reduction in the hepatic blood flow and this is most pronounced when associated with upper abdominal surgery. Although it is unlikely that this has any serious adverse effect in healthy individuals it is possible that those with pre- existing liver disease may be at greater risks from hypoxia (Gelman 1989).

Sepsis is an important cause of post-operative hepatitis since prompt recognition and treatment is imperative. The mechanism by which sepsis results in liver damage is multifactorial and mechanisms include haemolysis, septic shock with associated reduction in hepatic blood flow, endotoxaemia and release of cytokines, and direct invasion of the liver by the infecting organism. Serum bilirubin is the best predictor of outcome with the other liver tests having little discriminative value.

The role of drugs in post-operative liver dysfunction is discussed below.

DIAGNOSIS OF DRUG-RELATED LIVER DISEASE

In general the diagnosis of drug-related liver disease is one of exclusion and temporal association. The spectrum of liver damage induced by drugs is very broad and one drug may often be associated with several different manifestations of hepatotoxicity, ranging from mild derangement of liver tests to fulminant hepatic failure. It will be appreciated that it is very rarely possible to exclude all other causes of liver dysfunction. Furthermore, patients receiving anaesthesia often receive a variety of different therapeutic agents, thus making it difficult to establish which agent may be implicated in the pathogenesis of the hepatitis. It has been suggested that a challenge test should be performed. Although this has been done in a limited number of instances, challenge is hazardous and potentially fatal. Furthermore, the results of a positive test may be misleading as instanced by one study where patients with autoimmune chronic active hepatitis developed serological and immunological abnormalities when challenged with oxyphenisatin (a laxative which is known to induce chronic active hepatitis) even though the patient had never been exposed to the drug previously. Conversely, a negative test may not exclude the diagnosis.

It is important to appreciate the significance of attributing an episode of post-operative hepatitis to a particular drug: if for example, a patient has an episode of unexplained hepatitis following halothane anaesthesia, it is clearly prudent to advise the patient that he should not receive halothane again even though there may be some uncertainty as to the causal relationship between the anaesthetic agent and the hepatitis. In the author's experience, the majority of patients with fatal halothane hepatitis have suffered episodes of previous post-operative jaundice and these have been largely ignored. The incorrect labelling of an episode of post-operative liver dysfunction as halothane hepatitis does have some adverse consequence in that an anaesthetist may be required to use an agent with which he is less familiar, may be less suitable or may be more expensive, but this seems a small price to pay for the avoidance of a potentially fatal drug reaction.

Types of drug reactions

Adverse drug reactions affecting the liver are classically divided into two types, predictable and idiosyncratic (Table 9.2). Predictable drug reactions are usually dose-dependent and are typically illustrated by the case of paracetamol. Above a certain dose of paracetamol the patient will predictably develop liver cell damage. There may be some modifications to this principle, for example, patients receiving enzyme-inducing agents may be more prone to develop liver damage since there will be increased metabolism of the drug to a more toxic compound. These reactions are normally readily reproducible in animals and thus it may be possible to devise a logical strategy for treatment.

Table 9.2 Classification of drug hepatotoxicity

	Dose-dependent	Onset	Response to challenge	Animal model	Immune features
Predictable	+	Rapid (days)	Rapid	+	−
Idiosyncratic metabolic	+/−	Variable (up to 1 year)	Delayed	+/−	−
Immune-mediated	−	Variable (1 day to 12 weeks)	Rapid	−	+

In contrast to the predictable reactions are the idiosyncratic ones. These reactions do not have a simple dose-dependent relationship with toxicity. The interval between taking the drug and development of liver damage is more variable and may occur over a much wider interval. Idiosyncratic reactions may be due either to metabolic idiosyncracy or to immune involvement. Metabolic idiosyncracy may be due to a number of factors such as abnormalities of constitutive cytochrome or other drug metabolizing enzymes or interaction with other drugs which may affect drug metabolism. Involvement of immune reactions in the pathogenesis of liver damage is suggested by the occurrence of features such as pyrexia, peripheral eosinophilia, presence of circulating immune complexes, organ non-specific autoantibodies and hypergammaglobulinaemia. Some drugs have been associated with development of specific antibodies which react with the drug metabolizing enzymes (for example, in the case of the diuretic tienilic acid, the organ non-specific autoantibody reacts with the cytochrome P450 that metabolizes the drug). Idiosyncratic reactions tend to be seen more commonly in practice since those drugs with a predictable hepatotoxicity are given usually in a defined dose and liver damage is seen only after overdose, either iatrogenic or self-inflicted.

HALOTHANE HEPATITIS

Halothane (1,1,1, trichloro-2-fluoro-2-bromoethane) was first introduced into clinical practice in the early part of the 1950s and rapidly achieved a well deserved reputation as being a safe and easily administered anaesthetic and indeed became one of the commonest agents in use. However, occasional reports began to appear suggesting that halothane may cause severe liver damage, occasionally resulting in fulminant hepatic failure. Concern even spread to *Time Magazine* and was such that a large retrospective study was set up to analyse the incidence and causes of massive liver cell necrosis following anaesthesia. Anaesthetic records of 750 000 patients in selected hospitals in the United States were examined between 1959 and 1962 (National Halothane Study 1966). Eighty-two cases of massive liver cell necrosis were identified and in all but nine, the cause of liver failure could readily be identified as being due to shock, sepsis or pre-existing liver disease. Of the remainder, seven had received halothane. The incidence of otherwise unexplained massive liver cell necrosis following halothane anaesthesia was, thus, about 1 in 35 000 halothane exposures. In those where there was no history of previous exposure to halothane, the incidence was 1 in 80 000 but in those who had received the drug on more than one previous occasion the incidence was 1 in 3700 patients. The incidence of massive unexplained liver damage due to other agents is 1 in 16 000. This study can be criticized on many accounts (Neuberger & Kenna 1987). Not least is that the study was retrospective and it is possible that some of the hospitals were selected on the grounds that halothane hepatitis had been reported in that institution. Furthermore, the analysis was concerned only with cases of massive liver cell necrosis and serious but less major degrees of liver cell damage were not considered. Nevertheless, this study identified four important features which have since been confirmed by many other studies: first, severe liver cell damage following anaesthesia is rare; second, massive unexplained liver damage following halothane occurs more commonly than that seen following other anaesthetic agents; third, the incidence of hepatitis is greater in those who have received more than one exposure to halothane; and finally, more recent exposure to halothane is associated with a greater likelihood of developing liver cell damage.

Clinical patterns of halothane-related hepatitis

For the purposes of this chapter, halothane hepatitis will be arbitrarily defined as otherwise unexplained liver damage occurring within 28 days of halothane exposure in a patient with a previously normal liver.

Analysis of the many publications describing halothane hepatitis suggests that the spectrum of liver damage following halothane anaesthesia is wide, ranging from minor derangement of liver tests with few, if any, clinical symptoms, to massive liver cell necrosis, associated with fulminant hepatic failure and death. It remains uncertain whether these two extremes represent ends of a continuous spectrum or whether they represent two different manifestations of drug toxicity. Since it appears that the two extremes of halothane-associated liver damage may have a different mechanism the two types will be described separately.

Minor derangement of liver function

This type of reaction following halothane anaesthesia has been well described by a number of well controlled prospective studies. The conclusions from these studies are similar (Stock & Strunin 1985). Abnormalities of transaminase elevation occurs in up to 25% of patients following anaesthesia and rarely exceeds three times the upper limit of normal. The Oxford study (Trowell et al 1975) showed that elevation of serum transaminases were seen more frequently following halothane exposure than with the control anaesthetic and where the liver histology was available, this showed features of a focal hepatitis. An additional observation from the Southampton study (Wright et al 1975) was that abnormal liver function tests may not be detectable until way into the second post-operative week. Many of the other studies have performed liver tests only for the first post-operative week. An additional point from this study was that re-exposure to halothane in a patient who had already shown minor derangement of liver tests was not necessarily followed by derangement on re-exposure to halothane. In none of the studies was there any case of fulminant hepatic failure. A more recent study by Allan et al (1987) used a more sensitive marker of liver damage, gluthathione-S-transferase (GST). Three groups of patients were studied: two groups were given halothane in either 30% or 100% oxygen. The control group was given isoflurane in 30% oxygen. Elevations of serum GST above control levels were seen in none of the patients exposed to isoflurane, in 24% of the 17 patients given halothane in 100% oxygen and in one-third of the 37 patients given halothane in 30% oxygen. This study shows that halothane given under high oxygen tensions is associated with less liver damage than when given under lower oxygen tensions but at both concentrations is associated with more liver damage than isoflurane.

Severe hepatitis following halothane

An approximation of the incidence of severe halothane hepatitis has already been established by the National Halothane Study outlined above. An alternative approach to establishing the occurrence of halothane hepatitis was suggested by Trey et al (1968) who examined the cause of death in 150 patients dying with fulminant hepatic failure. Forty-one patients had died following surgery and in all but six, halothane had been the anaesthetic used. Of these 35 patients, 27 had received halothane on more than one occasion. This observation again reinforces the suggestion that halothane hepatitis is more likely to occur in patients who have received more than one exposure. Indeed, a recent study from London (Gimson & Williams 1983) suggests that halothane hepatitis is the third commonest cause of fulminant hepatic failure seen in the UK and represents the commonest iatrogenic cause of fulminant hepatic failure (Table 9.3). Fulminant hepatic failure due to halothane occurred twice as often as liver failure due to all other drugs seen in the series.

Table 9.3 Causes of fulminant hepatic failure (From Gimson & Williams 1983)

Paracetamol overdose	48%
Viral hepatitis	37%
Halothane hepatitis	5%
Pregnancy associated	5%
Drug sensitivity	2%
Others	3%

Table 9.4 Features of halothane hepatitis

Female:male	1.6:1
Previous exposure	78%
Drug allergy	15%
Eosinophilia	21%
Autoantibodies	29%

Analysis of the major published reports of the clinical and histopatho-logical features with halothane hepatitis is given in Table 9.4. It must be emphasized that not all the features listed were reported but characteristic features of the syndrome are the high incidence of females, the finding that the majority of patients had been noted to be exposed to halothane on more than one occasion and the high mortality. Some reports have drawn attention to the increased incidence of allergy to other drugs but this suggestion must be treated with some degree of caution. Thus, Fee et al (1978) have shown the incidence of drug allergy in a large group of patients undergoing anaesthesia to be similar to that seen in patients with halothane hepatitis. Rarely is the basis of the diagnosis of drug allergy defined. Other reports have drawn attention to the increased incidence of obesity in patients with halothane hepatitis but again obesity is rarely defined and compared with a control population. Other features of halothane hepatitis include peripheral eosinophilia and the presence of circulating auto-antibodies. These autoantibodies include anti-nuclear antibodies, anti-actin antibodies and anti-liver–kidney microsomal antibodies (anti-LKM).

Predisposing factors to the development of halothane hepatitis

If halothane hepatitis is a real entity, are there any features which would identify patients at risk (Table 9.5)? As illustrated above, the main feature that is present throughout all series is the high incidence of previous exposures to halothane. In our own study (Kenna et al 1987b) of 40 patients with severe halothane hepatitis, all patients had received at least one previous halothane anaesthetic. However, this is not true of all series but in many incidences the anaesthetic used for previous surgery was not documented. Indeed, even if halothane is not used, the anaesthetic agent can contaminate the anaesthetic equipment and significant levels of halothane metabolites can be detected in the urine of such patients (Varma et al 1985). A further feature of concern in our series was the observation that 11 patients had had previous documented adverse reactions to halothane. The mortality in this series was 30%.

Whether there is a genetic component to the development of halothane hepatitis remains unclear. Hoft et al (1981) describes severe hepatic necrosis after halothane anaesthesia in three pairs of closely related women,

Table 9.5   Risk factors for halothane hepatitis

High	Recent previous exposure
	Previous adverse reaction
Uncertain	Obesity
	Female
	Drug allergy
	Lymphocyte sensitivity to phenytoin
	Family history of halothane hepatotoxicity

all of whom shared a Mexican, Spanish or Indian background. More recently, Farrell et al (1985) showed that lymphocytes isolated from patients with halothane hepatitis are susceptible in vitro to a metabolite of phenytoin. This abnormality of lymphocyte function was also observed in a proportion of relatives of these patients.

Evidence of an association with a particular HLA phenotype is conflicting. Thus Eade et al (1978), in a study from two centres, were unable to identify any specific HLA phenotype associated with halothane hepatitis although the mixed ethnic background may have masked such an association. In Japan, Otsuka et al (1985) assessed HLA class I and class II antigens in 38 patients who had developed halothane hepatitis. Patients were subdivided into those with and without jaundice. There was a significant difference in the DR2 phenotype which was found in over half the patients with jaundice compared with one-third of the controls. Additionally, the phenotype frequency of AW24, BW52 and DR2 was higher in those patients with jaundice. These results must be treated with caution since in only six patients was hepatitis A viral infection excluded and hepatitis B viral infection was excluded only by the absence of surface antigen. There exists a subgroup of patients with hepatitis B in whom the disease can be detected only by the presence of IgM anti-core. Finally, no statistical correction was made for the number of antigens tested.

Whether concomitant use of enzyme-inducing agents predisposes to halothane hepatitis is uncertain. Greene (1973) was unable to show an increased incidence of liver damage in patients with epilepsy who were receiving phenobarbitone. However, a study from Japan (Nomura et al 1986) compared the effects of halothane anaesthesia in patients, some of whom had received phenobarbitone and other anticonvulsant medication. The incidence of post-operative unexplained hepatitis was 7% in those who had received phenobarbitone and 0.5% in those who had not. This incidence of post-operative hepatitis in both groups is startlingly high and differs greatly with that observed in other clinical practice. Although the cases, as described, fulfil the criteria for halothane hepatitis, it is difficult to reconcile these with other observations.

DIRECT TOXICITY OF HALOTHANE

Many early studies in a variety of laboratory animals showed no evidence of liver damage following halothane anaesthesia. However, subsequent models using enzyme induction demonstrated that halothane does have hepatotoxicity potential. Thus, investigations by Van Dyke et al (1964) showed that pretreatment of animals with the mixed function oxidase enzyme inducer, phenobarbitone, resulted in liver damage after halothane exposure. This liver damage could be further enhanced by exposing the rats to halothane in an hypoxic environment (Sipes & Brown 1976). The hepatotoxicity is reproducible and dose-dependent yet nevertheless, subsequent studies have shown there to be considerable differences between different species of animals, age and sex. Others (Shingu et al 1982) have suggested that the hypoxia was more important than enzyme induction in inducing hepatotoxicity since halothane, enflurane and isoflurane induced a degree of hepatotoxicity similar to intravenous agents such as thiopentone or fentanyl when given in 10% oxygen. Although the need for pretreatment with enzyme inducers would suggest that the metabolism was implicated in the pathogenesis of hepatotoxicity, enflurane and isoflurane are metabolized less extensively than halothane. Other models have been described using different enzyme inducers, triiodothyronine and chronic alcohol pretreatment with similar results. However, Lunam et al (1982) has revived interest in the guinea pig model since neither enzyme induction nor hypoxia were a prerequisite for hepatotoxicity. In this model, hypotension does occur but is less likely to be implicated in the pathogenesis of the hepatotoxicity since isoflurane, which induces a similar degree of hypotension, was not associated with a similar degree of liver damage.

How do these animal models relate to the clinical situation?

The features of halothane hepatitis in humans are that the syndrome is rare, occurs more commonly after multiple halothane exposures and is idiosyncratic. The possible involvement of obesity has already been discussed but obese animals do metabolize halothane differently from non-obese animals (Bierman et al 1989). Yet in the animal models, given the appropriate pretreatment, the toxicity is reproducible. There is uncertainty in humans as to whether phenobarbitone pretreatment enhances liver toxicity whereas this seems clearcut in animal studies. Pretreatment of humans with cimetidine (a weak enzyme inhibitor), does not prevent the subclinical halothane hepatotoxicity in man, using GST as a marker of hepatocellular damage (Ray et al 1989). None of the animals has demonstrated any evidence of immune involvement.

Immune-mediated toxicity

Many of the clinical laboratory features of halothane hepatitis detailed above suggests that immune mechanisms may be implicated in the pathogenesis of the disease. However, differentiation of primary and secondary immunological events is often difficult. Early studies failed to show any convincing evidence of sensitization to halothane but since the drug is a small molecule, it is possible that the drug itself is not the antigen but acts as a hapten. In order to circumvent the problems of selecting the appropriate antigen for testing, Vergani et al (1981) used isolated liver cells or liver homogenates isolated from rabbits previously exposed to halothane for in vitro testing. Early studies showed that lymphocytes from patients with halothane hepatitis were cytotoxic to halothane altered liver cells. Subsequent studies (Vergani et al 1981) showed that approximately three-quarters of patients with severe halothane hepatitis had circulating antibodies reacting with these halothane altered antigens. These techniques used both indirect immunofluorescence and an antibody-dependent cell-mediated cytotoxicity reaction. Results were subsequently confirmed using an enzyme linked immunoabsorbent assay and immunoblotting methods (Kenna et al 1987a, Kenna et al 1988b). Demonstration of circulating antibodies to halothane altered antigens in the serum of patients with halothane hepatitis does not prove that immune mechanisms are involved in the pathogenesis of the disease. Nevertheless, two pointers suggest that this may be the case: first, even in the early course of the disease, IgG class antibodies are present: if these antibodies were merely a response to a direct toxicity then early phase IgM antibodies might be anticipated although rapid switching from IgM to IgG can occur; second, patients who develop liver damage from other causes, such as malignant infiltration or viral hepatitis, do not have demonstrable antibodies present (Neuberger et al 1983).

Biotransformation of halothane

This subject has been well reviewed by Stock & Strunin (1985) and Farrell (1988). Following the early demonstration that chloroform was metabolized, it was shown that halothane was metabolized both in vitro and in vivo and that this was mediated by the mixed function oxidase system. Halothane is metabolized through two different pathways which involve the formation of free radicals which covalently bind to liver cell macro-molecules. The preferential route of metabolism is determined by the prevalent oxygen tension and the relative activities of the constituent P450 isoenzymes. At the oxygen tension prevailing during anaesthesia, halothane is metabolized in man through both routes. The oxidative route, which is preferentially stimulated at high oxygen tensions and by enzyme pre-treatment with inducers such as 3-methyl-cholanthrene, is associated with generation of trifluoroacetic acid. In contrast, the reductive route is pref-erentially stimulated at a low oxygen tension and by enzyme inducers such as phenobarbitone, and is associated with release of fluoride.

In animal models of hepatotoxicity, it seems likely that this mechanism of liver damage is mediated via the reductive route since both phenobarbitone pretreatment and administration of halothane in hypoxic conditions is associated with liver damage. Equally, as shown by Allan et al (1987), administration of halothane at low oxygen tensions is associated with an increased incidence of raised GST levels. However, conflicting evidence has come from studies using deuterated halothane which is metabolized preferentially by the reductive route: male guinea pigs given deuterated halothane have less severe liver damage (Lind et al 1989).

These observations contrast with the fact that the antigens to which the halothane antibodies react are associated with oxidative metabolism (Neuberger et al 1981).

Making the diagnosis of halothane hepatitis

As indicated above, the diagnosis of any drug reaction is essentially one of temporal association and exclusion of other causes. Nevertheless, the demonstration of halothane specific antibodies may offer an opportunity of making a positive diagnosis. Initial studies using immunofluorescence and antibody-dependent-cell-mediated cytotoxicity (Vergani et al 1981) showed that these antibodies were specific to patients with severe halothane hepatitis: antibodies were not detectable in patients who had been exposed to halothane and who had developed either no or minimal abnormality in liver function tests, in patients with other forms of liver disease, or in anaesthetists with normal liver function. These antibodies were present in approximately three-quarters of patients. Thus, whether or not these antibodies are involved in the mechanism of liver damage, their specificity suggests a possible diagnostic role.

However, these antibody tests are difficult to perform, time-consuming and cumbersome. Other techniques, therefore, have been developed to demonstrate the presence of these antibodies. An enzyme linked immuno-absorbent assay using hepatocyte microsomes from rabbits exposed to halothane was developed (Kenna et al 1987). Although cumbersome, this assay is quantitative and reproducible. Other methods have used immuno-blotting techniques. Again, these are reliable but impractical for general use. Recently, a simple ELISA method has been evaluated (Bird & Williams 1989) where the antigen used has been trifluoroacetic acid coupled to albumin (trifluoroacetic acid is the major product of oxidative metabolism of halothane).

Immunoblotting studies developed to characterize halothane-related antigens, have shown that serum from patients with halothane hepatitis contain antibodies that react to five different liver microsomal proteins (Mr100, 76, 59, 57 and 54 KD) which are covalently altered by the tri-fluoroacetyl metabolite of halothane (Kenna et al 1987a). These antigens are also present in human liver after halothane exposure in vivo (Kenna et al 1988a). A recent study by Martin et al (1990) compared three different ELISA assays to test for the presence of antibodies. Approximately 67% of patients with clinical diagnosis of halothane hepatitis had demonstrable antibodies when the test antigens were either trifluoroacetic acid, rabbit serum albumin or liver microsomes. This value was increased to just under 79% when purified trifluoroacetic acid-associated 57 KD, 76 KD and 100 KD proteins were used as antigens. Thus, the latter is the most sensitive method for detecting halothane antibodies. However, a significant number of patients with a clinical diagnosis are antibody negative. Whether this represents a form of antibody negative disease because antibody is

Table 9.6   Halothane exposure guidelines

Avoid halothane exposure if:
Previous exposure within 3 months
Previous adverse reaction to halothane
Family history of adverse reaction to halothane
Adverse reaction to other halogenated hydrocarbon anaesthetic
Pre-existing liver disease

present either in low titre or complexed to antigen, or whether other aetiological factors are implicated remains to be established.

Can halothane hepatitis be avoided?

It seems the most effective way to reduce the incidence of halothane hepatitis is to take a good clinical history. In the author's personal experience, in one-third of patients with halothane hepatitis there was a previous episode of unexplained post-operative jaundice following halothane exposure. Pre-operative screening for halothane antibodies is likely to be highly expensive and given the very low incidence of the disease is unlikely to be economical. Furthermore, there is no information on how long these antibodies persist and, thus, the value of pre-operative screening undertaken. The current guidelines given by the Committee on the Safety of Medicines is shown in Table 9.6.

If a patient is thought to be sensitive to halothane then clearly a different anaesthetic agent needs to be used. It has been shown (as discussed above) that enough halothane is absorbed on to the tubing of anaesthetic equipment to release halothane in sufficient dose to sensitize the patient. Ritchie et al (1988) showed that to decontaminate an anaesthetic machine effectively, 12 h of continuous flushing with oxygen at 8 l/min is required. This is clearly a difficult option and one alternative may be to use a dedicated machine (Martin et al 1988).

OTHER HALOGENATED ANAESTHETIC AGENTS

Halothane was the prototype of volatile halogenated anaesthetic agents. Since its introduction there have been several other agents which have been introduced, notably enflurane, isoflurane, sevoflurane and desflurane. Comparison of the anaesthetic properties and advantages of these different agents is beyond the scope of the author but they have recently been reviewed (Heijke & Smith 1990). The number of cases referred to the Committee on the Safety of Medicines is listed in Table 9.7. It must be stressed that reporting of a drug reaction does not necessarily prove causality and the number of cases reported may well represent a severe

Table 9.7   Adverse drug reactions reported to the Committee on Safety of Medicines

	Time	Cases	Fatal
Halothane	1961–1989	358	48
Enflurane	1973–1989	11	
Methoxyflurane	1971–1989	1	

underestimation. Indeed, of 40 patients recently reviewed by the author, only 12 had been referred to the Committee. Nevertheless, the results suggest that hepatitis following other anaesthetics is less common.

ENFLURANE HEPATITIS

Isolated reports of hepatic necrosis after enflurane anaesthesia began to appear in the early 1970s. The first large scale analysis was performed by Lewis et al (1985). Twenty-four cases of presumed enflurane-associated hepatitis were analysed. Fever occurred in 19 and jaundice occurred in a similar number. The mean onset of symptoms occurred eight days after the anaesthetic. Five of the reported cases died with hepatic failure. Of interest, 16 patients had previously been exposed either to halothane or enflurane. Comparison of these 24 cases with 900 patients with halothane-associated hepatitis from the literature showed a similar distribution of age, proportion of patients previously exposed either to halothane or enflurane and a similar proportion with peripheral eosinophilia. However, patients with enflurane had an approximately equal sex ratio and the mortality was less. This analysis was considered by Dykes (1984) who felt that on the evidence presented, it still remained uncertain as to whether enflurane was indeed hepatotoxic. The situation was compounded by a further retrospective analysis by Eger et al (1986). They reviewed 88 cases, comprising patients that had been published previously and additional cases referred either to the Food and Drug Administration or the Armed Forces Institute of Pathology. Review of these 88 cases revealed that in 30, data were, in the author's opinion, insufficient to make a proper evaluation; in 43 cases, factors other than anaesthetic toxicity could be implicated in the pathogenesis of hepatic injury and in 15 patients there were no other factors implicated. Cases were considered as being either possibly or unlikely a result of enflurane toxicity. Patients with a diagnosis of possible enflurane hepatotoxicity tended to be older, have a shorter interval between the anaesthetic and the onset of symptoms and have post-operative pyrexia. Encephalopathy was less prominent but nausea was more frequent. In addition, these patients had less renal failure, a lower peak LDH level, less major cavity surgery and less post-operative hypoxia. Twenty-four of the cases reviewed by Eger et al (1986) had also been reviewed by Lewis et al

(1985). It is of interest that there was only agreement in 13 cases. Of the 11 in whom there was disagreement about the diagnosis, Eger and colleagues felt that there was either too little information to make a judgement (three cases) or there were other reasons for excluding the anaesthetic as a cause of hepatotoxicity. These reasons included pre-existing liver disease, too long an interval between the anaesthetic and the onset of symptoms, occurrence of sepsis, hypotension, cardiac failure and pre-operative liver damage. Thus, it still remains uncertain as to whether enflurane causes significant hepatotoxicity.

Isoflurane hepatotoxicity

Compared with enflurane hepatotoxicity the number of reported cases of isoflurane hepatotoxicity is very limited. Stoelting et al (1987) reviewed 45 cases of hepatic dysfunction reported to the Food and Drug Administration between 1981 and 1984 as being due to isoflurane. All data were examined by four members of the Anaesthetic Life Support Advisory Committee of the FDA. For 29 (64%) patients, three or more members attributed non-anaesthetic causes to the liver dysfunction. These causes included hypoxia, sepsis and viral infection. Of the remaining 16 (36%), two or more members of the committee felt that isoflurane may have been a contributory factor. These patients tended to be younger but were otherwise not greatly different from those in whom isoflurane was not implicated. Thus, the overall conclusion was that the findings did not indicate a reasonable likelihood of an association between isoflurane administration and post-operative hepatic dysfunction cross-sensitization between halogenated anaesthetics.

It will be evident from the above that the association between both enflurane and isoflurane and liver damage is far less clear. It would appear that if the latter two agents do cause liver cell damage the incidence is far lower and this may relate to the differences in the extent of the metabolism. For example, between 15–25% of the metabolites can be recovered following halothane anaesthesia (Lewis et al 1985) compared with 2.4% for enflurane and 0.2% for isoflurane. Isoflurane, unlike halothane, in laboratory animals appears to protect the liver from the insults of ischaemia and reperfusion (Nagano et al 1990). Furthermore, enflurane and isoflurane can also produce acylated liver microsomal adducts similar to those produced by halothane, albeit at a lower level (Christ et al 1988).

While there has been evidence of cross-sensitization (for example, Sigurdsson 1985), these reports must be treated with a degree of caution. Nevertheless, as stated by Dykes (1984) the same caution should be applied to enflurane and isoflurane as halothane. Although this does not necessarily imply causality it concords with the usual medical doctrine (National Halothane Study 1966) that any treatment followed by ill effects should ordinarily not be repeated.

Acknowledgements

The assistance of Dr F. Bennetts and Dr L. Beeley is appreciated. The secretarial assistance of Miss M. Calcutt is gratefully acknowledged.

REFERENCES

Allan L G, Hussey A J, Howie J et al 1987 Hepatic glutathione-S transferase release after halothane anaesthesia. Lancet 1: 771–774

Bierman J S, Rice S A, Fish K J, Serra M T 1989 Metabolism of halothane in obese fisher 344 rats. Anesthesiology 71: 431–437

Bird G, Williams R 1989 Detection of antibodies to a halothane metabolite hapten in serum from patients with halothane associated hepatitis. J Hepatol 9: 366–373

Christ D D, Kenna J G, Kammerer W, Satoh H, Pohl L R 1988 Potential metabolic basis for enflurane hepatitis and the apparent cross-sensitization between enflurane and halothane. Drug Metab Dispos 1.6: 135–140

Chu C, Chang C, Liaw Y, Hseih M 1984 Jaundice after open heart surgery. Thorax 39: 52–56

Dykes M H M 1984 Is enflurane hepatotoxic? Anesthesiology 61: 235–237

Eade O E, Krawitt E L, Grice D, Wright R, Trowell J 1978 HLA antigens and halothane hepatitis. Lancet II: 1384–1385

Eger E I, Smuckler E A, Farrell I D, Godsmith C H, Johnson B H 1986 Is enflurane hepatotoxic? Anesth Analg 65: 21–30

Evans C, Evans M, Pollock A V 1974 The incidence and causes of post-operative jaundice. Br J Anaesth 46: 520–525

Farrell G, Prendergast D, Murray M 1985 Halothane hepatitis: detection of a constitutional susceptibility factor. N Engl J Med 313: 1310–1314

Farrell G C 1988 Mechanism of halothane induced liver injury. J Gastroenterol Hepatol 3: 465–482

Fee J P H, McDonald S R, Clarke R S J, Dundee J W, Pal P I C 1978 The incidence of atopy and allergy in 10,000 pre-anaesthetic patients. Br J Anaesth 50: 74

Gelman S 1989 Carbon dioxide and hepatic circulation. Anesth Analg 69: 149–151

Gimson A E S, Williams R 1983 Acute hepatic failure in: Thomas H C, MacSween R (eds) Recent advances in hepatology. Churchill Livingstone, Edinburgh, pp 57–70

Greene N M 1973 Halothane anaesthesia and hepatitis in a high risk population. N Engl J Med 289: 304–307

Heijke S, Smith G 1990 Quest for the ideal inhalational anaesthetic agent. Br J Anaesth 64: 3–6

Hoft R H, Bunker J P, Goodman H, Gregory P B 1981 Halothane hepatitis in 3 pairs of closely related woman. N Engl J Med 304: 1023–1024

Kenna J G, Neuberger J, Williams R 1987a Identification by immunoblotting of halothane induced microsomal polypeptide antigens recognised by antibodies in sera from patients with halothane associated hepatitis. J Pharmacol Exp Ther 8: 1635–1641

Kenna J G, Neuberger J, Williams R 1987b Specific antibodies to halothane induced liver antigens in halothane associated hepatitis. Br J Anaesth 59: 1286–1290

Kenna J G, Neuberger J, Williams R 1988a Evidence for expression in human liver of halothane induced antigens recognised by antibodies in sera from patients with halothane hepatitis. Hepatology 8: 1635–1641

Kenna J G, Satoh H, Christ D D, Pohl L R 1988b Metabolic basis for a drug hypersensitivity. J Pharmacol Exp Ther 245: 1103–1109

Lewis J H, Zimmerman H J, Ishak K G, Mollick F S 1985 Enflurane hepatotoxicity: a clinico-pathologic study. Ann Intern Med 98: 984–992

Lind R C, Gandolfi A J, Hall P 1989 Role of oxidative metabolism in the guinea pig model of halothane associated hepatology. Anesthesiology 70: 649–653

Lunam C A, Hall P, Cousins M 1982 Halothane hepatitis: a guinea pig model in the absence of enzyme induction or hypoxia. Clin Exp Pharmacol Physiol 9: 469–470

Martin J L, Kenna J G, Pohl L R 1990 Antibody assay for the detection of patients sensitized to halothane. Anesth Analg 70: 154–159

Martin P A, Cheshire M A, Perlie N 1988 Decontamination of halothane from anaesthetic machine by continuous flushing with oxygen. Br J Anaesth 60: 859–863

Nagano K, Gelman S, Parks D, Bradley E C 1990 Hepatic circulation and oxygen supply—uptake relationship after hepatic ischaemic insults during anaesthesia with volatile anaesthetic agents in miniature pigs. Anesth Analg 70: 53–62

National Halothane Study 1966 Summary of the National Halothane Study. JAMA 197: 121–134

Neuberger J, Kenna J G 1987 Halothane hepatitis. Clin Sci 72: 262–270

Neuberger J, Mieli Vergani G, Tredger J, Davis M, Williams R 1981 Oxidative metabolism of halothane in the production of altered hepatocyte membrane antigens in acute halothane induced necrosis. Gut 22: 669–672

Neuberger J, Gimson A E S, Davis M, Williams R 1983 Specific serological markers in the diagnosis of fulminant hepatic failure following halothane. Br J Anaesth 55: 15–19

Nomura F, Habaro H, Chrishi K, Akikusa B, Okuda K 1986 Effects of anti-convulsant agents on halothane induced liver injury in human subjects and experimental animals. Hepatology 6: 952–954

Otsuka S, Yamamoto M, Kasuya S et al 1985 HLA antigens in patients with unexplained hepatitis following halothane anaesthesia. Acta Anaesthesiol Scand 29: 497–501

Ray D C, Howie A P, Beckett G S, Drumond G B 1989 Pre-operative cimetidine does not prevent sub-clinical halothane hepatotoxicity in men. Br J Anaesth 63: 531–535

Ritchie P A, Cheshire M A, Pearce N 1988 Decontamination of halothane from anaesthetic machine by continuous flushing with oxygen. Br J Anaesth 60: 859–863

Shingu K, Eger E I, Johnson B H 1982 Hypoxia may be more important than reductive metabolism in halothane induced hepatitis injury. Anesth Analg 61: 824–827

Sigurdsson J 1985 Enflurane hepatitis. A report of a case with a previous history of halothane hepatitis. Acta Anaesthesiol Scand 29: 495–496

Sipes I G, Brown B B 1976 An animal model of hepatotoxicity associated with halothane anaesthesia. Anesthesiology 45: 622–628

Stock J G L, Strunin L 1985 Unexplained hepatitis following halothane. Anesthesiology 63: 424–439

Stoelting R K, Blitt C D, Cohen P, Merin R G 1987 Hepatic dysfunction after isoflurane anaesthesia. Anesth Analg 66: 147–153

Trey C, Lipworth L, Chalmers T C et al 1968 Fulminant hepatic failure: presumable contribution by halothane. N Engl J Med 279: 798–801

Trowell J, Peto P, Crampton-Smith A 1975 Controlled trial of repeated halothane anaesthetics in patients with carcinoma of the uterine cervix treated with radium. Lancet I: 823–824

Van Dyke R A, Chenoweth M B, Van Poznak A 1964 Metabolism of volatile anaesthetics I. Biochem Pharmacol 13: 1239–1247

Varma R A, Whitesell R C, Iskandarani M N 1985 Halothane hepatitis without halothane. Hepatology 5: 1159–1162

Vergani D, Mieli Vergani G, Alberti A et al 1981 Antibodies to the surface of halothane altered rabbit hepatocytes in patients with severe halothane associated hepatitis. N Engl J Med 303: 66–71

Wright R, Chisholm M, Lloyd B et al 1975 A controlled prospective study of the effect on liver function of multiple exposures to halothane. Lancet I: 821–823

10. Medical gases (2)—distribution

R. S. C. Howell

This chapter is the second of two dealing with medical gases (Howell 1990). It describes the methods of distribution of medical gases in the UK.

At present nearly all the medical gases in the UK are supplied by BOC Medical Gases (British Oxygen Company). Air Products Ltd, the second largest supplier of industrial gases in the UK, has at present elected to stay mostly out of the UK medical gases market, which is relatively unprofitable because of the position of the National Health Service as a near-monopoly consumer (House of Commons 1985).

This account therefore mainly describes the practice of BOC; much of this is valid in other countries.

Oxygen

Manufacturers

In the UK nearly all the oxygen used in medicine is made by BOC at their air separation plants in Belfast, Brinsworth (Sheffield), Fawley, Margam (Port Talbot), Middlesborough, Motherwell, Thame (Oxfordshire) and Widnes (Cheshire). In 1985 Air Products Ltd obtained a product licence for medical oxygen from their air separation plants in Bracknell, Carrington (Manchester), Cumbernauld, Ellesmere Port and Llanwern, although it does not appear to have used it yet.

Distribution of liquid oxygen

Liquid oxygen is taken from the manufacturing plants either directly to hospital liquid oxygen stores, or to regional distribution centres for cylinder filling. A certificate of analysis accompanies each shipment from the manufacturing plant.

Special transport vessels are used to maintain the liquid at cryogenic temperature. These tankers are subject to strict regulations, because if any liquid oxygen is spilt the gas which it forms is much heavier than air, and can accumulate in spaces beneath roads or floors, where it can damage the structure by expansion, as well as greatly increasing the combustion potential of any material which comes into contact with it.

As a result of these transportation problems liquid oxygen is not available for medical purposes on offshore islands such as the Isle of Man, the Isle of Wight and the Channel Islands.

Distribution of gaseous oxygen

Cylinders are filled at the distribution depot in a medical gases area, separate from industrial oxygen cylinders.

Liquid oxygen (the purity of which is checked daily) is pumped from a storage tank, vaporized in a high pressure vaporizer and put into the cylinders as described below.

Every hour gas from one of the cylinders is analysed with a paramagnetic oxygen analyser, or by the Orsat test (volumetric absorption of oxygen by ammoniacal cuprous chloride).

Nitrous oxide

Manufacturers

In the UK 99% of nitrous oxide is made by BOC at Brentford, Middlesex and Worsley, Manchester, using the aqueous ammonium nitrate feedstock method (Howell 1990). The only other UK manufacturer is Kingston Medical Gases Ltd, Hull, who use the traditional solid feedstock method; this company does not supply hospitals, only dentists and veterinary surgeons.

Distribution

Nitrous oxide is put into cylinders at the manufacturing plant and distributed from there. Brentford supplies the southeast of England, south Wales and Scotland, and Worsley supplies the remainder, including Northern Ireland.

Grant (1978) refers to an accident in France in 1966 in which a large nitrous oxide cylinder exploded when it fell from a truck; this uncommon occurrence is a reminder of the thermodynamic instability of nitrous oxide.

Other medical gases

These are put into cylinders either at the manufacturing plant (cyclopropane, Entonox® (50% nitrous oxide/oxygen gas mixture), medical air, pre-mixed gases) or at a distribution depot by transfer from a larger store (carbon dioxide, helium).

BULK GAS STORAGE SYSTEMS

Bulk storage in the gaseous phase (cylinder manifold)

This method is used for supplying the following gases to hospital pipeline distribution systems: nitrous oxide, Entonox®, oxygen (small installations) and air (small installations). A store of large, high pressure cylinders is divided into two groups (primary and secondary) which supply the pipeline alternately.

All the cylinders in each group are connected through non-return valves to a common pipe, the manifold, which is in turn connected through pressure regulators to the pipeline. All the cylinders' valves are open, so that all the cylinders in a group empty simultaneously.

When the primary group is nearly empty the supply is automatically changed to the secondary group by a device which is sensitive to decreasing pressure in the cylinders. An electrical signalling system alerts staff to the need to attach fresh full cylinders.

This arrangement is designed to maintain a continuous gas supply to the pipeline, and to ensure that at least 95% of the cylinder contents are discharged before the changeover occurs.

Further details can be found in Howell (1980).

Bulk storage in the liquid phase

In the UK this method is only used for oxygen; in some large North American hospitals it is also used for nitrous oxide. The gas must be stored at a temperature below its critical temperature.

Liquid oxygen is stored at about $-150°C$ (vapour pressure 10 bar), in a container which is insulated by a layer of vacuum, thus resembling a sealed and pressurized domestic vacuum flask.

The gas above the liquid is drawn off and replaced by gas formed from fresh vaporization of the liquid. In normal service the refrigeration of the store comes from the continual use of the latent heat of vaporization of the liquid.

The cold gas vaporized inside the container is warmed outside in a coil of copper tubing; this increases the pressure, which is then reduced and regulated before the oxygen is supplied to the hospital. In case of unexpected failure there is a reserve store of oxygen in a manifold of large cylinders.

The connector on the transfer hose from the liquid oxygen supply tanker is indexed to prevent a different cryogenic liquid (e.g. nitrogen) being added to a hospital store inadvertently: this has happened on several occasions in overseas countries (e.g. Sprague & Archer 1975).

In UK hospitals, liquid oxygen storage is usually more cost-effective than cylinders if a hospital uses more than $50 m^3$ (50 000 litres) of gaseous oxygen per week (BOC Gases 1985), but convenience of supply and the cost of transporting cylinders are also taken into account.

More detailed descriptions of liquid phase storage systems can be found in Dorsch & Dorsch (1984) and Howell (1980).

CYLINDERS

A gas cylinder (bottle, tank) is a portable container for compressed gas. It consists of a cylindrical body, a shoulder and a neck. A valve is inserted in the neck to form an integral part of the assembly.

To facilitate maintenance and testing, in the UK medical gas cylinders are usually the property of the gas supply company, who charge their customers rental for them.

Standards

The details of cylinder construction are specified in British Standard BS 5045:1982: this replaced five earlier Standards (BSS 399, 400, 1045, 1287 and 1288). Parts 1 and 3 of BS 5045:1982 apply to medical gas cylinders.

Medical gas cylinders are also covered by British Standard BS 1319:1976, which specifies features intended to prevent the coupling of incorrect cylinders to apparatus, and was first issued in 1946 in response to a request from the Medical Defence Union and the Association of Anaesthetists of Great Britain and Ireland.

Periodic testing of cylinders is covered by BS 5430:1977 (see below).

Many other countries have similar regulations. In the USA, where the standards are specified by the Compressed Gas Association, Feeley et al (1978) found that 1.2% of 14 500 medical gas cylinders delivered to the Beth Israel Hospital in Boston in the period 1972 to 1975 showed potentially hazardous breaches of standards.

Manufacture

Medical gas cylinders are made from a chromium molybdenum alloy of carbon steel which is lighter than pure carbon steel. The Association of Anaesthetists has encouraged its use for medical gas cylinders (Helliwell 1982), as it makes them easier to handle. Cylinders for domiciliary oxygen and for cyclopropane are made from aluminium alloy which is lighter than steel alloy (Table 10.1) but more expensive.

A cylinder is manufactured from a seamless tube which has been extruded from a solid block of alloy. The tube is cut to length and moulded at

Table 10.1 Medical gas cylinders: physical characteristics

					Cylinder size letter					
		B	C	D	E	F	AF	G	J
Dimensions, including valve (mm)		330 × 76	430 × 89	535 × 102	865 × 102	930 × 140	670 × 175	1320 × 178	1520 × 229
Tare weight (kg)		1.6	2.0	3.4	5.4	14.5	9.9	34.5	68.9
	State	Pressure (bar)	Nominal volume of gas contained(l), and type of valve fitted							
Oxygen	P	137		170 PI	340 PI	680 PI	1360 BN	1360 BN	3400 BN	6800 PI
Nitrous oxide	L	44		450 PI	900 PI	1800 PI	3600 HW		9000 HW	
Medical air	P	137				640 PI	1280 BN		3200 BN	6400 PI
Carbon dioxide	L	50		450 PI		1800 PI				
Helium	P	137			300 PI		1200 BN			
Cyclopropane	L	5	180 PI							
Entonox®	P*	137			500 PI		2000 PI		5000 PI	
Carbon dioxide/oxygen	P	137					1360 BN		3400 BN	
Helium/oxygen	P	137				600 PI	1200 BN			

P = permanent gas; L = liquefiable gas. Pressure is the nominal pressure of a full cylinder at 15°C.
PI = Pin-index valve; BN = bull-nose valve; HW = handwheel valve. *At temperatures above −7°C (see Howell 1990).
Data supplied by courtesy of BOC Gases.

each end to form the base and the shoulder and neck, respectively (see the series of photographs in Petty 1987). The formed cylinder is then hardened by treatment with heat and quenching, and carefully inspected to ensure the walls are uniformly thick, and to detect any folds in the neck or surface imperfections or cracks. A sample of the metal is subjected to tensile and bend tests to ensure that the composition of the alloy is satisfactory.

Medical gas cylinders up to size E normally have curved bases, while larger ones which are free-standing have flat ones. Internal tubes (dip tubes) are not normally fitted to medical gas cylinders other than the large cylinders for pipeline Entonox® (MacGregor et al 1972, Howell 1980).

Colour

In the UK medical gas cylinders are painted according to a two part colour code, consisting of the colour of the shoulder (valve end) of the cylinder and the colour of the body. These are defined in British Standard BS 1319:1976 and listed in Table 10.2. Before this code was introduced most cylinders were black, differentiated only by adhesive labels; this sometimes led to accidents (Sykes 1960). It is not permitted for cylinders to be re-painted in a different colour from the original.

Unfortunately, in spite of the efforts of the International Standards Organization (ISO) there is still no worldwide standard colour code. In the UK the standard colours for the shoulders of medical gas cylinders comply with the ISO specification, but the standard colours for cylinder bodies are sometimes different.

Internationally there are notable colour variations. In the USA, for example, the standard colour for oxygen is green, while in West Germany it

Table 10.2   Medical gas cylinders: standard colours and pin-index positions (BS 1319:1976)

	Colours			Pin-index positions	
	Body	Shoulder			
Oxygen	Black	White		2	5
Nitrous oxide	Blue	Blue		3	5
Air	Black	Black/white		1	5
Carbon dioxide	Grey	Grey		1	6
Helium	Brown	Brown		4	6
Cyclopropane	Orange	Orange		3	6
Pre-mixed gases					
Entonox®	Blue	Blue/white		Single pin	
Carbon dioxide/oxygen	Grey	Grey/white	CO_2 not $> 7\%$	2	6
			$CO_2 > 7\%$	1	6
Helium/oxygen	Black	Brown/white	He not $> 80\%$	2	4
			$O_2 < 20\%$	4	6

is blue, and in the UK only the valve end of an oxygen cylinder is white and the rest is black.

In some countries there is no compulsory colour coding standard, so that there is a possibility of confusion between different gases: Kumar & Mishra (1986) reported a serious accident which occurred in Iran when pure nitrous oxide was administered instead of pure oxygen because the cylinders for both gases were the same colour, differentiated only by markings written in Persian.

In the UK the colour of the cylinder is intended to be the secondary method of identifying the contents, the label being the primary identification (BS 1319:1976). Most people, understandably, identify cylinders by colour, but this can be misleading. In a recent incident in the UK an oxygen cylinder, colour coded for oxygen, was filled at a hospital with nitrogen to a pressure of more than 100 bar: a handwritten label reading '100% nitrogen' was attached to it and the cylinder was later found in the hospital cylinder store (Department of Health 1989). Fortunately no patient was affected. Conversely, Sawhney & Yoon (1983) in the USA described a cylinder which was colour coded for nitrous oxide but carried a 'compressed air' label: the cylinder actually contained nitrous oxide.

Industrial gas cylinder colours are: oxygen, black; nitrous oxide, silver body with yellow shoulder; air, grey; carbon dioxide, black; helium, brown; argon, blue; nitrogen, grey body with black shoulder; hydrogen, red. Non-standard gases are supplied in cylinders painted according to a special gas code, and carry an appropriate label.

Size

The size of a cylinder is expressed by a letter of the alphabet, starting with A for the smallest and extending to J for the largest (see Table 10.1). Each successive letter up to size F denotes an increase in the volume of contents of the cylinder of twice the preceding letter. The actual volume of contents is different for each gas: e.g. oxygen: size E = 680 l, size F = 1360 l; nitrous oxide: size E = 1800 l, size F = 3600 l.

In the UK, sizes A and H are not used for medical gases. Size AF denotes a size F aluminium alloy cylinder with carrying handle for domiciliary use.

Cylinder valves

Valves are made of brass and may also be chromium plated. The valve is screwed into the neck of the cylinder and acts as the mechanism for opening and closing the gas pathway. The joint between the neck and the valve is the weakest part of the cylinder assembly, and relatively easy to break, for example by dropping the cylinder on the valve. If the joint breaks when the cylinder contains compressed gas the cylinder body will behave like a released torpedo as the gas escapes (Feeley et al 1978).

Parts of a cylinder valve

Body, containing the mechanism. At the base of the body is a screw thread which joins the valve to the neck of the cylinder: the joint is made gas-tight with PTFE tape or similar material.

Spindle (or stem), operating the valve: the dimensions are specified in BS 1319:1976.

Seating, against which the spindle acts, usually made of a 'soft' material like PTFE.

Gland, a compressible plastic washer which acts as a packing around the spindle to make it gas-tight.

Gland nut, to exert pressure on the gland.

Outlet or port.

Safety relief valve (not normally fitted in the UK).

Pin-index valve

A pin-index valve is fitted to all medical gas cylinders up to and including size E, and to some others (Table 10.1).

The valve has a 7 mm diameter horizontal outlet, a vertical spindle (9.5×5.4 mm), and a 17.6 mm A/F gland nut. The outlet face of the body is drilled with two 4.75 mm diameter holes at a radius of 14.3 mm from the centre of the outlet. There are six possible positions for the holes, which are numbered 1 to 6; any two non-adjacent positions are allocated to each medical gas, providing ten possible combinations (see Table 10.2). For Entonox® a single 5.8 mm diameter hole pin-index is specified (BS 1319:1976; Wyant 1978). The holes mate with indexing pins in corresponding positions on the connector. If an attempt is made to connect the wrong cylinder to the connector, the pins will not locate and a gas-tight connection cannot be made. A compressible yoke sealing washer ('Bodok' seal) must be placed between the valve outlet and the apparatus to make a gas-tight joint. The chemical formula of the indexed gas is engraved on the body of the valve.

The pin-index system (Hogg 1973) is part of an ISO standard, and has been adopted by many countries. It is not foolproof, as it can be deliberately circumvented (Wyant 1978), or can fail accidentally for various reasons (MacMillan & Marshall 1981, Orr & Hamilton 1985, Jayasuriya 1986).

It is recommended in BS 1319:1976 that pin-index valves should be used for all medical gas cylinders irrespective of size, but this is not yet the case. Since 1985 size J pipeline cylinders of oxygen and medical air in the UK have been fitted with pin-index valves with horizontal spindles (Department of Health and Social Security 1984).

Bull-nose valve

This type of valve is found on cylinders which are normally connected directly to the pressure regulators on portable apparatus such as flowmeters or power drills (see Table 10.1).

It has a vertical outlet, with an inside, right hand thread, 15.87 mm (5/8 inch), BS pipe thread screw, and a conical seat which makes a gas-tight connection with the hemispherical connector on the apparatus (the 'bull-nose'). The spindle is horizontal, with a 7.14 mm square cross-section, and has a 27.4 mm A/F gland nut.

It is important to appreciate that the outlet of a bull-nose valve is the same for all the different gases, so it is possible for inadvertent cross-connection to occur.

Handwheel valve

This is usually found only on large nitrous oxide cylinders for pipelines (see Table 10.1). It has a horizontal outlet, with an outside, right-hand thread, 14.4 mm (11/16 inch), 0.127 mm pitch screw, and a removable protective metal cap. A circular metal handwheel is permanently attached to the vertical spindle.

This type of valve (with different outlet dimensions) is also fitted to some domiciliary oxygen cylinders because it is easy to use.

Engravings, marks and labels on cylinders

Engravings or stampings

Test pressure, on the body of the cylinder, or on the valve, or both: e.g. 'TP 220 BAR'; '2500 PSI'.

Dates of tests performed, on the body, or on the valve, or both; usually expressed as the year, or year and quarter, or month and year: e.g. '76'; '76 ④'; '6/87'.

Chemical formula of the gas on pin-index valves: e.g. 'N_2O'.

Tare weight (i.e. weight when empty) on the valve of cylinders of liquefied gases; on those dating from before about 1970 it is expressed in pounds and ounces, e.g. '7 12', but after that in kilograms, e.g. '3.250'.

Miscellaneous: these are usually of no practical relevance to anaesthetists: e.g. owner's identification and cylinder reference number, depot monogram (e.g. the back-to-back letter B for Brentford, or a W with a bar on top for Wolverhampton).

Cylinders complying with BS 5045: Part 1: 1982 show also: (a) BS compliance mark and code mark of material of construction, e.g. 'BS5045/1/CM" (= carbon manganese alloy steel); (b) design minimum water capacity in litres (liquefiable gases); (c) mass of cylinder in kilograms (permanent gases); (d) filling pressure at 15°C in bar (permanent gases); (e) identification mark of Independent Inspecting Authority.

Painted markings

Cylinders which do not carry a cylinder label (see below) have the following painted in stencilled letters (specified in BS 1319:1976):
   size of the cylinder (e.g. 'SIZE C');
   nominal gas capacity (e.g. '450 LITRE');
   name and formula of the gas (e.g. 'CARBON DIOXIDE CO_2')
   Proportions of constituent gases (pre-mixed gases) (e.g. 'He 79% O_2 21%').

Labels

   Cylinder label. On cylinders up to size E this rectangular label (135×80 mm) is attached to the body of the cylinder; on larger cylinders the label is arc shaped and attached to the shoulder (135×33 mm). The label is printed with the standard colours for the gas, and also states the chemical name and chemical symbol of the gas, the cylinder size letter, the nominal cylinder contents in litres, and the full pressure in bar at 15°C (a sight of this can be useful in an examination viva). They also show the appropriate Hazard Warning Sign and SI number, the product licence number for the gas, and specific gas and cylinder handling precautions, and instructions for use.
   Filling label (batch label). This is a circular (25 mm diameter), white or yellow, self-adhesive label attached to the valve. It shows the date of the last filling, a code number for the filling depot, and a filling number (or batch number) which permits the precise details of the manufacture of the gas to be traced.

Pressures in full and discharging cylinders

Permanent gases (oxygen, air, helium, Entonox®)

The pressure in a full cylinder is 137 bar at 15°C: this is an empirical value (equivalent to approximately 2000 pounds per square inch) which represents a compromise between optimum volume of contents and excessive internal pressure. Higher pressures are used outside medicine.
   During emptying the pressure falls in proportion to the volume of gas left in the cylinder providing the temperature remains constant (Boyle's law). When the temperature of the cylinder rises or falls the pressure inside also rises and falls, but this is of little significance in normal ambient conditions: e.g. full cylinder pressure at 15°C = 137 bar; at 40°C = 148 bar; at 0°C = 130 bar.

Liquefiable gases (nitrous oxide, carbon dioxide, cyclpropane)

The pressure in a cylinder is the *vapour pressure of the liquid*, as long as there is any liquid in the cylinder. The vapour pressure increases and decreases in proportion to the temperature of the liquid, and may be calculated by the Antoine equation (Rodgers & Hill 1978). When quoting the pressure the temperature should always be stated; failure to do this has sometimes led to inconsistencies in textbooks: e.g. N_2O vapour pressure at 15°C = 44 bar; at 20°C = 50 bar; at 0°C = 30 bar.

When a cylinder of liquefied gas is discharging continuously the liquid becomes colder than the ambient temperature because the energy used to convert the liquid into gas (the latent heat of vaporization) is taken from the liquid itself as heat, and the rate at which this occurs is usually greater than the rate at which the heat can be replaced from the surroundings through the wall of the cylinder. As the temperature of the liquid falls so the vapour pressure falls.

The liquid may become so cold that the outside wall of the cylinder may be colder than the dew point of the surrounding air, so that water vapour condenses on the cylinder and then freezes. The extent of this on the cylinder does not necessarily indicate the level of the liquid inside.

If the discharge of gas is stopped while there is still liquid in the cylinder, and the liquid is allowed to re-warm, its vapour pressure will increase again. (See Jones 1974 for a fuller discussion).

When all the liquid has been vaporized the pressure of the gas in the cylinder falls in accordance with Boyle's law.

Cylinder filling

Permanent gases

The cylinders are connected together in groups of six to 12, and attached to a filling manifold.

Prepare. The cylinder valves are all opened, and the cylinders are completely emptied through the manifold by a vacuum.

Fill. Gas is put in at a rate calculated to achieve rapid filling without producing excessive heat of compression (an average time for filling is 10 min). The filling stops when a predetermined pressure level is reached, dependent on the ambient temperature. The pressure gauges are checked against an independent reference standard once a month. The filling labels are attached, and then the valves are closed and the cylinders disconnected from the manifold. Complaints have been published of excessive tightness of closure of cylinder valves after filling (Bickford Smith 1983, Carter et al 1985).

Bond. The cylinders are allowed to cool for up to 2 h, and then inspected for leaks. Protective covers are fitted to prevent dirt or water entering the valve (Schiller 1986).

Liquefiable gases

The stages of the process are the same as for permanent gases, but the cylinders are handled individually.

Each cylinder is placed on an electronic weighing machine and connected to an automatic filling manifold. When the cylinder has been emptied by vacuum its tare weight is measured, and then a predetermined mass of liquid is decanted into the cylinder.

The liquid phase of a full cylinder normally occupies about 95% of the internal space of the cylinder and accounts for about 85% of the total gas content. The maximum permitted mass of liquid is determined by the filling ratio.

Filling ratio. This is defined as the mass of gas put into the cylinder divided by the mass of water at 15°C required to fill the empty cylinder completely (Gray & Richardson 1985): e.g. size E N_2O cylinder: filling ratio = 0.75, weight of water to fill cylinder = 4.5 kg, therefore weight of N_2O to be added = $4.5 \times 0.75 = 3.4$ kg.

The filling ratio is a safety precaution to limit the number of molecules of gas put into a cylinder in order to prevent an excessive rise in internal pressure at an increased temperature. Different filling ratios are specified for each liquefied gas (British Standard BS 5355:1976).

Tracey et al (1984) reported the explosion of a medical carbon dioxide cylinder which had been over-filled (Gray & Richardson 1985).

Storage and handling of cylinders

Main store. This is a specially designed, outdoor, locked store, where deliveries and collections take place. Medical gas cylinders are stored separately and segregated into different gases, both full and empty. Cylinders of liquefied gas and size F cylinders and larger are stored vertically, and size E and smaller are stored horizontally.

Ready use store. A small number (up to 24 h supply) of spare cylinders may be stored near to where they are used, e.g. in an operating department or intensive therapy unit.

Special considerations

Entonox® cylinders are protected from cold to prevent separation of the gases. With a small Entonox® cylinder (up to 5.5 l water capacity) the user should ensure that it has been adequately warmed, or keep the cylinder at a temperature above 10°C for 2 h before using it, and in any case should invert the cylinder three times before connecting it to the apparatus (BS 1319:1976). Large cylinders (more than 5.5 l water capacity, not normally used in clinical practice) may only be used after being stored horizontally at a temperature above 10°C for 24 h (BS 1319:1976).

Cyclopropane is not subject to the Highly Flammable Liquids and LPG Regulations, but storage and handling should 'meet the overall requirements of these Regulations and the Health and Safety Executive Guidance Notes' (Department of Health and Social Security 1985). As a general principle cyclopropane cylinders are kept away from cylinders containing oxidizing gases, but because only a small number is involved some compromise is permitted in the main store. However, only one cyclopropane cylinder may be kept in the ready use store.

Handling

Gas cylinders should always be handled carefully. Large cylinders (size F and larger) should only be moved on a trolley (British Standard BS 2718:1979). Cylinders of liquefied gas must be used vertically, with the valve uppermost, otherwise liquid may be discharged through the valve outlet.

Smoking and naked lights should be prohibited in the vicinity of gas cylinders. The intensification of combustion in the presence of oxygen or nitrous oxide is extremely dramatic. Unfortunately there are regular accidents involving patients who attempt to smoke while inhaling oxygen (Howard 1987).

Cylinders which are not being used should be turned off. A fireman was fatally injured in a fire in an Intensive Care Unit when gas escaped from cylinders which had been left in a storeroom with their valves open (Department of Health and Social Security 1982).

Lubricants must not be used on medical gas equipment, because they may be ignited by the heat generated by a sudden rise in pressure: the combination of this with the intensification of combustion by the gas can start a self-sustaining fire.

It is good practice to use one of the commercial labels or clips on the neck of a cylinder to indicate whether it is 'Full', 'In Use' or 'Empty' (Department of Health and Social Security 1987, Ward 1985).

Opening a cylinder

First the protective coloured wrapping ('Viskring') is removed from the valve outlet. Then the valve is opened momentarily to clear any debris from the outlet with a short blast of gas. Then the cylinder is connected to the apparatus with an appropriate compressible washer.

Rapid increases in pressure are dangerous because they generate heat, and can also damage the equipment downstream, so the valve should be opened slowly to its full extent. If there is any leakage of gas it may be coming from around the spindle, and can be corrected by tightening the gland nut. If this is not effective the valve should be closed, and the cylinder marked as faulty.

Further information on cylinder handling

1. Health Equipment Information HEI 163 'Code of practice: Safety and care in the storage, handling and use of medical gas cylinders on Health Authority premises' (Department of Health and Social Security 1987).

2. Safety Action Bulletin No 48 (Department of Health 1989).

3. 'Code of practice for the storage of medical, pathology and industrial gas cylinders' (Department of Health and Social Security 1985), which is based on national legislation such as the Highly Flammable Liquids and Liquefied Petroleum Gases Regulations 1972, and the Health and Safety at Work Act 1974.

Periodic tests

Cylinders are tested to detect any splits in their walls caused by the repeated expansions and contractions, which could cause them to burst under pressure. BS 5430:1977 states that the owners of cylinders are responsible for ensuring that they are tested every five years.

General inspection of the cylinder

The tare weight is checked, the outer surface is inspected and the cylinder is struck lightly to elicit a ringing sound. The inner surface is examined with an endoscope to detect any deformity or crack.

Hydraulic proof pressure test

This test has replaced the former 'stretch' test. The cylinder is filled with water and connected to a special test rig in which it is pressurized to at least 50% above its working pressure for 2 min, during which it is checked for any loss of pressure. The water is then removed and the inside of the cylinder is dried with nitrogen gas. Approximately one in ten cylinders fails the proof pressure test. (There are occasional reports of water being found in medical gas cylinders during use (e.g. Mowbray 1988, Schiller 1986), but this is an unlikely source.)

Nitrous oxide and cyclopropane cylinders may be tested hydraulically at intervals of up to 10 years, with only a general inspection every five years (BS 5430:1977).

Record of tests

The year in which the tests were performed is marked permanently on the cylinder.

A colour coded plastic test collar is inserted between the neck of the cylinder and the valve to denote the year in which the next tests are due.

Further information about cylinders

Other descriptions of cylinders can be found in Dorsch & Dorsch (1984), Halsey & White (1980), Parbrook et al (1985), Petty (1987) and Ward (1985).

ACKNOWLEDGEMENTS

The author acknowledges with gratitude the considerable help he has received from BOC Medical Gases. Thanks are also due to Air Products Ltd, Imperial Chemical Industries PLC, Kingston Medical Gases Ltd, Medigas Ltd, Puritan-Bennett Corporation, USA, Socsil-Inter S.A., Switzerland, and John M. Wynne of Anaquest, USA.

REFERENCES

Bickford Smith P J 1983 BOC cylinder valve keys and tight valves. Anaesthesia 38: 1232
BOC Gases 1985 Personal communication
British Standard BS 1319:1976 Medical gas cylinders, valves and yoke connections. British Standards Institution, 2 Park Street, London W1A 2BS
British Standard BS 2718:1979 Specification for gas cylinder trolleys. British Standards Institution, 2 Park Street, London W1A 2BS
British Standard BS 5045:1982 Transportable gas containers. Part 1. Specification for seamless steel gas containers above 0.5 litre water capacity. British Standards Institution, 2 Park Street, London W1A 2BS
British Standard BS 5355:1976 Filling ratios and developed pressures for liquefiable and permanent gases. British Standards Institution, 2 Park Street, London W1A 2BS
British Standard BS 5430:1977 Specification for periodic inspection, testing and maintenance of transportable gas containers (excluding dissolved acetylene containers). Part 1. Seamless steel containers. British Standards Institution, 2 Park Street, London W1A 2BS
Carter K B, Gray W M, Shaw A 1985 Overtightened cylinder valves. Anaesthesia 40: 498
Department of Health 1989 Safety Action Bulletin No 48. Medical Gas Cylinders: Safety and care in their storage, handling and use. SAB(89)28. Department of Health, 14 Russell Square, London WC1B 5EP
Department of Health and Social Security 1982 Safety Information Bulletin SIB(6)1. Medical gas cylinders: Fire hazard. Department of Health and Social Security, 14 Russell Square, London WC1B 5EP
Department of Health and Social Security 1984 Notice WKO(84)3. Pin-indexing of 'J' size cylinders of medical air and oxygen. Department of Health and Social Security, Euston Tower, 286 Euston Road, London NW1 3DN
Department of Health and Social Security 1985 Notice WKO(85)1. Code of practice for the storage of medical, pathology and industrial gas cylinders. Department of Health and Social Security, Euston Tower, 286 Euston Road, London NW1 3DN
Department of Health and Social Security 1987 Health Equipment Information HEI 163: Code of practice: Safety and care in the storage, handling and use of medical gas cylinders on Health Authority premises. Department of Health and Social Security, 14 Russell Square, London WC1B 5EP
Dorsch J A, Dorsch S E 1984 Understanding anesthesia equipment. Construction, care and complications, 2nd edn. Williams & Wilkins, Baltimore
Feeley T W, Bancroft M L, Brooks R A, Hedley-Whyte J 1978 Potential hazards of compressed gas cylinders. A review. Anesthesiology 48: 72–74
Grant W J 1978 Medical gases. Their properties and uses. H.M. & M., Aylesbury
Gray W M, Richardson W 1985 Filling CO_2 cylinders. Anaesthesia 40: 504
Halsey M J, White D C 1980 Gas and vapour supply. In: Gray T C, Nunn J F, Utting J E (eds) General anaesthesia, 4th edn. Butterworth, London, pp 943–949

Helliwell P J 1982 The Association of Anaesthetists of Great Britain and Ireland 1932–82. Fifty years of service to the specialty of anaesthesia. Anaesthesia 37: 913–923

Hogg C E 1973 Pin-indexing failures. Anesthesiology 38: 85–87

House of Commons 1985 Twelfth Report from the Committee of Public Accounts, Session 1984–85: British Oxygen Company and the National Health Service (HC 67). HMSO, London

Howard P 1987 Oxygen therapy. Wright, Bristol

Howell R S C 1980 Piped medical gas and vacuum systems. Anaesthesia 35: 676–698

Howell R S C 1990 Medical gases 1—manufacture and uses. In: Kaufman L (ed) Anaesthesia review 7. Churchill Livingstone, Edinburgh, pp 87–103

Jayasuriya J P 1986 Another example of Murphy's law—mix up of pin index valves. Anaesthesia 41: 1164

Jones P L 1974 Some observations on nitrous oxide cylinders during emptying. Br J Anaesth 46: 534–538

Kumar P, Mishra L D 1986 Deviation from international colour codes. Anaesthesia 41: 1055–1056

MacGregor W G, Bracken A, Fair J A 1972 Piped premixed 50% nitrous oxide and 50% oxygen mixture (Entonox®). A study of the behaviour of the mixture when supplied from a bank of cylinders fitted with internal tubes. Anaesthesia 27: 14–24

MacMillan R R, Marshall M A 1981 Failure of the pin index system on a Cape Waine Ventilator. Anaesthesia 36: 334–335.

Mowbray A 1968 Oxygen cylinder contamination. Today's Anaesthetist 3: 86–88

Orr I A, Hamilton L 1985 Entonox® hazard. Anaesthesia 40: 496

Parbrook G D, Davis P D, Parbrook E O 1985 Basic physics and measurement in anaesthesia, 2nd edn. Heinemann, London

Petty C 1987 The anesthesia machine. Churchill Livingstone, New York

Rodgers R C, Hill G E 1978 Equations for vapour pressure versus temperature: derivation and use of the Antoine Equation on a hand-held programmable calculator. Br J Anaesth 50: 415–424

Sawhney K K, Yoon Y K 1983 Erroneous labeling of a nitrous oxide cylinder. Anesthesiology 59: 260

Schiller D J 1986 Rusty water in an oxygen flowmeter. Anaesthesia 41: 1061

Sprague D H, Archer G W 1975 Intraoperative hypoxia from an erroneously filled liquid oxygen reservoir. Anesthesiology 42: 360–362

Sykes W S, 1960 Essays on the first hundred years of anaesthesia, Volume II. Churchill Livingstone, Edinburgh

Tracey J A, Kennedy J, Magner J 1984 Explosion of a carbon dioxide cylinder. Anaesthesia 39: 938–939

Ward C S 1985 Anaesthetic equipment. Physical principles and maintenance, 2nd edn. Bailliere Tindall, London

Wyant G M 1978 Mechanical misadventures in anaesthesia. University of Toronto Press, Toronto

11. Audit in anaesthesia

J. Secker-Walker

Medical audit can be defined as a systematic process by which a group of clinicians agree upon levels of excellence in practice, monitor whether they are being achieved, and then resolve any deficits found. Failure to resolve deficits discovered and bring about change in clinical practice effectively negates the whole purpose of audit.

Recognition by the medical profession of the need to put some measure on the success and failure of medical care started some years ago in this country (Dudley 1974, Shaw 1980) and considerably before that in North America; indeed the idea of audit probably dates from the 'end result idea of hospital organization' concept of the American Dr Ernest A Codman in about 1900 at the Massachusetts General Hospital (Roberts et al 1987). It was probably largely due to this remarkable man and his friendship with Dr Edward Martin that the American College of Surgeons held a conference on Hospital Standardization in October 1917 and two months later on 20 December formally established the Hospital Standardization Program. By October 1919, 692 hospitals of over 100 beds had been surveyed and only 82 had met the required standards.

MINIMUM STANDARDS

The five minimum standards, which are as valid today in the UK as 70 years ago in the USA (American College of Surgeons 1924), required all doctors allowed to practice in a hospital to be organized as a group, that all members of the group should be properly qualified, and should be competent in their respective fields and worthy in character. The third requirement was that the doctors should adopt rules, regulations and policies governing the professional work of the hospital and should hold monthly meetings to review and analyse their clinical experience. The fourth standard required that accurate and complete records should be kept for all patients and should be filed in an accessible manner. The fifth standard demanded diagnostic and therapeutic facilities under competent supervision to include a chemical serological and bacteriological laboratory and an X-ray department.

In 1951 the American College of Physicians joined the Surgeons to form the Joint Commission on Accreditation of Hospitals. By 1970 the Commission had altered the requirement from minimum standards to the optimal achievable standard which they published in 1971 (Joint Commission on Accreditation of Hospitals 1971). Today there is little doubt that the requirements of the Joint Commission are a major driving force behind medical quality assurance in the USA. The whole process is based on the concept of setting standards of practice against which actual performance is measured.

No such accreditation of hospitals took place in the UK, probably because from 1948 all hospitals were effectively nationalized and presumed to be of a common (high) standard. Despite this, the Royal College of Obstetricians and Gynaecologists set up the Confidential Enquiry into Maternal Deaths in the 1930s and the DHSS acknowledged this as a formal audit in 1952.

The Royal Colleges have reviewed departments of hospitals for suitability for junior staff training since 1976 and the recent acceleration of the importance of medical audit has been largely due to the Royal Colleges, inspired by the report of a Confidential Enquiry into Perioperative Deaths (CEPOD) in 1987 (Buck et al 1987) and the 1982 report by Lunn & Mushin (1982) on mortality associated with anaesthesia. Surgical audit had been carried out by some pioneers prior to this, Irving & Temple (1976) and Gough et al (1980) amongst them. In 1989 the Royal College of Physicians and the Royal College of Surgeons of England each published recommendations concerning the need for medical audit and now require evidence that audit takes place as a criterion for the renewal of training approval in postgraduate medical education. The UK Government of the late 1980s appeared to have a policy of making establishment monopolies more accountable for their actions and the publication of the White Paper 'Working for patients' (Department of Health 1989) to reorganize the NHS laid great stress on the importance of medical audit. It could be said that the White Paper appeared to confuse audit with hospital accreditation. The fundamental difference between the two is that the former is an activity carried out locally by individual firms and departments reviewing their activity and setting their own standards, whilst accreditation is the requirement to meet national standards of performance and quality.

The primary aim of medical audit is to set standards and monitor and improve the quality of patient care. At the same time it should be an educational activity and will often indicate areas where patient care can be delivered more efficiently. The word efficiently inevitably involves examination of the cost of care whether in terms of time, staff or money. In a cash limited environment one profligate doctor deprives another's patient of the resources for medical care.

Medical practice can be considered in terms of the structure, process and outcome of medical care. The *structure* is the organization within which we practice, be that the district, hospital, anaesthetic department, or operating

Table 11.1   Structure of a
department of anaesthesia

- Administration
- Guidelines
- Call rota
- Safety checks
- Equipment
- Recovery facilities

theatre. There are areas in all of these aspects of our work where we can attempt to set standards to change our working environment for the better so that patient care and safety improves and that our staff are encouraged to function to the best of their abilities.

The *process* of medical care is the area that receives most attention when audit is discussed since it focuses on the interaction between doctor and patient. It is not uncommon when first embarking on medical audit to assume that the collection of large quantities of data will of itself produce useful results, and the temptation to purchase a computer and software before considering the questions that need to be addressed by that software is usually overwhelming.

Finally, *outcome* of care is the area most difficult to measure in most fields of medicine (although much talked about) and there is still much work to be done in this area. One outstanding example of the audit process improving outcome comes from the Lothian surgeons (Gruer et al 1986) who demonstrated that by concentrating specialist work into the fields where individual surgeons had the least morbidity, outcomes for patients improved. In anaesthesia the area of outcome is perhaps easier to measure since the vast majority of patients recover from anaesthesia, the mortality rate is extremely low, and major complications are rare.

STRUCTURE

Table 11.1 indicates aspects of the structure of a department of anaesthesia that can be considered in audit, and these will be considered in turn.

Administration

Investigation of critical incidents, principally the work of Cooper (1984) at Harvard University has shown that poor anaesthetic organization was a factor responsible for 33% of incidents that led to *substantive negative outcomes* and this illustrates the importance that an efficiently run department has on the care of the patient.

One of the important features of a well run department is a clearly explicit mechanism by which the department is managed day-to-day on the one hand, and strategic planning for the future is undertaken on the other.

This requires the election of a Director (or chairman of Division) who is ultimately responsible to the District General Manager for the safe and efficient supply of anaesthetic services. The Director then appoints colleagues to undertake different aspects of the task. In larger hospitals the day-to-day rota management is often deputed to a senior registrar, whilst care of postgraduate teaching, ensuring a balanced training programme for junior staff, the equipment replacement programme, pastoral care of junior staff etc., is delegated to consultant colleagues.

It is the responsibility of the Director to ensure that the hospital management provide appropriate staff to assist anaesthetists to perform in safety where and when necessary (Association of Anaesthetists of Great Britain and Ireland 1988b).

The quality of postgraduate education and training is fundamental to excellence in a department. The consultant responsible should aim to motivate consultants and junior staff to keep abreast of new developments, and postgraduate education is a field where it is easy to set standards and monitor attainment. Such standards might involve encouraging all staff to take maximum study leave with records of courses attended, ensuring that weekly programmes relate to the training needs of the junior staff, keeping records of attendance at lectures, and using questionnaires to measure the perceived quality of teaching. The Association of Anaesthetists of Great Britain and Ireland (1988c, 1989) has published handbooks on the duties of Chairmen of Divisions of Anaesthesia and on consultant:trainee relationships and whilst each department should set its own standards these publications provide an invaluable starting point.

Guidelines

It is important that a department has clear guidelines and policies on how to deal with certain situations. AIDS and hepatitis pose a risk to anaesthetists and audit can play a part in ensuring that agreed policies, perhaps following the guidelines suggested by the Association of Anaesthetists of Great Britain and Ireland (1988a) are followed. Gaba et al (1987) advises written protocols for rapidly propagating incidents such as malignant hyperpyrexia and cardiac arrest. Adequate knowledge within the department of how to react to a major disaster or a fire in the operating theatre need to be tested from time to time, as does a clear understanding of the 'three wise men' and 'sick doctor' procedures.

Call rota

An important feature of the structure of an anaesthetic department is the organization of the call rota. This requires that junior staff get adequate exposure to emergency cases without having to work hours that are excessive for either their own health or that of the patient. Surprisingly, neither the Lunn & Mushin (1982) nor the CEPOD report (Buck et al 1987) indicate that fatigue of the anaesthetist has much relation to anaesthetic mortality; anaesthetic audit, however, may in time point to other less serious negative outcomes that are associated with fatigue. There is no easy solution to arrive at the ideal balance, especially in view of present government initiatives, but that does not mean that a department cannot set a standard of the optimum number of hours that any member of staff should be expected to work without proper sleep or food. The fact that the achievement of the standard cannot be reached because of outside constraints in no way negates the standard, rather it provides ammunition in the battle for better staffing or resources.

Safety checks

There is evidence that patient safety is enhanced if the anaesthetic equipment, machine, ventilator and monitors are subject to a routine series of checks (as in aircraft) before a patient is anaesthetized (Cundy & Baldock 1982, Heath 1983, Ward 1985). Craig & Wilson (1981) felt failure of 'cockpit drill' was the commonest associated human failure relating to their survey of anaesthetic misadventures. The Lunn & Mushin report (1982) showed that in 17.8% of the cases they considered, the anaesthetic machine was not tested before use, whilst Cooper et al (1984) felt equipment inspection prior to use was a key strategy in mishap prevention. Anaesthesia audit should ensure that the relevant protocols are in place and measure from time to time the extent to which those protocols are followed.

Equipment

Although equipment failure is a relatively small factor as a cause of anaesthetic mortality (Buck et al 1987) and only accounts for 14% of critical incidents (Cooper et al 1978), there is evidence that equipment design is a factor associated with human error as a cause of anaesthetic incidents (Cooper et al 1984). The development of a rational equipment programme with a suitable budget is the responsibility of the director of the department or his or her appointed deputy. The programme needs to take into account proper training of anaesthetic staff on all equipment in use, standards required for monitoring, regular servicing, the depreciation cost of equipment, the likely useful life and the need for uniformity, simplicity and safety of design on the one hand and diversity for teaching on the other. In addition to the increased safety of having uniform equipment in each theatre, there are cost advantages. Bulk buying of equipment almost invariably allows considerable discounts to be obtained and servicing costs tend to be less with one company servicing ten pieces of equipment rather than ten companies each servicing one.

Table 11.2   Process of anaesthetic care

- When to call
- Premedication visits
- Clinical manoeuvres
- Monitoring
- Supervision
- Drug usage
- Post-operative care

Recovery facilities

It is the responsibility of the department of anaesthesia to ensure that the health authority provides safe recovery facilities up to the standard recommended by the Association of Anaesthetists of Great Britain and Ireland (1985, 1988d) that these are available whenever required, and have adequate equipment and monitoring systems. Gaba et al (1987) suggest that such equipment should be subject to regular inspection and testing. The recovery room is an invaluable source for research and audit into outcome in anaesthesia and many American hospitals assign junior residents to this area as part of their training as demonstrated by the 1987/88 report from Yale University (Annual Report 1987/88).

PROCESS

It is the process and outcome of anaesthesia that can be analysed after the collection of data on anaesthetic. Methods of data collection will be described later in this chapter, but the collection of quantities of facts without a standard against which to measure them will elicit the 'so what?' response. Table 11.2 provides an illustration of the areas in the process of anaesthetic care that can be considered as part of medical audit where standards can be set by the department.

When to call

There is a need for explicit guidelines, known to all members of the department, about the expected levels of responsibility. These will probably be related to the age of the patient and should take into account the recommendations of the 1989 Report of the National Confidential Enquiry into Perioperative Deaths (NCEPOD 1990): what grade of staff can anaesthetize a neonate; is a consultant anaesthetist contacted whenever a child is scheduled for surgery?; the physical status of the patient should be assessed perhaps using the ASA scale (Saklad 1941); the type of operation or even perhaps the surgeon! Subsequent analysis of the audit data may then show, for example, that a particular member of staff is ignoring the guidelines and undertaking cases inappropriate to his or her experience.

Pre-operative visits

It is generally accepted that a pre-operative visit by an anaesthetist is good practice, is appreciated by the patient, and allows a risk assessment, a subject which has been fully reviewed by Derrington & Smith (1987). Lack of pre-operative assessment is an associated factor in up to 30% of anaesthetic incidents (Cooper et al 1984). It is explicitly a part of the workload for consultant anaesthetists approved by the College of Anaesthetists and the DHSS (Association of Anaesthetists of Great Britain and Ireland 1983) and is also a requirement for General Professional Training (Faculty of Anaesthetists 1987). The department of anaesthesia needs to establish the ground rules for premedication since although ideally a patient should be seen by the doctor who will give the anaesthetic there are many instances where this is impossible due to either geography or time. For certain types of patients, such as small children or in obstetrics, it may be appropriate for the department to have premedication protocols.

Clinical manoeuvres

Some countries practice anaesthesia in a way that requires adherence to a protocol for any particular anaesthetic problem, and Cooper et al (1984) and Gaba et al (1987) both suggest the development of protocols as a means of preventing anaesthetic accidents. Up until now the NHS has allowed doctors to practise as they saw fit being accountable to their patients and the General Medical Council with the defence societies paying the cost of any resulting litigation. As a result, rigid protocols of what technique and what drugs to use for any particular situation are very uncommon. Some generally accepted protocols exist, such as the treatment of the child with a bleeding tonsillar bed, failed intubation at Caesarian section or the practice of crash induction.

The change on 1 January 1990 whereby the employing authorities in the NHS became financially responsible for the costs of medical litigation against their medical employees may have a profound effect on medical practice, since if medical audit shows that certain procedures or treatments are associated with increased complications, morbidity or litigation, then it is likely that the Authority will require that doctors conform to practices that the Authority considers safe. Indeed the relationship between medical audit and risk management is inevitably close and will probably lead to anaesthetic departments having to be more specific about what techniques should be used for each eventuality. Even before this happens it is probably beneficial for junior staff to have clear protocols for certain situations. Three of these have already been mentioned. Others might include best anaesthetic practice for emergency surgery of aortic aneurysm rupture, transposition of free flaps in reconstructive surgery, drainage of subdural haematoma and safe techniques for hypotension and when hypotension is appropriate. To arrive at a standard for the department for any particular situation requires a literature search and discussion of available material before the optimum technique is chosen, an exercise that must have considerable educational benefits for all concerned.

Monitoring

The Lunn & Mushin report (1982) recommended that minimal standards of monitoring should be an ECG, a means of taking blood pressure, and a device to measure the volume of ventilation for artificially ventilated patients. Since that time Harvard Medical School has published its standards for patient monitoring during anaesthesia (Eichorn et al 1986), adoption of which has led to a decrease in malpractice claims and subsequent reduction in the rate of increase of malpractice insurance premiums for those working in suitably equipped departments. The American Society of Anesthesiologists adopted the Harvard Standards in 1986 (American Society of Anesthesiologists 1986) and Cass et al (1988) from Australia published standards in 1988, the same year that the Association of Anaesthetists published its recommendations. Anaesthetic audit systems should be able to log the monitoring associated with each case and individual departments should either adopt the Association standards which require 'clinical observations augmented, *where appropriate*, by the use of continuously-acting monitoring devices' or go beyond them to set a departmental standard requiring the use of automatic monitors on all patients in addition to clinical observations. It has yet to be demonstrated in the UK that improved monitoring has reduced litigation costs although it would seem probable that it will in due course. However, monitoring can help reduce the cost of an anaesthetic. Use of capnography allows control of minute volume in ventilated patients to maintain a normal CO_2. This often requires a minute volume as little as 3 l, with a subsequent reduction in volume of expensive isoflurane or enflurane that is vaporized.

Supervision

Both the Lunn & Mushin (1982) and the CEPOD (Buck et al 1987) reports comment that peri-operative mortality is to some degree related to the level of supervision of trainees in anaesthesia, especially in the very sick, urgent or emergency cases. Cooper et al (1984) demonstrated that lack of supervision was the single most frequent factor in anaesthetic mishaps and suggested improved supervision to be a key strategy in mishap prevention. The assessors in anaesthesia in the CEPOD report were surprised that no consultant was responsible for some elective lists and felt it was 'rubbish' to state that no one was responsible for what trainees do. It is clear from the reports that the majority of non-routine cases at night and weekends are carried out by trainees. The Royal College of Surgeons has recently published guidelines on consultant responsibility in invasive surgical procedures (Commission on the Provision of Surgical Services 1990) which recommend explicit consultant responsibility for every procedure under-taken. The College of Anaesthetists' general professional training guide requires a *minimum* of three lists a week to be carried out in the presence of a consultant which is approximately 33% of routine work. Bearing in mind comments from these sources, it is up to the individual department to decide what is a proper degree of supervision for its junior staff. What is appropriate for a senior registrar is not obviously for a new SHO. Once the standard is set for the amount of supervision in each grade, it is not difficult to analyse audit data on a monthly basis to ascertain whether or not the standard is achieved.

Drug usage

Resource management and budgets are related to medical audit albeit indirectly. An anaesthesia department's budget usually has a drug usage component and although this, in real terms, is a small proportion of the total budget, changes and improvements in anaesthetic drugs can make a significant difference to budget management (Lethbridge & Secker-Walker 1986). The cost of propofol is nearly five times that of thiopentone, and isoflurane about twice that of enflurane and whilst there are undoubtedly specific indications for both of the more expensive drugs, considerable savings can be made by using the cheaper drugs unless specific indications are actually satisfied. The savings made can then be used in ways that may indirectly benefit other patients, as in postgraduate courses or new and safer equipment purchase. This process requires that the department decides the criteria that need to be satisfied before using certain types of drug and then monitors through the audit that staff are following those criteria.

Post-operative care

Like pre-operative care, post-operative care is included in the pattern of workload for consultant anaesthetists (Association of Anaesthetists of Great Britain and Ireland 1983) and is a requirement for General Professional Training (Faculty of Anaesthetists 1987). Holland (1987) identifies inadequate post-operative care as a contribution to anaesthetic mortality. For logistical reasons it is often very difficult for an anaesthetist to follow up all patients; however, a department should decide what is good practice in the interests of the patient and the trainee and attempt to tailor the organization of rotas to allow the maximum effective post-operative care. Discussions with the surgeons are essential to demarcate whose responsibility is what. American practice of allocating a trainee to the recovery room for a period, with the added task of following up the patients

Table 11.3   Outcome of anaesthesia

- Mortality
- Clinical morbidity
- Adverse events/critical incidents
- Prolonged hospital stay
- Unanticipated admission to ICU
- Hospital admission after day-stay

who pass through it onto the wards for the first 48 h after operation has much to commend it.

OUTCOME

Table 11.3 indicates areas that can be considered when auditing the outcome of anaesthesia. Departments of anaesthesia have traditionally held *mortality* and *morbidity* meetings to discuss major complications and these are a valid means of audit, provided recommendations are made to prevent the preventable occurring again, together with a means of measuring whether it does. Nine out of ten patients have no complications at all, 0.45% suffer a major complication, and of the minor complications, nausea, sore throat and headache are the commonest, as demonstrated by Cohen et al (1986) in a review of 112 000 anaesthetics in one teaching hospital.

The total death rate due to surgery and anaesthesia quoted by the CEPOD report is 0.7%. In 14.1% of these deaths, anaesthesia was felt to have played some part and in only three of nearly half a million operations was anaesthesia totally to blame for the death of the patient. Prior to this report there had been at least three previous surveys of deaths related to anaesthesia. Edwards et al (1956) looked at 1000 deaths over a five and a half year period whilst Dinnick (1964) reviewed a further 600 cases. Both these surveys were unable to measure the total cases performed and therefore gave no death rate or incidence. Both felt that a major factor in the great majority of deaths was departure from accepted anaesthetic practice and the CEPOD report found that failure to apply knowledge was associated with 75% of deaths. The Lunn & Mushin report (1982) gave the incidence of death related to anaesthesia alone (1 in 10 000) and showed that 1 in 166 (0.6%) patients died within six days of surgery, but like the previous works was not able to combine the influence of surgery on the outcome.

The department of anaesthesia will need to decide what time interval between anaesthesia and death will count as an 'anaesthetic death', bearing in mind the difficulty of keeping track of patients in hospitals with short lengths of stay and high throughput. It is unlikely that most departments will have many deaths or cases of serious morbidity to review each year, but each needs to be carefully researched and presented with a view to the degree of risk assessment prior to the operation. An index could be used as suggested by Goldman et al (1977); was the death preventable, were the anaesthetic notes of proper standard and what can be done in future to improve practice.

Adverse events

It is sensible to consider adverse events under two headings; complications that arise during anaesthesia because of the anatomy, physiology or pathology of the patient and critical incidents that arise from human error or mechanical or electrical failure, or a combination.

Complications during anaesthesia

Several papers have reported the presence of more than one identifiable complication in relation to an anaesthetic death (Cooper et al 1984, Holland 1987, Strunin et al 1988) which bears out the feeling most anaesthetists have that the actual disasters or near misses they experience are due to several, often minor factors all occurring at about the same time. Recording of complications arising during anaesthesia is notoriously difficult although it must be an essential part of anaesthetic audit. A single ventricular ectopic can be classified as an arrhythmia but hardly constitutes a complication. Thus it is important to have clear definitions, in this case perhaps a complication would be an arrhythmia requiring some form of treatment. Some complications may only become apparent to the patient after the post-operative visit of the anaesthetist; the painful thrombosed vein on the back of the hand that may last for several weeks, the headache after the day case returns home. The anaesthetist may forget to log a complication that was minor and quickly rectified or may deliberately not log it for fear of possible litigation or embarrassment before colleagues, although this can be improved by a third party keeping the audit record (Cooper et al 1984). The issue of audit records remaining undiscoverable by a litigant has been raised (Secker-Walker et al 1989) but the problem is not yet resolved. In addition to recording the fact that a complication occurred, it is important to grade its severity, and this applies equally to critical incidents. Scoring can be done on a simple 4 point scale as in the Bloomsbury Anaesthetic Audit; 1, a complication unnoticed by the patient with no action required; 2, an event that is potentially harmful to the patient but which is successfully remedied; 3, an event causing actual harm to the patient; and 4, an event that causes serious harm to the patient. Lack (personal communication, 1990) suggests a different 5 point classification which includes death, whilst another 3 point scale has been suggested by Derrington & Smith (1987). For inter-hospital comparison it would be useful to arrive at nationally agreed definitions.

Critical incidents

The logging of critical incidents is now considered to be an important factor in research into and prevention of anaesthetic accidents, and the first report of the audit committee of the College of Anaesthetists (personal communication, November 1989) suggests a register of critical incidents as part of the audit process. The work of Cooper et al (1978) from Harvard has undoubtedly made an enormous contribution to knowledge in this field together with research into human factors in aircraft accidents from the Institute of Aviation Medicine and Army Personnel Research Establishment. Cooper showed that 82% of preventable incidents involved human error, with breathing circuit disconnections, inadvertant changes in gas flow and errors with drug syringes being the most frequent. Straightforward equipment failure accounted for only 14% of the total number of preventable incidents, but equipment design was partially involved with many of the human errors. The importance of choosing the most appropriate equipment in terms of function and design cannot be over emphasized and needs to have a major priority in the deliberations of every anaesthetic department.

Cooper et al (1978) also showed that contrary to popular belief the majority (42%) of incidents occur during the middle of the surgical procedure with 26% during induction, 17% at the beginning of the procedure and 9% at the end. Craig & Wilson (1981) showed that human error was responsible for 65% of anaesthetic mishaps with 12% being a combination of human and equipment failure and Cooper et al (1984) reviewed 1089 incidents (which resulted in 70 substantive negative outcomes) and suggested a list of key strategies for mishap prevention. He indicated that critical incidents were more likely to lead to a substantive negative outcome in patients graded ASA III or worse, a substantive negative outcome being defined as death, cardiac arrest, cancelled operative procedure or extended stay in recovery ICU, or hospital. Allnut (1987) points out that the memory of participants in an accident starts to decay rapidly after the event and with absolute integrity the individual starts to report not what happened but what must have happened.

An audit system needs to pick up critical incidents, as they occur, as part of the overall data on each case. With a suitable relational database it is possible to pick out patterns of events that may lead to changes that prevent further similar incidents occurring. The Joint Commission on Accreditation of Healthcare Organizations (1988) have published their potential anaesthesia care clinical indicators in which they list 14 adverse events that should always trigger a review of that particular case in the audit meeting, and these include injury to teeth and eyes, headache after epidural or spinal anaesthesia, aspiration pneumonitis, cardiac arrest, myocardial infarction, pulmonary oedema or respiratory arrest within a period of time after anaesthesia specified by the department. In addition, peripheral neurological deficit and injury to the brain or spinal cord need to be reviewed. Other examples of unexpected outcome in anaesthesia are unplanned admission to ICU, admission after day-stay surgery and cancellation of

Table 11.4   Possible agenda for anaesthetic audit meetings

1. Those attending
2. Topics
   —Departmental organization
   —Anaesthetic process. Review of monthly reports
   —Outcomes, morbidity, adverse advents, mortality
3. Conclusions and recommendations reached

surgery due to anaesthetic problems. Departments designing or purchasing audit systems should look for the ability of the system to log these types of event.

METHODS OF AUDIT

Manual

Having decided which areas are suitable for setting standards for medical audit purposes and having decided the type of agenda (Table 11.4) and frequency of the audit meetings, the next task is to decide by what means to review data (although it usually happens the other way round!). There are several ways to achieve this objective. The first requires no computer but dedication and time, and involves random or triggered access to patients' notes with the emphasis in the audit meeting on the quality of the notes, the appropriateness of the technique, the degree of monitoring and any problems with outcome. The trigger can be any untoward occurrence, most of which have already been discussed. The disadvantage of this system is that it does not collect quantities of data from which to build up patterns of events or complications, nor does it allow records of the degree of super-vision and experience of trainees.

Computer datasets

Other methods are more likely to be used in the future and rely on computers to store and analyse large quantities of information that satisfy the needs of audit, record a trainee's pattern of experience and perhaps maintain the business plan for the department. An audit system needs to address details of the time and date of the operation, where it took place and the code number of the anaesthetists, indicating who was supervising. There need to be some patient detail, their ASA grade and the rating of the urgency of their operation as suggested by the CEPOD report (1987). Details of the surgical speciality and the grade and supervision of the operator allow audit across surgical firms, and provide anaesthetic trainees with a pattern of their experience, both in terms of type of surgery, whether routine or emergency, at what time of day, how sick the patient was and whether they were supervised. A section on administrative problems is

IN CONFIDENCE   NOT TO BE INCLUDED IN PATIENT'S NOTES
BLOOMSBURY ANAESTHETIC AUDIT

Anaesthetic location code [   ]   Audit N°.

Date Of Procedure: [:   :   ]

Emergency List[1] ☐   Day Case? Y[1] ☐   N[2] ☐

Day :   Mon [1] ☐ Tue [2] ☐ Wed [3] ☐ Thu [4] ☐ Fri [5] ☐ Sat [6] ☐ Sun [7] ☐

Time of Starting [:   ] (24 hr)

Anaesthetists   i.d. Code: Hrs cont. duty   Primary Anaes   Supervisor
   form-filler →   [   ]   [   ]   ☐   ☐
                     [   ]   [   ]
                     [   ]   ☐   ☐
                                                             ☐   ☐

Patient   Date Of Birth: [:   :   ]

Weight [   ]Kg   White[1] ☐   Non-White[2] ☐

Sex   M[1] ☐ F[2] ☐   CEPOD: Emergency 1 ☐   Obstetric: Scheduled 5 ☐
                                    Urgent 2 ☐   Immediate 6 ☐
ASA Grade [   ]   Scheduled 3 ☐
                                    Elective 4 ☐

Surgical Specialty
   Gen Surg 1 ☐   ENT   7 ☐   Dental/Oral 13 ☐   Endoscopy 20 ☐
   Vascular 2 ☐   Gynaecology 8 ☐   Cardiac 14 ☐ Haematology 21 ☐
   Paed. Surg 3 ☐   Obstetric 9 ☐   Thoracic 15 ☐   Oncology 22 ☐
   Orthopaedic 4 ☐   Plastic 10 ☐   Neuro 16 ☐ Radiotherapy 23 ☐
   Urology 5 ☐   Burns   11 ☐   Ophthalm. 17 ☐   Pain 24 ☐
  Renal Trans. 6 ☐   Max Fac 12 ☐   A/E 18 ☐   ECT 25 ☐
                                     X-ray/Imaging 19 ☐   Other* 26 ☐

            C[1] SR[2] C Ast[3] Reg[4] SHO[5] HO[6] Studt.[7] Anaes only[8] Other[*9]
   1[0] Operator ☐ ☐   ☐   ☐   ☐   ☐   ☐   ☐   ☐

   Supervisor ☐ ☐   ☐   ☐   ☐   ☐   ☐   ☐   ☐

Administrative Problems

Pt not seen pre-theatre?   AA ☐   Inadequate anaesth. seniority?   AF ☐
List details / order incorrect? AB ☐   Full case notes not available?   AG ☐
Trained assistant not avail?   AC ☐   Premed not given as written?   AH ☐
List delayed?   AD ☐   Other*   AI ☐
Results/xmatch unavailable?   AE ☐

Special Survey 1   2   3   4   5   6   7   8   9   10 11   12   13   14   15
  16   17   18   19   18   20   21   22   23   24   25   26   27   28   29   30   31 32
  33   34   35   36   37   38   39   40   41   42   43   44   45   46 47   48   49 50
            * **Enter details in "further reporting" overleaf**

Fig. 11.1   Bloomsbury audit card.

The Anaesthetic

GA ^{1}☐   Region^2☐   GA and Reg ^{3}☐   Other Procedure *^{4}☐
Epidural^1☐   Spinal^2☐   Caudal ^{3}☐   Bier's^4☐   Nerve ^{5}☐   Other*^{6}☐
Local ^{1}☐   Opiate^2☐
Intubated ^{1}☐   Facemask ^{2}☐ Lar mask ^{3}☐   Trach. ^{4}☐   Other*^{5}☐
Spont resp^1☐   Ventilated^2☐ Other *^{3}☐

Fent ^{1}☐   Alfent ^{2}☐   Papav ^{3}☐   Peth ^{4}☐   Other*^{5}☐
Thio ^{1}☐   Propofol ^{2}☐ Methohex^3☐   Other ^{4}☐
Sux ^{1}☐   Atrac ^{2}☐   Vec ^{3}☐   Panc ^{4}☐   Curare ^{5}☐   Other* ^{6}☐
Halothane^1☐   Enflurane^2☐ Isoflurane^3☐

Monitoring

ECG ^{1}☐   Cuff BP^2☐   SpO$_2$ ^{3}☐
E$_T$CO$_2$ ^{4}☐   Pa/w ^{5}☐   VentAlarm^6☐   FiO$_2$ ^{7}☐
Temp ^{8}☐   ArtBP ^{9}☐   CVP ^{10}☐   Wedge ^{11}☐
EEG ^{12}☐   N/M ^{13}☐   Inhal% ^{14}☐   Other* ^{15}☐
None ^{16}☐

Time of Finishing ☐ : ☐

**Adverse Events   None^1☐

	enter score**			enter score**
Inadequate Preop	↓			↓
Sedation	BA ☐	Laryngospasm	BT	☐
Resuscitation	BB ☐	Bronchospasm	BU	☐
Investigation	BC ☐	Accidental one-lung intubation	BV	☐
Local Anaesthetics		Aspiration	BW	☐
Dural Tap	BD ☐	Other*	BX	☐
Incomplete Block	BE ☐	**Difficult Intubation**		
Excess Spread	BF ☐	Successfully achieved	BY	☐
Hypotension	BG ☐	Assistance summoned	BZ	☐
Fitting	BH ☐	Abandoned*	CA	☐
Other*	BI ☐	**Patient Injury**		
Cardiovascular		Eyes	CB	☐
Arrhythmia	BJ ☐	Teeth	CC	☐
Myocardial ischaemia	BK ☐	Diathermy burn	CD	☐
Haemorrhage	BL ☐	Other*	CE	☐
Hypotension	BM ☐	**Prolonged recovery period**	CF	☐
Hypertension	BN ☐	**Critical Incident**		
Arrest	BO ☐	Br. Circuit disconnect	CG	☐
Other*	BP ☐	I.V. disconnect	CH	☐
Atypical Drug Reaction	BQ ☐	Other Technical Failure*	CI	☐
Respiratory		Wrong Drug/Dose	CJ	☐
Resp. Depression	BR ☐	Regurgitation	CK	☐
Inadequate Reversal	BS ☐	Patient unattended *Reason	CL	☐
		Death	CM	☐
		Unforseen Admiss. ITU	CN	☐

**Adverse Event Severity Scores

1 = No action required   2 = Potentially harmful to patient but successfully remedied
3 = Actual Harm to patient   4 = Serious harm to patient

*Details and Further Reporting : (Give box reference)

important to enable audit of such things as availability of the patient's notes or of trained assistance (Assistance for the Anaesthetist 1988), appropriate seniority of anaesthetist or proper premedication. There should be space to record details of the anaesthetic drugs and technique and what monitors were used. It is essential to log the occurrence of adverse advents with a severity index. Space for amplification of answers to set questions and free text are important, as is space for research or special surveys.

Having designed or obtained a suitable dataset, there are then two problems to consider. The first is how to get the information from the anaesthetist into the computer and the second is to decide the most appropriate software to receive it.

Methods of data transfer

Card systems

There are several means of getting the information into the computer. Cards can be filled at the time of operation and transcribed into the database by the anaesthetic secretary. This method developed by Lack (personal communication, 1990) has been in use in Salisbury for three years and has been modified and expanded in Bloomsbury Health Authority as reported to the Annual Scientific Meeting, Association of Anaesthetists, Swansea 1989. Figure 11.1 illustrates the current Bloomsbury Audit Card which gathers much of the available information about every anaesthetic including most of the relevant material described previously, and also allows space for free text and special survey research exercises. It does not have the name or hospital number of the patient to preserve anonymity, nor does it have the name of the operation. The reason for this omission is that for coding purposes and comparison the name of the operation must be exact, repeatable and consistent from week to week and surgeon to surgeon. This is extremely difficult to maintain.

Optical mark readers

A more sophisticated version of the card is the optically mark-read anaesthetic sheet in use by the Anaesthetic Department of the Southern Derbyshire Health Authority. The great advantage of this technology is that there is no requirement of a secretary's time to input the data, and the data can be produced as monthly reports almost automatically. The disadvantage of this system is that quite a lot of the anaesthetic audit sheet is taken up by space for recording date, time, date of birth and the anaesthetist's code number. This leaves less space for recording other data, and does not allow any free text. There is also a significant rate of refusal of sheets by the optical mark reader which then have to be manually entered.

Data loggers

Some departments have opted for the use of data loggers, computer style personal organizers like the Psion Organizer. Here the data is entered on the device in the theatre and then down-loaded onto the departmental computer at the end of the day thus avoiding any transcription onto and off paper. The disadvantage of this method is that the devices are small and fragile and easily 'mislaid'. There would have to be one for each theatre or perhaps each member of the department. The spread of this technology however is such that it is quite conceivable that in a short time all doctors will own and use these devices in much the same way as all doctors own a stethoscope.

Laptop computers

Laptop computers are becoming relatively cheap, they can be used in theatre and they collect and also process data and so can be loaded with the department's chosen software for anaesthetic audit.

Software

To be dogmatic in a book about a particular type of software, or for that matter hardware, makes little sense. The state of the industry is developing and changing so fast that today's choice may have been superseded in a year's time. The development of fourth generation languages and multi-user operating systems may significantly alter available products in the future. The choice of suitable software for anaesthetic audit will need to be determined by six factors: ease of use for clinicians and secretaries including a word processing facility; ability to create graphical reports, alone or batched on a monthly basis; ability to relate all facets of the data one with another (a relational database); ability to interrogate the database on a one-off basis; ability to integrate the system into the overall district information system in due course; and finally cost. The choice needs to be made in the knowledge that the system will be replaced by something superior in a fairly short time. The system in use in Bloomsbury at present is written in Paradox, a relational database working under MS DOS. As far as the future is concerned, a likely development in information technology in the NHS is towards Ingres systems working under the Unix operating system allowing integration of the various intelligent terminals and development of distributed processing where the power to gather and manipulate information, just like the information itself, is distributed throughout the system.

REFERENCES

Allnut M F 1987 Human factors in accidents. Br J Anaesth 59: 856–864

American College of Surgeons 1924 The minimum standard. Bulletin of the American College of Surgeons 8: 1–4

American Society for Anesthesiologists 1986 Standards of basic intraoperative monitoring. Newsletter 50: 9

Annual Report 1987/88. Department of Anesthesiology 1988 Yale University School of Medicine, New Haven, Connecticut

Association of Anaesthetists of Great Britain and Ireland 1983 Workload for consultant anaesthetists. London

Association of Anaesthetists of Great Britain and Ireland 1985 Post anaesthetic recovery facilities. London

Association of Anaesthetists of Great Britain and Ireland 1988a AIDS and hepatitis B. Guidelines for anaesthetists. London

Association of Anaesthetists of Great Britain and Ireland 1988b Assistance for the Anaesthetist. London

Association of Anaesthetists of Great Britain and Ireland 1988c Guidelines on the duties of Chairmen of Divisions of Anaesthesia. London

Association of Anaesthetists of Great Britain and Ireland 1988d Recommendations for standards of monitoring during anaesthesia and recovery. London

Association of Anaesthetists of Great Britain and Ireland 1989 Consultant: Trainee relationships. A guide for consultants. London

Buck N, Devlin H B, Lunn J N 1987 Report of a Confidential Enquiry into Perioperative Deaths (CEPOD) Nuffield Provincial Hospitals Trust/King's Fund, London

Cass N M, Crosby W M, Holland R B 1988 Minimal monitoring standards. Anaesth Intensive Care 16: 110–113

Cohen M H, Duncan P G, Pope W D B et al 1986 A survey of 112 000 anaesthetics at one teaching hospital. Can Anaesth Soc J 33: 22

Commission on the Provision of Surgical Services 1990 Consultant responsibility in invasive surgical procedures. Royal College of Surgeons of England, London

Cooper J B, Newbower R S, Long C D et al 1978 Preventable anesthesia mishaps. Anesthesiology. 49: 399–406

Cooper J B, Newbower R S, Kitz R J 1984 An analysis of major errors and equipment failures in anesthesia management: considerations for prevention and detection. Anesthesiology 60: 34–42

Craig J, Wilson M E 1981 A study of anaesthetic misadventures. Anaesthesia 36: 933–936

Cundy J, Baldock G J 1982 Safety check procedures to eliminate faults in anaesthetic machines. Anaesthesia 37: 161

Department of Health 1989 Working for patients. HMSO, London

Derrington M C, Smith G 1987 A review of studies of anaesthetic risk, morbidity and mortality. Br J Anaesth 59: 815–833

Dinnick O P 1964 Anaesthetic deaths. Anaesthesia 19: 125

Dudley H A F 1974 Necessity for surgical audit. Br Med J 1: 275–277

Edwards G, Morton H J V, Pask E A et al 1956 Deaths associated with anaesthesia. Anaesthesia 11: 194

Eichorn J H, Cooper J B, Cullen D J et al 1986 Standards for patient monitoring during anesthesia at Harvard Medical School. JAMA 256: 1017–1020

Faculty of Anaesthetists 1987 General professional training guide. Faculty of Anaesthetists. Royal College of Surgeons of England, London

Gaba D M, Maxwell M, DeAnda A 1987 Anesthetic mishaps: breaking the chain of accident evolutions. Anesthesiology 66: 670–676

Goldman L, Caldera D L, Nussbaum S R et al 1977 Multifactorial index of cardiac risk in non-cardiac surgical procedures. N Engl J Med 297: 845

Gough M H, Kettlewell M G W, Mark C G et al 1980 Audit: an annual assessment of the work and performance of a surgical firm in a regional teaching hospital. Br Med J 281: 913–918

Gruer R, Gordon D S, Gunn A A et al 1986 Audit of surgical audit. Lancet 1: 23–26

Heath M L 1983 Safety check procedures to eliminate faults in anaesthetic machines. Anaesthesia 38: 297

Holland R 1987 Anaesthetic mortality in New South Wales. Br J Anaesth 59: 834–841

Irving M, Temple J 1976 Surgical audit: one year's experience in a teaching hospital. Br Med J 2: 746–747

Joint Commission on Accreditation of Healthcare Organisations 1988 Potential anaesthesia care clinical indicators. News about the agenda for change: 2 (1), Chicago

Joint Commission on Accreditation of Hospitals 1971 Accreditation manual for hospitals 1970. Chicago

Lethbridge J R, Secker-Walker J 1986 Cost of anaesthetic drugs and clinical budgeting. Br Med J 293: 1587–1588

Lunn J N, Mushin W W 1982 Mortality associated with anaesthesia. Nuffield Provincial Hospitals Trust, London

NCEPOD 1990 National Confidential Enquiry into Perioperative Deaths Report 1989. NCEPOD, London

Roberts J S, Coale J G, Redman R R 1987 A history of the Joint Commission on Accreditation of Hospitals. JAMA 258: 936–940

Royal College of Physicians 1989 Medical audit. London

Royal College of Surgeons of England 1989 Guidelines to clinical audit in surgical practice. London

Saklad M 1941 Grading of patients for surgical procedures. Anesthesiology 2: 281

Secker-Walker J, Purser H, Crown J 1989 Editorial. Development of clinical audit. Br J Hosp Med 42: 169

Shaw C O 1980 Looking forward to audit. Br Med J 28: 1509–1511

Strunin L, Forrest J B, Lunn J N et al 1988 Towards excellence in anaesthesia. Can J Anaesth 35: 278–286

Ward C S 1985 Anaesthetic equipment. 2nd edn. Bailliere Tindall, London

12. Pain

L. Kaufman

The quest for pain relief for a variety of disorders has been with us for many centuries. Many potions and mixtures have been devised in the past for the relief of pain from toothache, trauma, backache, carcinoma as well as the many ill-defined causes. There are many developments in the range of analgesic agents available for administration during operation or in the post-operative period, as well as the use of extradural and spinal techniques. This chapter only reviews some of the recent papers on the subject which is considered also in the Symposium on Aspects of Pain (Symposium on Aspects of Pain 1989).

MECHANISMS OF PAIN

The peripheral mechanisms of somatic pain are discussed in detail by Raja et al (1988). Release of chemicals following tissue injury includes bradykinin, substance P, histamine, prostaglandins, thromboxanes and leukotrienes. The clinical implications of prostaglandin formation are discussed by Oates et al (1988a, b). The metabolites of arachidonic acid are prostaglandins and thromboxane A_2 which stimulate platelet activation. Prostacyclin (prostaglandin I_2) is a vasodilator which stimulates the release of renin but inhibits the aggregation of platelets. Prostaglandin (D_2) is produced by mast cells resulting in bronchoconstriction while prostaglandin E_2 is a vasodilator, inducing diuresis and loss of sodium. The synthesis of prostaglandin and thromboxane A_2 depends on hydroperoxidase and cyclooxygenase. Aspirin blocks the biosynthesis of prostaglandin and thromboxane A_2 by acetylating the cyclooxygenase and, as the link is covalent, its action is irreversible. However, the actions of other non-steroidal anti-inflammatory drugs (NSAIDs) are reversible and they may affect the circulation, renal function, electrolyte control, the ductus arteriosus, gastric acid secretion and also the asthmatic. Indomethacin, by inhibiting prostaglandin formation, may potentiate the action of analgesic agents and epidural analgesia (Schulze et al 1988).

Thromboxane (B_2) and prostaglandin levels increase during hip surgery which might contribute to the increase in post-operative thromboembolism. The levels are also increased during spinal and epidural analgesia (Kaukinen et al 1989). However, in patients who received 200 mg of indomethacin daily, prostaglandin and thromboxane levels were unaltered (Oettinger & Beger 1987).

Lembeck (1988) has reviewed experimental work on the discovery of substance P in afferent neurons which are capsaicin-sensitive. Substance P was initially discovered by von Euler & Gaddum in 1931. Substance P also exists in many organs and tissues of the body and not only in the dorsal horn or the hypothalamus. The receptors for substance P and related neurokinins are discussed by Regoli et al (1989). There is a relationship between substance P and 5-HT, controlling the nociceptive stimuli in the dorsal horn (Rodriguez & Rodriguez 1989). During surgery there was no significant increases in CSF concentrations of substance P, although levels were high post-operatively when post-operative pain was severe. Surprisingly, during patient-controlled analgesia in which only a small amount of analgesia was required, CSF levels of substance P increased but for those who needed a large amount of pethidine, levels were decreased (Sjostrom et al 1988). CSF levels of substance P were also low in patients with chronic pain disorders (Almay et al 1988).

Substance P has been shown to affect the pain threshold in the brain, the spinal cord and peripherally. In the brain it increases pain threshold whereas in the cord and peripherally it is decreased. There are substance P antagonists but it remains to be proven that they have analgesic properties (Vaught 1988). In recent years there have been developments not only in information on afferent pathways but also on the central influence of nociceptive response in the dorsal horn (Willis 1988).

Capsaicin not only releases substance P but stimulates the secretion of mucus in the bronchial tract, an effect which is antagonized by morphine which in itself is antagonized by naloxone. Although morphine is contra-indicated in asthmatic conditions and chronic bronchitis, Rogers & Barnes (1989) have shown a possible indication for its use.

Pain relief from opioids appears to be mediated through complicated interactions between the mu, delta and kappa receptors. Centrally the mu-receptors appear to be important, although these receptors have been subdivided into mu_1 and mu_2 sites. Peripherally morphine appears to act at delta and kappa sites (Pasternak 1988) and this has also been reviewed by Yaksh (1987). It has been suggested that beta-endorphin acts primarily at mu receptors, enkephalin at delta receptors and dynorphin at kappa receptors but they may be active at any of the receptors.

There are numerous papers on opioid peptides and metabolism, and in humans beta-endorphin produces hyperglycaemia by stimulating glucagon release. It also increases plasma insulin, an effect which is dose-dependent. A bolus dose of beta-endorphin increases plasma insulin whereas lower doses inhibit its release. In obesity plasma levels of beta-endorphin are also increased. There may well be a link between beta-endorphins and type II diabetes (Giugliano et al 1988).

In patients with liver disease, there are increased levels of enkephalins but not beta-endorphin. Many of the symptoms of biliary cirrhosis, e.g. pruritus, were improved with the use of the opioid antagonist, nalmefene which is more potent than naloxone (Thornton & Losowsky 1988).

In animals, kappa-opioid agonists affect fluid loss by altering glomerular filtration resulting in an increase in reabsorption of sodium and potassium (Ashton et al 1990).

Smith & Lee (1988) reviewed the pharmacology of dynorphin, showing that many of its actions are complex. It appears that there is little analgesic activity of its own but it potentiates morphine analgesia. In certain circumstances it may even antagonize morphine. In contrast to these effects which occur when the ligand is given centrally, dynorphin is a potent analgesic when administered intrathecally. Dynorphin lowers blood pressure and heart rate and causes respiratory depression. Morphine can cause hypothermia while dynorphin increases temperature, but when given together the result is potentiation of hypothermia. Dynorphin suppresses oxytocin release, an effect which is antagonized by naloxone. Dynorphin levels increase in response to chronic pain, trauma and it has even been shown to have an anticonvulsant action. Dynorphin also modulates the bradycardia produced by morphine. It should be noted that some of these actions may depend on the length of the dynorphin chain; dynorphin A and B have been described by Glatt et al (1987). Blockade of neuronal calcium may account for analgesia or dynorphin A in the spinal cord (Wang et al 1989).

Spiradoline is a potent kappa-agonist whose analgesic reaction is detected by the use of naloxone. It is also active but least so at the mu-receptor. These activities may be synergistic or antagonistic (VonVoigtlander & Lewis 1988). Advancement of highly selective and potent peptide ligands continues, and developments are taking place in producing those with similar selectivities and potencies at kappa-opioid receptors, although no effective antagonist at this site is yet available (Hruby & Gehrig 1989).

Dopamine inhibitory mechanisms may be involved in the regulation of beta-endorphin, ACTH and prolactin in normal subjects undergoing extracellular fluid volume expansion produced by water immersion (Coruzzi et al 1988).

ANALGESIC AGENTS

Morphine

Lipid solubility is an important factor in the mode of action of opioids, and there may be a central membrane effect in addition to interaction at receptor sites (Stone & DiFazio 1988). The more lipid soluble drugs such as buprenorphine, fentanyl, methadone and heroin are absorbed more effectively sublingually than the less lipophilic drugs such as morphine, oxycodone and hydromorphone. The pH is also an important factor and when the mouth was buffered to pH 8.5, methadone absorption was increased to 75% (Weinberg et al 1988). Premedication with 30 mg buccal morphine was less effective than that produced by 10 mg given intra-muscularly; plasma concentrations were lower with the buccal route as absorption was poor, resulting in inadequate pre-operative sedation and post-operative pain relief (Simpson et al 1989). Meptazinol, although equipotent with morphine has an increased incidence of vomiting (Frater et al 1989).

Sear et al (1989a) have studied morphine disposition at operation and found that peak concentration of morphine-6-glucuronide was higher compared with the control group, and it was felt that this was due to the decrease in renal blood flow and glomerular filtration rate during halothane anaesthesia. In a further study Sear et al (1989b) confirmed that impaired renal function does not damage the clearance of morphine in the anaesthetized patient, but it does that of the morphine-6-glucuronide metabolites. In hepatic cirrhosis, glucuronidation is surprisingly spared, although there may be an extrahepatic site for morphine metabolism (Crotty et al 1989). Adrenalectomy potentiates the action of subcutaneous morphine (Miyamoto et al 1989).

Morphine may cause hypotension, possibly due to a central effect or peripheral vasodilatation. Intravenous morphine reduced myocardial depression in animals during hypothermia at 30°C. During hypothermia plasma and CSF levels of morphine were elevated while histamine release was enhanced (Alcaraz et al 1989). In addition, animal studies have indicated that morphine reduces the development of digoxin-induced arrhythmias and this effect is mediated by the parasympathetic nervous system (Rabkin 1988).

There have been suggestions that morphine stored in syringes for use in the treatment of chronic pain by epidural routes readily deteriorates. Hung et al (1988) demonstrated that there was < 3% degradation of morphine to pseudomorphine, and the shelf-life of the drug was 20 to 33 weeks. However, some leaching may occur from contaminants from the syringe.

The effects of morphine in patients with severe liver damage such as cirrhosis has been investigated by Hasselstrom et al (1990), who found that the metabolism of morphine whether given orally or intravenously was severely impaired. There was a high level of oral bioavailability, lower plasma clearance and a long elimination half-life.

Alfentanil

The pharmacokinetics and metabolism of alfentanil have been reported in man by Meuldermans et al (1988); the main metabolite is noralfentanil

(30%) and the other major metabolite is the glucuronide of N-(4-hydroxyphenyl) propanamide.

Tolerance to alfentanil can develop rapidly even an hour after subsequent bolus injections (Doorley et al 1988). An interesting study by Gesink-Van Der Veer et al (1989) suggested that alfentanil requirement was greater in patients with Crohn's disease and although the alpha-1 acid glycoprotein (AAG) was also raised, there was no correlation between the increased level and the dose of alfentanil. Patients with Crohn's disease are often treated with salazopyrine and steroids which might influence the requirements for anaesthetic agents.

Cardiopulmonary bypass (CPB) affects the binding of alfentanil to plasma proteins and in assessing the effects of CPB on drug plasma concentrations, it is felt that it is necessary to monitor the unbound as well as the bound fractions (Kumar et al 1988). During and after CPB lower infusions of alfentanil than those given prior to the onset appeared to be effective in obtunding responses to stimulation.

Alfentanil may have significant actions on myocardial function and metabolism during CPB, and induction with fentanyl produced the greatest stability of the cardiovascular parameters without associated myocardial lactate production. Sufentanil produced a greater degree of myocardial depression while alfentanil produced the greatest myocardial depression and increase in myocardial lactate production (Miller et al 1988). Thus the safest analgesic under these circumstances is fentanyl.

Scheinin et al (1989) administered alfentanil (75 µg/kg) prior to induction with thiopentone and suxamethonium, and found that it modulated the response to laryngoscopy and intubation. Prolongation of the QT interval was reduced and it is worthy of note that the changes in QT interval were directly related to changes in plasma noradrenaline concentration. Unfortunately some patients developed chest wall rigidity.

The place of alfentanil infusion for patients requiring intensive care has been outlined by Bodenham & Park (1988). There may be difficulties in predicting the response of individual patients who are critically ill and factors such as age, obesity, liver dysfunction, sex, plasma protein concentration and regional changes in blood flow may be involved. Alfentanil does not produce sedation and therefore other drugs such as benzodiazepine may also be required.

Fentanyl

Studies are in progress to evaluate the analogues of fentanyl and recent research affecting the anilino aromatic ring is reported by Casy & Huckstep (1988). Many of the analogues are more potent than morphine although the phenacyl analogues are of lower potency or inactive. Fentanyl also increases the concentrations of dopamine metabolites within the brain (Finlay et al 1988).

Attempts have been made to reduce chest wall rigidity with midazolam but when given in a dose of 0.075 mg/kg, it is only partially successful. Rigidity of the chest wall leads to an increase in central venous and pulmonary capillary wedge pressure with a rise in P_{CO_2} (Neidhart et al 1989). Klausner et al (1988) have described delayed muscular rigidity and respiratory depression following fentanyl in a dose of 55–75 µg/kg. The patients had appeared to recover satisfactorily from operation but there may have been increased plasma levels from fat, muscle and the gastrointestinal tract, leading to a secondary rise in plasma concentration. Factors which might influence this are hypothermia, rewarming and acidosis. Treatment included endotracheal intubation, ventilation and/or naloxone. Opioid-induced rigidity may be confused with seizures, but EEG failed to confirm epileptiform activity (Smith et al 1989).

In depressive patients, intravenous fentanyl increases plasma cortisol and plasma noradrenaline but reduces growth hormone when compared with controls. This study suggests that there may be a relationship between the neuroreceptors and alpha-2 adrenoceptors in depressive patients (Matussek & Hoehe 1989).

It has been felt that respiratory depression occurred more readily with opioids in infants compared with adults. Hertzka et al (1989) showed that infants older than three months were tolerant to large doses of fentanyl and did not exhibit significant post-operative respiratory depression. Frecska et al (1988) measured the endocrine response to an intravenous bolus of fentanyl in a dose of 100 µg. There was a diurnal variation, in that there was a marked elevation in prolactin and thyrotropin in the evening but a reduced response in the morning.

Sufentanil

The pharmacological properties of sufentanil have been reviewed in detail by Monk et al (1988). Sufentanil is more potent than alfentanil, having a shorter distribution time and elimination half-life compared with fentanyl. Although it appears to have little effect on the cardiovascular system during anaesthesia, post-operative respiratory depression has been reported although Bailey et al (1990) found that it produced less respiratory depression than fentanyl. It is claimed to be up to 4000 times more potent than morphine and 5–15 times more than fentanyl, and surprisingly the duration of action was not prolonged in cirrhotic patients (Chauvin et al 1989). It is highly lipophilic and highly protein-bound. It has been used epidurally (10–100 µg) during labour, producing rapid onset of analgesia of shorter duration than morphine. Chest wall rigidity has also been reported.

Nefopam

Nefopam is a rapidly acting analgesic causing apparently no respiratory depression. McLintock et al (1988) reported favourably on its use in post-operative pain and when given pre-operatively (20 mg) and immediately following surgery, it reduced the morphine requirements post-operatively by 50%.

Baclofen

Baclofen is a GABA agonist but the mechanism of producing analgesia differs from that of opioids. Analgesic due to morphine is reduced by giving phenoxybenzamine, tolazoline and nadolol while analgesia due to baclofen is increased by tolazoline, propranolol and nadolol (Tamayo et al 1988).

Pentazocine

Pentazocine has lost popularity because of its cardiovascular effects. It has agonist–antagonist analgesic activity at kappa-receptors and this can be potentiated with low dose naloxone. The analgesia produced is more effective than high dose morphine (Levine et al 1988).

Adenosine agonists

Herrick-Davis et al (1989) have shown that in animals adenosine agonists are potential analgesics acting through a central mechanism. The responses are antagonized by theophylline.

Transdermal absorption

The administration of drugs by the subdermal route has attracted attention and Sebel et al (1987) have demonstrated that sufentanil and fentanyl are readily absorbed via the skin, although the amount of drug available compared with intravenous use is only 30%. Sufentanil appears to be absorbed faster than fentanyl. Transdermal fentanyl reduced the requirements for morphine following major surgery on the shoulder, but it did increase the incidence of vomiting as well as reducing the respiratory rate (Caplan et al 1989).

The administration of drugs via the transdermal route raises the possibility of its use for the treatment of post-operative and chronic pain. Roy & Flynn (1988, 1989) confirmed that pethidine, fentanyl and sufentanil were rapidly absorbed through the skin and suggested that this method may provide pain relief at drug levels below that which produces sedation. The absorption characteristics of fentanyl have been described by Varvel et al (1989) indicating that transdermal fentanyl produced constant serum fentanyl concentrations for some time in patients undergoing major orthopaedic surgery. It also reduces the hypertensive post-operative response (Leading article, Lancet 1989).

Chronic pain

Kerr et al (1988) have reported favourably on continuous infusions of pethidine, morphine and hydromorphone using programmable portable pumps as a means of providing adequate analgesia in patients with chronic pain due to cancer. Spinal cord stimulation has been found to have little value for cancer pain, although it may be indicated in pain of vascular origin or in post-herpetic neuralgia (Meglio et al 1989).

POST-OPERATIVE PAIN
(see also individual agents and spinal and epidural analgesia)

Morphine is considered by many to be the best post-operative analgesic agent, despite being given intramuscularly at repeated intervals. Some advocate intravenous infusion or intrathecal or extradural administration.

Dextromoramide has been used as a post-operative analgesic and is 2–3 times more potent than morphine. Its pharmacokinetics have been reviewed by Pagani et al (1989) who showed that the absorption is rapid, resulting in an early onset of analgesia but of short duration.

Picenadol which is a racemic mixture with the d-isomer being a potent opioid agonist and the l-isomer being an opioid antagonist, produce pain relief similar to that of codeine. Their side effects are similar (Brunelle et al 1988).

Dexamethasone suppressed the post-operative increase in circulating levels of beta-endorphin but increased post-operative pain following dental extraction (Hargreaves et al 1987). However, their findings on post-operative dental pain are in variance with other studies involving larger dose of dexamethasone (4 mg). It also reduces post-operative sweating. Small dose of proglumide, a cholecystokinin antagonist, potentiates the magnitude and duration of morphine analgesia for relief of pain following extraction of impacted third molars (Lavigne et al 1989).

El-Naggar et al (1989) have reported favourably on the use of intra-pleural injection of 30 ml of 0.75 bupivacaine with adrenaline. In patients who underwent cholecystectomy intrapleural analgesia resulted in pro-longed pain relief with minimal requirements for further analgesia.

Spinal and extradural analgesia

Spinal analgesia was considered in detail in *Anaesthesia Review 5* (McClure & Wildsmith 1988, pp. 269–285), but there are still aspects of intrathecal techniques appearing in the literature to be considered. The anatomy of the lumbar epidural space on CT examination is complex, with divisions and transverse connective tissue planes not previously noted. This might be responsible for the failure of drugs to act satisfactorily and the failure of correct positioning of epidural catheters (Savolaine et al 1988). Wulf &

Striepling (1990) reported the non-specific actions following continuous epidural analgesia and that inflammatory actions with fibrous tissues may interfere with the spread of drugs in the epidural space.

Lumbar puncture

Untoward complications may occur even after lumbar puncture. Kar et al (1987) described the occurrence of a cerebrospinal fistula following lumbar puncture which failed to respond to epidural blood patch, subcutaneous suturing and it was finally cured by absolute bed rest in the prone position with daily cisternal punctures. Norris et al (1989) have re-affirmed the importance of having the bevel of the needle parallel to the longitudinal fibres of the dura in case of inadvertent dural tear during epidural anaesthesia.

Epidural haematoma

Lumbar puncture often leads to some degree of bleeding as revealed by percutaneous epiduroscopy and this might be reduced by the paramedian approach (Blomberg & Olsson 1989). However, epidural haematoma is a major concern and in some centres the use of heparin, other anticoagulants or dextran is viewed with caution. Baron et al (1987) in a retrospective study of 912 patients who had continuous epidural analgesia for vascular surgery, could not find any neurological complication that could be ascribed to the use of heparin. In their study heparin was given at operation after the epidural catheter had been inserted. Bunt et al (1987) also favoured continuous epidural anaesthesia for aortic surgery but made no reference to the use of heparin.

Intrathecal and extradural analgesia (bupivacaine)

The factors affecting the spread of isobaric and hyperbaric bupivacaine had been studied by Pitkanen (1987) who found that the height and weight of body mass exerted very little influence. A high spread of analgesia was associated with a diminution in peak expiratory flow rate but blood gas tensions remained normal. Diaphragmatic function is depressed following upper abdominal surgery, possibly due to depression of phrenic nerve activity and this effect is partially reversed by thoracic epidural blockade (Mankikian et al 1988). Surprisingly, spinal analgesia even up to analgesic level of T_4 only produced a complete sympathetic blockade in the feet in 60% of patients (Malmqvist et al 1987). (For mechanisms of differential blockade see Fink (1989).)

There have been many studies on the pharmacokinetics of local anaesthetics. Bupivacaine, etidocaine and lignocaine are rapidly absorbed into the systemic circulation following lumbar epidural administration, to be followed by a much slower phase of absorption. However, following spinal injection of lignocaine and bupivacaine, the initial phase of absorption is much slower and the next phase is similar to that following epidural administration (Burm 1989). It has been suggested that there is an increased incidence of neonatal jaundice in obstetric analgesia following bupivacaine, but Gale et al (1988) were unable to demonstrate any association between bupivacaine given epidurally and neonatal jaundice.

Studies have suggested that in the post-operative period there was an increased elimination half-life of bupivacaine given epidurally, even though plasma levels on the fourth post-operative day did not support this (Wulf et al 1988). They also concluded that more studies would be needed on the phase of action of bupivacaine, especially as their results indicated an increase in protein binding in relation to surgery. The duration of sensory loss during continuous epidural bupivacaine infusion is significantly longer in patients with chronic pain compared with the acute pain following surgery, and it appears that the trauma of surgery may result in an increase in afferent impulses, render the spinal cord more excitable or result in an increased elimination of bupivacaine from the epidural space (Mogensen et al 1988).

Intrathecal analgesia (spinal or epidural) has often been advocated for total hip replacement. Intra-operative and post-operative blood loss were less in patients who had epidural analgesia compared with patients who had general anaesthesia, either with spontaneous or controlled ventilation (Modig & Karlstrom 1987). Spinal analgesia appears to enhance blood flow in the lower limb and in a detailed study of clotting factors, also during hip replacement, there was less intra-operative activation of fibrinolysis (Davis et al 1987). Fibronectin, a plasma glucoprotein involved in wound healing and coagulation, is depressed following surgery irrespective of the type of anaesthesia, but the restoration to normal levels is more prolonged following epidural anaesthesia. This may be due to the suppression of adrenocortical response to surgical stimulation (Hesselvik et al 1987). The use of a larger volume of 0.1% in preference to the equivalent dose of 0.25% bupivacaine is not beneficial as assessed by oxygen consumption, oxygen content and arterial venous difference (Bernard et al 1989). The serum potassium fell following epidural analgesia with mepivacaine and adrenaline, presumably due to the action of adrenaline (Hahn 1987).

Temeck et al (1989) reported on the successful use of epidural analgesia with bupivacaine in high risk cases undergoing thoracic surgery. Possible hazards of spinal techniques in abdominal surgery have included a reduction in splanchnic blood flow by causing hypotension and increased intestinal activity. In experimental haemorrhage, epidural analgesia improves survival rate possibly due to its effects in reducing circulating catecholamines (Shibata et al 1989). Lundberg et al (1989) have demonstrated that an infusion of dopamine maintains the systemic blood pressure and inhibits intestinal activity.

Hazards

Neurological complications

The neurotoxicity of spinal agents has been reviewed by Coombs & Fratkin (1987) who were concerned that agents used, either by bolus or single injection, should be completely safe. There are many possible mechanisms of toxicity including vasoconstriction, vascular injury, or alteration in the blood flow to the spinal cord. Spinal cord damage had been reported following 2-chloro-procaine and even hypertonic saline (Kim et al 1988). Although there have been advances in materials aimed at improving the safety of epidural catheters, Hutchison (1987) has drawn attention to the danger of the 18-gauge radio-opaque catheter which could sever much easier than the non-radio-opaque one of the same gauge. Foreign matter such as glass or plastic fragments could contaminate the solution to be injected and this does not appear to be influenced by the type of syringe, whether it is glass or plastic, or by the container, whether it is ampoule or vial. Bacterial filters do decrease the amount of possible glass fragments but they themselves increase the amount of filter debris in the form of cotton-like fragments (Eriksen 1988).

An unusual episode of paralysis developed in a patient who was given spinal anaesthesia in the presence of an undiagnosed spinal cord arterio-venous malformation. The patient developed signs of anterior spinal artery syndrome but the paralysis was only temporary, lasting for no more than six days (Warner et al 1987).

Svensson et al (1988) showed that intrathecal papaverine was beneficial in preventing spinal cord complications following prolonged periods of cross-clamping of the aorta. A dose of 3 ml of 1% preservative-free papaverine hydrochloride in 10% dextrose was injected at 3–5 min intervals (pH 3.5–5). The papaverine appears to act by dilating the anterior spinal arteries. Other techniques and drugs recommended to minimize paraplegia following aortic occlusion include barbiturates, superoxide dismutase and infusions of cool crystalloid solutions (Kirshner et al 1989).

Cardiac arrest

Unexpected cardiac arrest has been reported in 14 healthy young patients who were either ASA 1 or ASA 2 following spinal anaesthesia (Caplan et al 1988). Records were studied from insurance claims for major anaesthetic mishaps and in this group of patients six suffered severe neurological damage and died in hospital. Of the others only one recovered sufficiently from neurological damage to have an independent existence. One of the factors which is likely to lead to the complication was the use of intra-operative sedation including fentanyl, diazepam, droperidol or thiopentone, resulting in the patients appearing to be asleep but also unable to communicate with the anaesthetist. Cardiac arrest was preceded by cyanosis suggesting some degree of under-ventilation. Hypotension and bradycardia associated with high spinal anaesthesia could also be augmented by the use of fentanyl. Another feature was the failure to appreciate the results of sympathetic blockade from high spinal anaesthesia. Despite the use of external cardiac massage and intravenous fluids, atropine and ephedrine, Caplan et al (1988) felt that adrenaline was a much more potent alpha-agonist than ephedrine which is less effective in producing peripheral vasoconstriction.

Distension of the main pulmonary artery leads to distal pulmonary hypertension and in animal studies, total spinal anaesthesia was shown not to affect this response indicating that the hypertensive response does not involve central pathways (Pearl et al 1988).

Intrathecal opioids

A nationwide study in the use of intrathecal opioids in the management of post-operative pain relief was undertaken by Rawal et al (1987), who found that morphine had been given to 14 000 patients extradurally and intra-thecally to 11 000 patients in 1984. However, Gustafsson & Wiesenfeld-Hallin (1988) urged caution in the use of intrathecal opioids and suggested that more control studies were necessary. The commonest complications were pruritus and urinary retention, especially after morphine. Urinary retention appears to be associated with inhibition at mu- and delta- but not kappa-receptors, and it has been suggested that pentazocine or methadone might be preferable to morphine in preventing urinary retention (Dray 1988). In patients who have spinal cord lesions with hyperactive detrusor reflexes and low capacity of the bladder, intrathecal morphine led to an increase in bladder capacity with reduced liability to incontinence and frequent catheterization (Herman et al 1988). Itching is much more common after spinal than epidural opioids and is possibly due to local excitation within the spinal cord itself (Ballantyne et al 1988).

Attempts have been made to use intrathecal opioids for operative procedures in conscious patients. Pethidine seemed to be the ideal choice as it also has local anaesthetic properties, but Sangarlangkarn et al (1987) found that the complication rate was comparable with lignocaine, except that pethidine often led to intra-operative drowsiness, respiratory depression, bronchospasm and itching.

The possibility of other opioids such as fentanyl and sufentanil for epidural administration have been considered by van den Hoogen & Colpaert (1987). Animal studies suggest that sufentanil provides much better pain relief with less side effects when compared with lofentanil, carfentanil, fentanyl and alfentanil (Meert et al 1988). Intrathecal fentanyl inhibits the flexor withdrawal reflexes at spinal cord level, as a result of the inhibition of A-delta and C-fibres but sparing the spinal reflexes under the influence of large diameter I–A afferent fibres (Chabal et al 1989).

Factors influencing the spread of spinal opioids

There are many factors during surgery which affect the absorption of morphine from the CSF and these include metabolic acidosis, a fall in body temperature, and also the haemodynamic changes that occur at operation; these may affect CSF flow and the ionization of morphine. Free morphine could not be measured in the plasma but morphine-3-glucuronide was detected after 5 min. After 16 h it also could not be detected. Hanna et al (1990) in fact found that intrathecal morphine-6-glucuronide was a more effective analgesic than morphine.

The physical factors of the solution may well affect the outcome of analgesia following spinal opioids. The effects of temperature and specific gravity were considered in *Anaesthesia Review 2* (Williams 1984, pp. 148–161). Surprisingly, when the opioid is dissolved in saline, the baricity may well depend upon the saline and not the amount of drug given. The chloride ion may well be responsible for some of the C-fibre blockade (King et al 1972).

Payne (1987) discussed the factors which influence the clearance of opioids administered into the CSF. The factors include age, position, anatomy, lipid solubility, ionization and baricity. The lipid soluble opioids have an affinity for delta and/or kappa opioid receptors; therefore a small dose of lipid soluble opioid would be rapidly taken up by the cord, limiting the spread in the CSF and distribution via the blood stream to the brain. This is further amplified by Gourlay et al (1987) who showed that the major factor affecting absorption into CSF following epidural administration is the physicochemical characteristics of opioids, namely lipophilicity. The more lipophilic the opioid, the more likely they are to diffuse into the lipid-rich tissues of the spinal cord, reducing the amount that is available for rostral spread. Respiratory depression, occurring immediately or delayed, is not a feature seen following epidural pethidine administration. However, given intrathecally the CSF levels rise progressively and it appears that there is systemic absorption with redistribution into the CSF (Maurette et al 1989). Methadone is more lipophilic than pethidine and may be the drug of choice in preventing respiratory depression; 1 mg is less potent than the equivalent dose of morphine (Jacobsen et al 1989).

Little is known about the factors which affect the drugs reaching and leaving the nerve tissue (Cousins 1987). Sjostrom et al (1987a, b) have in fact shown that pethidine was removed faster than morphine from the CSF following epidural administration. Blood levels of alfentanil were comparable whether the drug was given intramuscularly or epidurally, while the analgesia was found to be superior to that of morphine. Intramuscular alfentanil produced respiratory depression which lasted for 30 min, whereas if given epidurally it lasted 90 min suggesting rostral spread (Penon et al 1988). Morphine, whether given epidurally or intravenously resulted in similar plasma concentrations, but the epidural group produced more prolonged analgesia (Alexander et al 1990).

There was an inverse relationship between lipid soluble drugs and potency (McQuay et al 1989). Thus to achieve equivalent analgesia following the intrathecal route of morphine 0.5 mg, the dose for pethidine would be 5 mg and 8.5 mg for methadone. When the drugs are given extradurally, to achieve equivalent analgesia to 5 mg of morphine, a dose of lipid soluble opioid may have to be on the higher side (McQuay et al 1989).

The pharmacokinetics of fentanyl has been compared following lumbar epidural and intravenous administration. There was little uptake of fentanyl in the blood stream but there was a rapid penetration into the dura mater, and it travelled towards the brain as a result of passive CSF flow (Gourlay et al 1989).

Abdominal surgery

Ionescu et al (1988) recommended the use of intrathecal morphine (0.05 mg/kg) for elective abdominal aortic surgery, and commented that this produced excellent post-operative analgesia without side effects or complications. The effect achieved did not appear to depend on the age or sex of the patient. Intrathecal morphine (0.75 mg) should also decrease anaesthetic requirements as it reduces the MAC for halothane from 0.81% to 0.48% (Drasner et al 1988).

For pain control post-operatively following transurethral resection of the prostate, Kirson et al (1989) found that 0.1 or 0.2 mg of intrathecal morphine were effective and the lower dose was not associated with nausea and vomiting. Yamaguchi et al (1989) found that a mixture of morphine (0.04–0.08 mg) and 12–14 mg of tetracaine made post-operative systemic analgesia unnecessary in 60–70% of patients undergoing hysterectomy.

Thoracic surgery

Intrathecal morphine was also effective in reducing analgesia and antihypertensive drug therapy in the post-operative period following coronary artery bypass surgery, although there may be hazards of haematoma when patients are also given heparin (Vanstrum et al 1988).

Epidural opioids

Respiratory depression remains a source of concern following the administration of epidural or intrathecal opioids. The incidence of delayed respiratory depression was 0.09% for extradural morphine and 0.36% following spinal morphine (Rawal et al 1987). There are many factors which influence the spread of the drug, including rapid absorption via epidural veins. Nordberg et al (1987) felt that spread centrally could be eliminated by reducing the volume of fluid injected.

Respiratory depression is not encountered following the use of diamorphine (which is lipophilic) when it is given intrathecally to conscious patients for pain relief. When it is administered following induction of anaesthesia for major abdominal procedures, apnoea or respiratory depression seen at the end of operation is often due to a low $P\text{CO}_2$ as a result of hyperventilation (Kaufman 1988). Etches et al (1989) also agreed that spinal morphine could cause delayed respiratory depression, but any respiratory depression that occurred with lipophilic drugs developed soon after the administration.

Intrathecal diamorphine prolonged the duration of post-operative analgesia following the use of intrathecal bupivacaine for major orthopaedic operations, and although respiratory depression did not occur in the post-operative period, there was a high incidence of nausea and vomiting and urinary retention (Reay et al 1989). However, Jacobson et al (1989) were less impressed when diamorphine was mixed with bupivacaine and given intrathecally for operations involving knee replacement. Epidural diamorphine was found to be more effective than ketamine for post-operative analgesia following hysterectomy (Peat et al 1989).

Age appears to affect the dose of epidural morphine and therefore the dose should be reduced in the elderly (Ready et al 1987). The addition of local anaesthetics such as 25 µg of bupivacaine or 200 µg of lignocaine increased the intensity and prolonged the duration of spinal morphine (Akerman et al 1988).

Epidural morphine

Continuous epidural morphine in a dose of 0.005 mg/kg provided excellent post-operative pain relief in patients undergoing radical gynaecological surgery for malignancy. Side effects included nausea, vomiting and pruritus (25%), but it was considered that the benefits of haemodynamic stability and the ease with which patients participated in post-operative physiotherapy outweighed the disadvantages (Planner et al 1988). However, Thoren et al (1989) found that the duration of post-operative ileus after hysterectomy was shorter following epidural bupivacaine compared with epidural morphine, and if anything pain relief was superior following the use of bupivacaine. Bisgaard et al (1990) found that lumbar epidural bupivacaine plus morphine was more effective than epidural morphine alone for the relief of pain following major abdominal surgery.

An interesting finding of Schulze et al (1988) was that following chole-cystectomy, post-operative pain was eliminated after epidural bupivacaine and morphine when supplemented by systemic indomethacin. Despite adequate pain relief, this regime had little effect on suppressing the metabolic changes associated with surgical stimulation. Epidural clonidine (150 µg) was considered unsuitable for the treatment of post-operative pain by Lund et al (1989a). Despite being more effective than morphine in the first 2 h, it caused hypotension and had little effect in attenuating the increased cortisol levels associated with surgical stimulation. Despite adequate pain relief, epidural morphine does not affect the monosynaptic H reflexes leading Willer et al (1988) to conclude that epidural morphine produces 'selective spinal analgesia'.

Nalbuphine, a partial agonist at the mu-receptor and an agonist at the kappa-receptor, reverses the respiratory depression and pruritus associated with epidural morphine in a dose of 0.3 ml/kg intravenously without reducing analgesia (Penning et al 1988). This effect is not surprising as its action is similar in some respects to that of naloxone, even in producing the withdrawal syndrome (Preston et al 1989).

Long term treatment with intrathecal opioids

Arner et al (1988) in a nationwide survey on the use of epidural and intrathecal opioids for chronic severe pain, found that 750 patients have been treated with epidural morphine over a 5-year period in Sweden. The highest daily dose for morphine was 480 mg given epidurally and 50 mg given intrathecally. There apparently appeared to be no major problems with respiratory depression nor with pruritus and urinary retention. For non-cancer pain, spinal opioids did not appear to give satisfactory results. Downing et al (1988) were able to manage patients with chronic pain from carcinoma as out-patients with epidural morphine, and to teach the patients and their families to administer the drugs themselves via a catheter equipped with a filter.

Epidural steroid injections have been used to predict whether surgical treatment is advisable for pain relief from lumbar nerve root compression. The patients who improved with epidural methylprednisolone responded to chymopapain (Warfield & Crews 1987). However, epidural steroids combined with morphine failed to relieve the chronic back pain still present following laminectomy ('failed back syndrome') (Rocco et al 1989).

Other intrathecal agents

A variety of other drugs besides opioids have been used including ketamine, midazolam, baclofen and clonidine. Baclofen, a gamma-aminobutyric acid agonist, has been used to treat spinal spasticity resulting from multiple sclerosis or spinal cord injury; it acts pre-synaptically by preventing the influx of calcium and inhibiting transmitter release. If there is no response to oral baclofen then resource may be made to the use of intrathecal baclofen by continuous infusion. In a trial conducted by Penn et al (1989), excellent results were reported with a reduction of muscle tone and muscle spasm, so that near normal daily activities could be undertaken. There were no complications such as drowsiness or confusion. This has been confirmed by Ochs et al (1989) who found that an infusion of 50–800 μg/day of baclofen completely abolished spasticity.

Spinal opioid analgesia is complicated by the fact that other receptors are involved, as alpha-2 agonists appear to augment the analgesic effects of opioids (see Kitahata 1989, Solomon et al 1989). Epidural clonidine alleviates the pain in patients with cancer (Lund et al 1989b), producing post-operative analgesia of faster onset than epidural morphine, although it is less effective in reducing pain scores (Van Essen et al 1990).

Somatostatin has been given epidurally and was effective not only in controlling intractable pain from cancer but also in post-operative pain relief. Respiratory depression was not evident. However, it has a short duration of action and needs to be given by continuous infusion (Carli et al 1989). On the other hand, Desborough et al (1989) while noting that intrathecal somatostatin reduced plasma levels of growth hormone and insulin, failed to demonstrate any post-operative analgesia.

REFERENCES

Alcaraz C, Bansinath M, Turndorf H, Puig M M 1989 Cardiovascular effects of morphine during hypothermia. Arch Int Pharmacodyn Ther 297: 133–147
Alexander J I, Kong K L, Black A M S 1990 Epidural and intravenous infusions of diamorphine. Eur J Anaesthesiol 7: 309–315
Akerman B, Arwestrom E, Post C 1988 Local anesthetics potentiate spinal morphine antinociception. Anesth Analg 67: 943–948
Almay B G L, Johansson F, Von Knorring L, Le Greves P, Terenius L 1988 Substance P in CSF of patients with chronic pain syndromes. Pain 33: 3–9
Arner S, Rawal N, Gustafsson L L 1988 Clinical experience of long-term treatment with epidural and intrathecal opioids—a nationwide survey. Acta Anaesthesiol Scand 32: 253–259
Ashton N, Balment R J, Blackburn T P 1990 Kappa-opioid-receptor agonists modulate the renal excretion of water and electrolytes in anaesthetized rats. Br J Pharmacol 99: 181–185
Bailey P L, Streisand J B, East K A et al 1990 Differences in magnitude and duration of opioid-induced respiratory depression and analgesia with fentanyl and sufentanil. Anesth Analg 70: 8–15
Ballantyne J C, Loach A B, Carr D B 1988 Itching after epidural and spinal opiates. Pain 33: 149–160
Baron H C, LaRaja R D, Rossi G, Atkinson D 1987 Continuous epidural analgesia in the heparinized vascular surgical patients: a retrospective review of 912 patients. J Vasc Surg 6: 144–146
Bernard J M, Hommeril J L, Bourreli B, Gunst J P, Drouet J C 1989 The comparative effects of bupivacaine epidural analgesia on postoperative rewarming. In: Lomax P, Schonbaum E (eds), Thermoregulation: Research and Clinical Applications. Karger, Basel: 1989: 24–25
Bisgaard C, Mouridsen P, Dahl J B 1990 Continuous lumbar epidural bupivacaine plus morphine versus epidural morphine after major abdominal surgery. Eur J Anaesthesiol 7: 219–225
Blomberg R G, Olsson S S 1989 The lumbar epidural space in patients examined with epiduroscopy. Anesth Analg 68: 157–160
Bodenham A, Park G R 1988 Alfentanil infusions in patients requiring intensive care. Clin Pharmacokinet 15: 216–226
Brunelle R L, George R E, Sunshine A, Hammonds W D 1988 Analgesic effect of picenadol, codeine, and placebo in patients with postoperative pain. Clin Pharmacol Ther 43: 663–667
Burm A G L 1989 Clinical pharmacokinetics of epidural and spinal anesthesia. Clin Pharmacokinet 16: 283–311
Bunt T J, Manczuk M, Varley K 1987 Continuous epidural anesthesia for aortic surgery: thoughts on peer review and safety. Surgery 101: 706–714
Caplan R A, Ward R J, Posner K, Cheney F W 1988 Unexpected cardiac arrest during spinal

anesthesia: a closed claims analysis of predisposing factors. Anesthesiology 68: 5–11

Caplan R A, Ready L B, Oden R V, Matsen F A III, Nessly M L, Olsson G L 1989 Transdermal fentanyl for postoperative pain management—A double-blind placebo study. JAMA 261: 1036–1039

Carli P, Ecoffey C, Chrubasik J, Benlabed M, Gross J B, Samii K 1989 Spread of analgesia and ventilatory response to carbon dioxide following epidural somatostatin. Eur J Anaesthesiol 6: 257–263

Casy A F, Huckstep M R 1988 Structure-activity studies of fentanyl. J Pharm Pharmacol 40: 605–608

Chabal C, Jacobson L, Little J 1989 Intrathecal fentanyl depresses nociceptive flexion reflexes in patients with chronic pain. Anesthesiology 70: 226–229

Chauvin M, Ferrier C, Haberer J P et al 1989 Sufentanil pharmacokinetics in patients with cirrhosis. Anesth Analg 68: 1–4

Coombs D W, Fratkin J D 1987 Neurotoxicology of spinal agents. Anesthesiology 66: 724–726

Coruzzi P, Ravanetti C, Muslari L, Biggi A, Vescovi P P, Novarini A 1988 Circulating opioid peptides during water immersion in normal man. Clin Sci 74: 133–136

Cousins M J 1987 Comparative pharmacokinetics of spinal opioids in humans: a step toward determination of relative safety. Anesthesiology 67: 875–876

Crotty B, Watson K J R, Desmond P V et al 1989 Hepatic extraction of morphine is impaired in cirrhosis. Eur J Clin Pharmacol 36: 501–506

Davis F M, McDermott E, Hickton C et al 1987 Influence of spinal and general anaesthesia on haemostasis during total hip arthroplasty. Br J Anaesth 59: 561–671

Desborough J P, Edlin S A, Burrin J M, Bloom S R, Morgan M, Hall G M 1989 Hormonal and metabolic responses to cholecystectomy: comparison of extradural somatostatin and diamorphine. Br J Anaesth 63: 508–515

Doorley B M, Knight V V, Spaulding T C 1988 Development of acute tolerance to the cardiorespiratory effects of alfentanil after subsequent bolus injection in conscious rats. Life Sci 43: 365–372

Downing J E, Busch E H, Stedman P M 1988 Epidural morphine delivered by a percutaneous epidural catheter for outpatient treatment of cancer pain. Anesth Analg 67: 1159–1161

Drasner K, Bernards C M, Ozanne G M 1988 Intrathecal morphine reduces the minimum alveolar concentration of halothane in humans. Anesthesiology 69: 310–312

Dray A 1988 Epidural opiates and urinary retention: new models provide new insights. Anesthesiology 68: 323–324

El-Naggar M A, Schaberg F J Jr, Phillips M R 1989 Intrapleural regional analgesia for pain management in cholecystectomy. Arch Surg 124: 568–570

Eriksen S 1988 Particulate contamination in spinal analgesia. Acta Anaesthesiol Scand 32: 545–548

Etches R C, Sandler A N, Daley M D 1989 Respiratory depression and spinal opioids. Can J Anaesth 36: 165–185

Fink B R 1989 Mechanisms of differential axial blockade in epidural and subarachnoid anesthesia. Anesthesiology 70: 851–858

Finlay J M, Jakubovic A, Phillips A G, Fibiger H C 1988 Fentanyl-induced conditional place preference: lack of associated conditional neurochemical events. Psychopharmacology 96: 534–540

Frater R A S, Moores M A, Parry P, Hanning C D 1989 Analgesia-induced respiratory depression: comparison of meptazinol and morphine in the postoperative period. Br J Anaesth 63: 260–265

Frecska E, Arato M, Banki C M et al 1988 Diurnal variation in fentanyl-induced hormone responses and side effects. Neuropsychopharmacology 1: 235–238

Gale R, Vreman H J, Ferguson J E II, Stevenson D K 1988 Effect of bupivacaine hydrochloride on bilirubin production in neonatal rats. Biol Neonate 54: 45–48

Gesink-Van Der Veer B J, Burm A G L, Hennis P J, Bovill J G 1989 Alfentanil requirement in Crohn's disease. Anaesthesia 44: 209–211

Giugliano D, Torella R, Lefebvre P J, Onofrio F D 1988 Opioid peptides and metabolic regulation. Diabetologia 31: 3–15

Glatt C E, Kenner J R, Long J B, Holaday J W 1987 Cardiovascular effects of dynorphin A

(1–13) in conscious rats and its modulation of morphine bradycardia over time. Peptides 8: 1089–1092

Gourlay G K, Cherry D A, Plummer J L, Armstrong P J, Cousins M J 1987 The influence of drug polarity on the absorption of opioid drugs into CSF and subsequent cephalad migration following lumbar epidural administration: application to morphine and pethidine. Pain 31: 297–305

Gourlay G K, Murphy T M, Plummer J L, Kowalski S R, Cherry D A, Cousins M J 1989 Pharmacokinetics of fentanyl in lumbar and cervical CSF following lumbar epidural and intravenous administration. Pain 38: 253–259

Gustafsson L L, Wiesenfeld-Hallin Z 1988 Spinal opioid analgesia. A critical update. Drugs 35: 597–603

Hahn R G 1987 Decrease in serum potassium concentration during epidural anaesthesia. Acta Anaesthesiol Scand 31: 680–683

Hanna M H, Peat S J, Woodham M, Knibb A, Fung C 1990 Analgesic efficacy and CSF pharmacokinetics of intrathecal morphine-6-glucuronide: comparison with morphine. Br J Anaesth 64: 547–550

Hargreaves K M, Schmidt E A, Mueller G P, Dionne R A 1987 Dexamethasone alters plasma levels of beta-endorphin and postoperative pain. Clin Pharmacol Ther 42: 601–607

Hasselstrom J, Eriksson S, Persson A, Rane A, Svensson J O, Sawe J 1990 The metabolism and bioavailability of morphine in patients with severe liver cirrhosis. Br J Clin Pharmacol 29: 289–297

Herman R M, Wainberg M C, delGiudice P F, Willscher M K 1988 The effect of a low dose of intrathecal morphine on impaired micturition reflexes in human subjects with spinal cord lesions. Anesthesiology 69: 313–318

Herrick-Davis K, Chippari S, Luttinger D, Ward S J 1989 Evaluation of adenosine agonists as potential analgesics. Eur J Pharmacol 162: 365–369

Hertzka R E, Gauntlett I S, Fisher D M, Spellman M J 1989 Fentanyl-induced ventilatory depression: effects of age. Anesthesiology 70: 213–218

Hesselvik F, Brodin B, Hakanson E, Rutberg H, von Schenck H 1987 Influence of epidural blockade on postoperative plasma fibronectin concentrations. Scand J Clin Lab Invest 47: 435–440

Holland I S, Seymour R A, Ward-Booth R P, Ord R A, Lim K L M 1988 An evaluation of different doses of soluble aspirin and aspirin tablets in postoperative dental pain. Br J Clin Pharmacol 26: 463–468

Hruby V J, Gehrig C A 1989 Recent developments in the design of receptor specific opioid peptides. Med Res Rev 9: 343–401

Hung C T, Young M, Gupta P K 1988 Stability of morphine solutions in plastic syringes determined by reversed-phase ion-pair liquid chromatography. J Pharm Sci 77: 719–723

Hutchison G L 1987 The severance of epidural catheters. Anaesthesia 42: 182–185

Ionescu T I, Drost R H, Roelofs J M M et al 1988 The pharmacokinetics of intradural morphine in major abdominal surgery. Clin Pharmacokinet 14: 178–186

Jacobson L, Kokri M S, Pridie A K 1989 Intrathecal diamorphine: a dose-response study. Ann R Coll Surg Engl 71: 289–292

Jacobson L, Chabal C, Brody M C, Ward R J, Ireton R C 1989 Intrathecal methadone and morphine for postoperative analgesia: a comparison of the efficacy, duration, and side effects. Anesthesiology 70: 742–746

Kar A M, Pradhan S, Mittal P 1987 Cerebrospinal fluid fistula after lumbar puncture. Br Med J 295: 528

Kaufman L 1988 Intraspinal diamorphine; epidural and intrathecal. In: Scott D B (ed), Diamorphine—Its Chemistry, Pharmacology and Clinical use. Woodhead–Faulkner, London, pp 82–96

Kaukinen S, Ojanen R, Kaukinen L, Seppala E, Vapaatalo H 1989 Plasma thromboxane B$_2$ levels and thromboxane B$_2$ production by platelets are increased in patients during spinal and epidural anesthesia. Prostaglandins Leukotrienes Essential Fatty Acids 37: 83–88

Kay B, Lindsay R G, Mason C J, Healy T E J 1988 Oral nalbuphine for the treatment of pain after dental extractions. Br J Anaesth 61: 313–317

Kerr I G, Sone M, DeAngelis C, Iscoe N, MacKenzie R, Schueller T 1988 Continuous narcotic infusion with patient-controlled analgesia for chronic cancer pain in outpatients. Ann Intern Med 108: 554–557

Kim R C, Porter R W, Choi B H, Kim S W 1988 Myelopathy after the intrathecal administration of hypertonic. Neurosurgery 22: 942–945

King J S, Jewett D L, Sundberg H R 1972 Differential blockade of cat dorsal root C fibers by various chloride solutions. J Neurosurg 36: 569–583

Kirshner D L, Kirshner R L, Heggeness L M, DeWeese J A 1989 Spinal cord ischemia: an evaluation of pharmacologic agents in minimizing paraplegia after aortic occlusion. J Vasc Surg 9: 305–308

Kirson L E, Goldman J M, Slover R B 1989 Low-dose intrathecal morphine for postoperative pain control in patients undergoing transurethral resection of the prostate. Anesthesiology 71: 192–195

Kitahata L M 1989 Spinal analgesia with morphine and clonidine. Anesth Analg 68: 191–193

Klausner J M, Caspi J, Lelcuk S et al 1988 Delayed muscular rigidity and respiratory depression following fentanyl anesthesia. Arch Surg 123: 66–67

Kumar K, Crankshaw D P, Morgan D J, Beemer G H 1988 The effect of cardiopulmonary bypass on plasma protein binding of alfentanil. Eur J Clin Pharmacol 35: 47–52

Lavigne G J, Hargreaves K M, Schmidt E A, Dionne R A 1989 Proglumide potentiates morphine analgesia for acute postsurgical pain. Clin Pharmacol Ther 45: 666–673

Leading Article 1989 Epidural morphine, hypertension, and aortic surgery. Lancet II: 598–599

Lembeck F 1988 The 1988 Ulf von Euler Lecture. Substance P: from extract to excitement. Acta Physiol Scand 133: 435–454

Levine J D, Gordon N C, Taiwo Y O, Coderre T J 1988 Potentiation of pentazocine analgesia by low-dose naloxone. J Clin Invest 82: 1574–1577

Lund C, Qvitzau S, Greulich A, Hjortso N C, Kehlet H 1989a Comparison of the effects of extradural clonidine with those of morphine on postoperative pain, stress responses, cardiopulmonary function and motor and sensory block. Br J Anaesth 63: 516–519

Lund C, Hansen O B, Kehlet H 1989b Effect of epidural clonidine on somatosensory evoked potentials to dermatomal stimulation. Eur J Anaesthesiol 6: 207–213

Lundberg J, Biber B, Delbro D, Martner J, Werner O 1989 Effects of dopamine on intestinal hemodynamics and motility during epidural analgesia in the cat. Acta Anaesthesiol Scand 33: 487–493

McClure J H, Wildsmith J A W 1988 Aspects of spinal anaesthesia. In: Kaufman L(ed) Anaesthesia review 5. Churchill Livingstone, Edinburgh, pp 269–285

McLintock T T C, Kenny G N C, Howie J C, McArdle C S, Lawrie S, Aitken H 1988 Assessment of the analgesic efficacy of nefopam hydrochloride after upper abdominal surgery: a study using patient controlled analgesia. Br J Surg 75: 779–781

Malmqvist L A, Bengtsson M, Bjornsson G, Jorfeldt L, Lofstrom J B 1987 Sympathetic activity and haemodynamic variables during spinal analgesia in man. Acta Anaesthesiol Scand 31: 467–473

Mankikian B, Cantineau J P, Bertrand M, Kieffer E, Sartene R, Viars P 1988 Improvement of diaphragmatic function by a thoracic extradural block after upper abdominal surgery. Anesthesiology 68: 379–386

McQuay H J, Sullivan A F, Smallman K, Dickenson A H 1989 Intrathecal opioids, potency and lipophilicity. Pain 36: 111–115

Matussek N, Hoehe M 1989 Investigations with the specific μ-opiate receptor agonist fentanyl in depressive patients: growth hormone, prolactin, cortisol, noradrenaline and euphoric responses. Neuropsychobiology 21: 1–8

Maurette P, Tauzin-Fin P, Vincon G, Brachet-Lieman A 1989 Arterial and ventricular CSF pharmacokinetics after intrathecal meperidine in humans. Anesthesiology 70: 961–966

Meert T F, Lu H R, van Craenndonck H, Janssen P A J 1988 Comparison between epidural fentanyl, sufentanil, carfentanil, lofentanil and alfentanil in the rat: analgesia and other in vivo effects. Eur J Anaesthesiol 5: 313–321

Meglio M, Cioni B, Rossi G F 1989 Spinal cord stimulation in management of chronic pain. A 9-year experience. J Neurosurg 70: 519–524

Meuldermans W, Van Peer A, Hendrickx J et al 1988 Alfentanil pharmacokinetics and metabolism in humans. Anesthesiology 69: 527–534

Miller D R, Wellwood M, Teasdale S J et al 1988 Effects of anaesthetic induction on myocardial function and metabolism: a comparison of fentanyl, sufentanil and alfentanil. Can J Anaesth 35: 219–233

Miyamoto Y, Ozaki M, Yamamoto H 1989 Effect of adrenalectomy on correlation of analgesia with tissue content of morphine. Eur J Pharmacol 167: 11–20

Modig J, Karlstrom G 1987 Intra- and post-operative blood loss and haemodynamics in total hip replacement when performed under lumbar epidural versus general anaesthesia. Eur J Anaesthesiol 4: 345–355

Mogensen T, Scott N B, Lund C, Bigler D, Hjortso N-C, Kehlet H 1988 The roles of acute and chronic pain in regression of sensory analgesia during continuous epidural bupivacaine infusion. Anesth Analg 67: 737–740

Monk J P, Beresford R, Ward A 1988 Sufentanil—a review of its pharmacological properties and therapeutic use. Drugs 36: 286–313

Neidhart P, Burgener M C, Schwieger I, Suter P M 1989 Chest wall rigidity during fentanyl- and midazolam–fentanyl induction: ventilatory and haemodynamic effects. Acta Anaesthesiol Scand 33: 1–5

Norberg G, Hansdottir V, Kvist L, Mellstrand T, Hedner T 1987 Pharmacokinetics of different epidural sites of morphine administration. Eur J Clin Pharmacol 33: 499–504

Norris M C, Leighton B L, DeSimone C A 1989 Needle bevel direction and headache after inadvertent dural puncture. Anesthesiology 70: 729–731

Oates J A, FitzGerald G A, Branch R A, Jackson E K, Knapp H R, Roberts L J II 1988a Clinical implications of prostaglandin and thromboxane A_2 formation (first of two parts). N Engl J Med 319: 689–698

Oates J A, FitzGerald G A, Branch R A, Jackson E K, Knapp H R, Roberts L J II 1988b Clinical implications of prostaglandin and thromboxane A_2 formation (second of two parts). N Engl J Med 319: 761–767

Ochs G, Struppler A, Meyerson B A et al 1989 Intrathecal baclofen for long-term treatment of spasticity: a multi-centre study. J Neurol Neurosurg Psychiatry 52: 933–939

Oettinger W, Beger H G 1987 Prostaglandin, and thromboxane release in critical states. In: Baethmann A, Messmer K (eds), Surgical Research: current concepts and results. Springer-Verlag, Berlin: pp 31–38

Pagani I, Barzaghi N, Crema F, Perucca E, Ego D, Rovei V 1989 Pharmacokinetics of dextromoramide in surgical patients. Fundamental Clin Pharmacol 3: 27–35

Pasternak G W 1988 Multiple morphine and enkephalin receptors and the relief of pain. JAMA 259: 1362–1367

Payne R 1987 CSF distribution of opioids in animals and man. Acta Anaesthesiol Scand 31 (suppl 35): 38–46

Pearl R G, McLean R F, Rosenthal M H 1988 Effects of spinal anesthesia on response to main pulmonary arterial distension. J Appl Physiol 64: 742–747

Peat S J, Bras P, Hanna M H 1989 A double-blind comparison of epidural ketamine and diamorphine for postoperative analgesia. Anaesthesia 44: 555–558

Penn R D, Savoy S M, Corcos D et al 1989 Intrathecal baclofen for severe spinal spasticity. N Engl J Med 320: 1517–1521

Penning J P, Samson B, Baxter A D 1988 Reversal of epidural morphine-induced respiratory depression and pruritus with nalbuphine. Can J Anaesth 35: 599–604

Penon C, Negre I, Ecoffey C, Gross J B, Levron J-C, Samii K 1988 Analgesia and ventilatory response to carbon dioxide after intramuscular and epidural alfentanil. Anesth Analg 67: 313–317

Pitkanen M T 1987 Body mass and spread of spinal anesthesia with bupivacaine. Anesth Analg 66: 127–131

Planner R S, Cowie R W, Babarczy A S 1988 Continuous epidural morphine analgesia after radical operations upon the pelvis. Surg Gynecol Obstet 166: 229–232

Preston K L, Bigelow G E, Liebson I A 1989 Antagonist effects of nalbuphine in opioid-dependent human volunteers. J Pharmacol Exp Ther 248: 929–937

Rabkin S W 1988 The interrelationship of morphine and the parasympathetic nervous system in digoxin-induced arrhythmias in the guinea-pig. Clin Exp Pharmacol Physiol 15: 565–573

Raja S N, Meyer R A, Campbell J N 1988 Peripheral mechanisms of somatic pain. Anesthesiology 68: 571–590

Rawal N, Arner S, Gustafsson L L, Allvin R 1987 Present state of extradural and intrathecal opioid analgesia in Sweden. A nationwide follow-up survey. Br J Anaesth 59: 791–799

Ready L B, Chadwick H S, Ross B 1987 Age predicts effective epidural morphine dose after abdominal hysterectomy. Anesth Analg 66: 1215–1218

Reay B A, Semple A J, Macrae W A, MacKenzie N, Grant I S 1989 Low-dose intrathecal diamorphine analgesia following major orthopaedic surgery. Br J Anaesth 62: 248–252

Regoli D, Drapeau G, Dion S, D'Orleans-Juste P 1989 Receptors for substance P and related neurokinins. Pharmacology 38: 1–15

Rocco A G, Frank E, Kaul A F, Lipson S J, Gallo J P 1989 Epidural steroids, epidural morphine and epidural steroids combined with morphine in the treatment of post-laminectomy syndrome. Pain 36: 297–303

Rodriguez F D, Rodriguez R E 1989 Intrathecal administration of 5, 6-DHT or 5, 7-DHT reduces morphine and substance P–antinociceptive activity in the rat. Neuropeptides 13: 139–146

Rogers D F, Barnes P J 1989 Opioid inhibition of neurally mediated mucus secretion in human bronchi. Lancet 1: 930–932

Rowbotham D J, Wyld R, Peacock J E, Duthie D J R, Nimmo W S 1989 Transdermal fentanyl for the relief of pain after upper abdominal surgery. Br J Anaesth 63: 56–59

Roy S D, Flynn G L 1988 Solubility and related physicochemical properties of narcotic analgesics. Pharm Res 5: 580–586

Roy S D, Flynn G L 1989 Transdermal delivery of narcotic analgesics: comparative permeabilities of narcotic analgesics through human cadaver skin. Pharm Res 6: 825–832

Sangarlangkarn S, Klaewtanong V, Jonglerttrakool P, Khankaew V 1987 Meperidine as a spinal anaesthetic agent: a comparison with lidocaine–glucose. Anesth Analg 66: 235–240

Savolaine E R, Pandya J B, Greenblatt S H, Conover S R 1988 Anatomy of the human lumbar epidural space: new insights using CT-epidurography. Anesthesiology 68: 217–220

Scheinin B, Scheinin M, Vuorinen J, Lindgren L 1989 Alfentanil obtunds the cardiovascular and sympathoadrenal responses to suxamethonium-facilitated laryngoscopy and intubation. Br J Anaesth 62: 385–392

Schulze S, Roikjaer O, Hasselstrom L, Jensen N H, Kehlet H 1988 Epidural bupivacaine and morphine plus systemic indomethacin eliminates pain but not systemic response and convalescence after cholecystectomy. Surgery 103: 321–327

Sear J W, Hand C W, Moore R A, McQuay H J 1989a Studies on morphine disposition: influence of general anaesthesia on plasma concentrations of morphine and its metabolites. Br J Anaesth 62: 22–27

Sear J W, Hand C W, Moore R A, McQuay H J 1989b Studies on morphine disposition: influence of renal failure on the kinetics of morphine and its metabolites. Br J Anaesth 62: 28–32

Sebel P S, Barrett C W, Kirk C J C, Heykants J 1987 Transdermal absorption of fentanyl and sufentanil in man. Eur J Clin Pharmacol 32: 529–531

Shibata K, Yamamoto Y, Murakami S 1989 Effects of epidural anesthesia on cardiovascular response and survival in experimental hemorrhagic shock in dogs. Anesthesiology 71: 953–959

Simpson K H, Tring I C, Ellis F R 1989 An investigation of premedication with morphine given by the buccal or intramuscular route. Br J Clin Pharmacol 27: 377–380

Sjostrom S, Hartvig P, Persson M P, Tamsen A 1987a Pharmacokinetics of epidural morphine and meperidine in humans. Anesthesiology 67: 877–888

Sjostrom S, Tamsen A, Persson M P, Hartvig P 1987b Pharmacokinetics of intrathecal morphine and meperidine in humans. Anesthesiology 67: 889–895

Sjostrom S, Tamsen A, Hartvig P, Folkesson R, Terenius L 1988 Cerebrospinal fluid concentrations of substance P and (met)enkephalin-ARG^6-PHE^7 during surgery and patient-controlled analgesia. Anesth Analg 67: 976–981

Smith A P, Lee N M 1988 Pharmacology of dynorphin. Ann Rev Pharmacol Toxicol 28: 123–140

Smith N Ty, Benthuysen J L, Bickford R G et al 1989 Seizures during opioid anesthetic induction—are they opioid-induced rigidity? Anesthesiology 71: 852–862

Solomon R E, Brody M J, Gebhart G F 1989 Pharmacological characterization of alpha adrenoceptors involved in the antinociceptive and cardiovascular effects of intrathecally administered clonidine. J Pharmacol Exp Ther 251: 27–38

Stone D J, DiFazio C A 1988 Anesthetic action of opiates: correlations of lipid solubility and spectral edge. Anesth Analg 67: 663–666

Svensson L G, Stewart R W, Cosgrove D M III et al 1988 Intrathecal papaverine for the prevention of paraplegia after operation on the thoracic or thoracoabdominal aorta. J Thorac Cardiovasc Surg 96: 823–829

Symposium on Aspects of Pain 1989 Br J Anaesth 63: 135–226

Tamayo L, Rifo J, Contreras E 1988 Influence of adrenergic and cholinergic mechanisms in baclofen induced analgesia. Gen Pharmacol 19: 87–89

Temeck B K, Schafer P W, Park W Y, Harmon J W 1989 Epidural anesthesia in patients undergoing thoracic surgery. Arch Surg 124: 415–418

Thoren T, Sundberg A, Wattwil M, Garvill J-E, Jurgensen U 1989 Effects of epidural bupivacaine and epidural morphine on bowel function and pain after hysterectomy. Acta Anaesthesiol Scand 33: 181–185

Thornton J R, Losowsky M S 1988 Opioid peptides and primary biliary cirrhosis. Br Med J 297: 1501–1504

van der Hoogen R H W M, Colpaert F C 1987 Epidural and subcutaneous morphine, meperidine (pethidine), fentanyl and sufentanil in the rat: analgesia and other in vivo pharmacologic effects. Anesthesiology 66: 186–194

Van Essen E J, Bovill J G, Ploeger E J, Schout B C 1990 A comparison of epidural clonidine and morphine for post-operative analgesia. Eur J Anaesthesiol 7: 211–218

Vanstrum G S, Bjornson K M, Ilko R 1988 Postoperative effects of intrathecal morphine in coronary artery bypass surgery. Anesth Analg 67: 261–267

Varvel J R, Shafer S L, Hwang S S, Coen P A, Stanski D R 1989 Absorption characteristics of transdermally administered fentanyl. Anesthesiology 70: 928–934

Vaught J L 1988 Substance P antagonists and analgesia: a review of the hypothesis. Life Sci 43: 1419–1431

VonVoigtlander P F, Lewis R A 1988 Analgesic and mechanistic evaluation of spiradoline, a potent kappa opioid. J Pharmacol Exp Ther 246: 259–262

Wang J F, Han S P, Lu Z, Wang X J, Han J S, Ren M F 1989 Effect of calcium ion on analgesia of opioid peptides. Int J Neurosci 47: 279–285

Warfield C A, Crews D A 1987 Epidural steroid injection as a predictor of surgical outcome. Surg Gynecol Obstet 164: 457–458

Warner D O, Danielson D R, Restall C J 1987 Temporary paraplegia following spinal anesthesia in a patient with a spinal cord arteriovenous malformation. Anesthesiology 66: 236–237

Weinberg D S, Inturrisi C E, Reidenberg B et al 1988 Sublingual absorption of selected opioid analgesics. Clin Pharmacol Ther 44: 335–342

Willer J C, Bergeret S, De Broucker T, Gaudy J-H 1988 Low dose epidural morphine does not affect non-nociceptive spinal reflexes in patients with postoperative pain. Pain 32: 9–14

Williams A R 1984 The pharmacist's approach to spinal analgesia. In: Kaufman L (ed) Anaesthesia review 2. Churchill Livingstone, Edinburgh, pp 148–161

Willis Wm D Jr 1988 Anatomy and physiology of descending control of nociceptive responses of dorsal horn neurons: comprehensive review. in: Fields H L, Besson J M (eds) Progress in Brain Research Vol 77. Elsevier Science Publishers B V, Amsterdam, pp 1–29

Wulf H, Striepling E 1990 Postmortem findings after epidural anaesthesia. Anaesthesia 45: 357–361

Wulf H, Winckler K, Maier Ch, Heinzow B 1988 Pharmacokinetics and protein binding of bupivacaine in postoperative epidural analgesia. Acta Anaesthesiol Scand 32: 530–534

Yaksh T L 1987 Opioid receptor systems and the endorphins: a review of their spinal organization. J Neurosurg 67: 157–176

Yamaguchi H, Watanabe S, Fukuda T, Takahashi H, Motokawa K, Ishizawa Y 1989 Minimal effective dose of intrathecal morphine for pain relief following transabdominal hysterectomy. Anesth Analg 68: 537–540

13. Complications of central venous catheterization

S. A. Ridley

Although it was as long ago as 1912 that Bleichroder first described central venous catheterization it is only in recent years that the technique has been adopted for the management of patients for major surgical operations and also for intravenous alimentation.

Despite the relative ease of cannula insertion, there is an incidence of morbidity and mortality, which prompted the Medical Protection Society to issue a booklet outlining some of the possible hazards (Taylor 1989).

This review will briefly cover catheter materials and design, indications and contraindications for central venous catheterization together with some aspects of insertion. The complications associated with the various types of central venous catheters will be discussed in detail.

CATHETERS

Catheter types

Despite the large array of specialized cannulae, catheters may be classified as either external or internal. External catheters, which have their proximal end emerging through the skin, are the most commonly used and may be divided into single, double or triple lumen catheters. Multilumen catheters were developed in the early 1980s and are useful for simultaneous monitoring and multiple infusion therapy. Recent improvements in catheter design include in-line valves, such as the 'Vygon' triple lumen catheter, and special injection ports to decrease infective complications (Segura et al 1987).

Internal catheters, such as 'Port-A-Cath', consist of an intravascular catheter ending in an extravascular but subcutaneous proximal chamber which is buried at a convenient site for the patient and into which drugs or nutritional support may be injected. Such catheters are cosmetically more attractive and allow the patients greater freedom (Gyves et al 1982). They have been used to good effect in paediatric oncology patients where, compared to external catheters, they proved more acceptable to the patients and their parents and became less frequently infected (Ross et al 1988).

Catheter materials

Catheters may be manufactured from polythene, polyurethane, polyvinyl chloride and silicone, all of which have differing physical properties. For example, polyurethane does not absorb nitrates while polyvinyl chloride does (Cote & Torchia 1982). Silicone elastomer catheters are soft (Stenqvist et al 1983) and relatively non-thrombogenic (Borow & Crowley 1985) despite having a rougher surface than polyurethane on electron microscopy (Curelaru et al 1983). Any glueing or welding required during manufacture is more difficult with silicone. Cervera et al (1989) recently demonstrated that polyurethane catheters, especially unused ones, are less flexible than silicone catheters and that polyvinyl chloride catheters actually become more rigid with manipulation. Varying flexibility may contribute to arterial laceration, tearing of the intima, and other mechanical complications.

Surface coatings

Heparin can be chemically bonded to the catheter plastics and is initially very effective. Hoar et al (1981) compared ten heparin bonded catheters to ten non-heparin bonded catheters and reported that during cardiopulmonary bypass no sleeve clot was seen in the heparin bonded catheters while all the other catheters showed evidence of sleeve clot. However, heparin bonding quickly loses its efficacy, as Bennegrad et al (1982) noted that clot was seen on all heparin bonded catheters after 1 to 11 days. Also, heparin coated catheters have induced thrombocytopenia by heparin associated antiplatelet antibodies (Laster et al 1989). Hydromer, produced by the interaction of polyvinylpyrolidine and an isocyanate prepolymer, absorbs water and so may become more slippery on contact with blood. Catheters coated with hydromer are claimed to be easier to insert but this is probably of minor significance. Other catheters (e.g. 'Cook' catheters) are coated with a cationic surfactant which may then bind anionic antibiotics, such as penicillin, with the aim of reducing catheter infection. However, the surfactant–antibiotic complex is degraded by sterilization (Donetz et al 1984) and its efficacy has only been proved in rats (Trooskin et al 1985).

INDICATIONS FOR CATHETERIZATION

The indications for central venous catheterization are increasing and may be broadly classified as follows:

Cardiorespiratory measurements

One of the commonest indications for central venous catheterization is vascular pressure measurement and derivation of cardiorespiratory parameters in peri-operative or critically ill patients. Manipulation of oxygen delivery, systemic vascular resistance and cardiac output, as proposed by Shoemaker et al (1982), depends upon the satisfactory placement of a pulmonary artery catheter.

Vascular access

Double lumen catheters, such as those made by 'Kimal', now allow temporary renal support without an arteriovenous shunt. Similarly, central venous catheters provide vascular access for plasmaphoresis and blood sampling without the need for frequent venepuncture.

Long term infusion

Critical illness or prolonged malabsorption states have increased the requirement for both long and short term parenteral nutrition. Special non-irritant silicone elastomer catheters, such as 'Nutricath S' (Vygon), have been developed and this together with the advances in infection control enable catheters to remain infection free for considerable periods of time (see below). Chemotherapy, antibiotics, hypertonic or irritant drugs are best infused into a large central vein so that peripheral vascular complications are reduced.

Resuscitation

In very low cardiac output states, direct administration of resuscitative drugs in the central circulation is appropriate. Specialized pulmonary artery catheters are manufactured with a pacing port so that a temporary pacing wire may be used (Lavie & Gersh 1988). Unfortunately during cardiopulmonary resuscitation, difficulty in catheter placement can lead to an increased complication rate (20% versus 6%) (Puri et al 1980).

CONTRAINDICATIONS

There are no absolute contraindications to central venous catheterization if the need for access is sufficiently great. However complications are more likely in the presence of coagulopathy. If this can not be corrected by clotting factors or platelets, then surgical cut down may be the most appropriate because it allows the direct compression of the vessel should bleeding occur (Takasugi & O'Connell 1988). Because the subclavian vessels cannot be directly compressed, direct subclavian approaches are probably best avoided in the presence of a coagulopathy. Davis et al (1984) reported that in experienced hands both percutaneous catheterization and cut-down have a low and comparable morbidity. Arrighi et al (1989) performed a randomized prospective study and found that the only difference between percutaneous catheterization and basilic cut-down was that the surgical approach was lengthier (14 versus 8 min).

ASPECTS FOR INSERTION

Approaches and sites for central venous access

Many approaches and techniques have been described for cannulating the central veins; one textbook describes over 26 approaches (Rosen et al 1981) and algorithms for pulmonary artery and central venous catheterization have recently been published (Armstrong et al 1990). Access via the superior vena cava is commonest but recent reports suggest that inferior vena cava cannulation may be just as safe and effective (Curtas et al 1989, Emerman et al 1990). The internal jugular and subclavian veins are the most frequently catheterized veins and there appears to be little difference in complication rate for each site when cannulation is performed by experienced personnel (Hoshal 1985). However, pneumothorax is more likely after subclavian vein catheterization while arterial puncture is more common during internal jugular vein cannulation (Puri et al 1980, Sise et al 1981). The external jugular and arm veins have the lowest rate of complications of all approaches with no serious complications being reported regularly, although the number of successful cannulations may be lower when compared to other approaches. New approaches are being developed to avoid the major complications associated with established routes. For example, the 'Half-Way' catheter is inserted via an arm vein and advanced only as far as the first rib. This has been proposed as an effective route to the central circulation avoiding damage to intra-thoracic structures (Gustavsson et al 1985). Similarly the axillary approach to the central veins avoids the hazards of pneumothorax and arterial puncture but is easy to perform (Nickalls 1987). The efficacy of this technique has been confirmed in a study of 102 patients (Taylor & Yellowlees 1990).

Side of insertion

On the right side, the route to the superior vena cava and the right atrium is straighter than on the left. However, anatomical variation is great, with the length of the superior vena cava varying between 3 and 10 cm (Brandt et al 1970). Insertions on the left side may be complicated by erosion of the superior vena cava wall by a rigid cannula (Ghani & Berry 1983, Eichold & Berryman 1985). Ellis et al (1989) reported a series of ten patients suffering from central venous catheter vascular erosions. In seven patients the catheter was placed in the left subclavian vein and three of the catheter tips abutted against the lateral wall of the superior vena cava. In these circumstances the combination of hyperosmolar solutions and mechanical damage may act synergistically to erode through the wall. Although infrequently reported, damage to the thoracic lymph duct is also more likely on the left (Gramulin et al 1986).

Insertion technique

Refinements to insertion technique may improve safety. The more sophisticated catheters, such as 'LeaderCath' (Vygon) now have soft 'J' guide wires which assist insertion and help reduce the complication rate. However it is important that such guide wires have soft flexible tips as vascular perforation by a straight guide wire has caused a mediastinal haematoma during subclavian vein catheterization for haemodialysis (Masud & Tapson 1989). Also, Hilton et al (1988) showed that replacement catheters inserted using a guide wire over which the existing cannula had been withdrawn were more likely to become infected compared to newly inserted catheters (22% versus 2%).

Belani et al (1980) reported that when the combination of a short 18-gauge needle and flexible guide wire was used to puncture the internal jugular vein, the rate of successful cannulations was higher and the frequency of arterial puncture was only one-third of the rate when direct puncture of the vein with a 14 cm 14-guage 'over the needle' cannula was used. Schartz et al (1979) in a retrospective study of 1021 patients under-going internal jugular catheterization before cardiac bypass surgery found that there was no morbidity associated with arterial puncture when a 20-gauge needle was used for vein location. The only death in this study was attributed to carotid artery laceration after the introduction of an 8-gauge catheter.

Catheter length and position

The catheter length is important; for central venous catheters, the tip should lie above the reflection of the pericardium on the superior vena cava to prevent cardiac tamponade should the catheter tip erode the vein wall. In adult patients of normal stature, the catheter length should be between 10 to 15 cm and this will mean that some of the longer multilumen catheters need not be inserted to their full length.

Correct placement is important and difficult to guarantee without in-jection of radio-opaque dye under fluoroscopic control. A low osmolarity and non-ionic dye such as 'Iopomidol' is probably the most suitable as this limits tissue damage should the catheter not be intravascular. Indeed the use of venography in patients undergoing repeated cannulations and in whom the procedure is becoming more difficult, allows detection of any stenosis or other obstruction. Under these circumstances, when the insertion is performed under fluoroscopic visualization of the vein, a high success rate was achieved (Selby et al 1989). In paediatric patients where the distances involved are much smaller and positioning more critical,

Hauser et al (1989) reported that 46% of pulmonary artery catheters required repositioning after the initial check chest radiograph. .

If the catheter is inserted under local anaesthesia, the patient may complain of a painful or unpleasant sensation if the guide wire or catheter is being misdirected but this is not always a reliable sign. Correct positioning during insertion may be checked by using a catheter filled with a conducting medium as an exploring electrode and watching the changes in the 'P' wave on the ECG (Hoffman et al 1989). This is a very simple technique and the 'P' wave changes are easily observed and reproducible. The position of the catheter once in place may also be checked by ultrasound (Lee et al 1989).

COMPLICATIONS ASSOCIATED WITH PARTICULAR CATHETERS TYPES

Pulmonary artery catheters

The most frequent and serious complications occur with pulmonary artery catheters (PAC) and include dysrhythmias, pulmonary vascular damage, thrombosis and embolism. Gore et al (1987) demonstrated an increased mortality in myocardial infarction victims who had a PAC inserted compared to those who had not. This report prompted Robin (1987) to suggest that a moratorium of PAC use for such patients would be appropriate.

Cardiac dysrhythmias

Cardiac arrhythmias are usually associated with insertion of PAC but may also occur on removal (Damen 1985). Ventricular and atrial arrhythmias or conduction abnormalities may all complicate PAC placement. Sprung et al (1980) reported premature ventricular contractions in 15 of 28 patients undergoing pulmonary artery catheterization. These arrhythmias are more likely to occur in critically ill patients who are hypoxic and acidotic (Iberti et al 1985). Profound shock, a large right ventricle, dilated pulmonary arteries and marked pulmonary hypertension may all increase the difficulty and duration of PAC insertion (Patel et al 1986). Sprung et al (1983) has shown that prophylactic lignocaine reduces the incidence of arrhythmias if catheterization is completed within 17 min. However, as prolonged catheterization itself tends to be arrhythmogenic, it is difficult to determine whether the protective effect of the lignocaine was due to the drug itself or simply the shorter insertion time.

Atrial arrhythmias, which are usually atrial fibrillation or flutter, are less common. Patel et al (1986) reported a 22% incidence of atrial dysrhythmias but premature ectopic atrial contractions are relatively infrequent (1.3%) (Shah et al 1984).

Bundle branch block complicates PAC insertion in about 5% of patients (Sprung et al 1980). Right bundle branch block is usually transient and Shah reported three cases all of which resolved spontaneously in 10 to 24 h. Thomson et al (1979) reported a progression to complete heart block during PAC placement in 5% of patients who had suffered a myocardial infarct complicated with left bundle branch block. In such circumstances, he recommended the prophylactic placement of a temporary pacing line. However, a more recent study by Morris et al (1987) revealed that, although 7 of 47 patients with pre-existing left bundle branch block developed complete heart block, this occurred either before catheterization (1 patient) or some time after the PAC was in place (1 to 16 days). The authors concluded that the incidence of complete heart block on PAC insertion in patients with left bundle branch block was very low and they could not recommend temporary pacing. During PAC insertion, the spontaneous development of complete heart block without pre-existing myocardial pathology is very rare.

Pulmonary artery damage

Pulmonary artery damage may result in rupture or false aneurysm formation. Pulmonary artery rupture is infrequent. In two retrospective (McDaniel et al 1981, Hannan et al 1984) and three large prospective studies (Elliott et al 1979, Sise et al 1981, Boyd et al 1983), the reported incidence varied between 0.1 to 0.2%. Nevertheless although infrequent, massive haemoptysis results and in the 28 cases reported in one review, mortality was 50% (McDaniel et al 1981).

Pulmonary artery rupture may be caused by the tip of the PAC being propelled through the arterial wall by forward migration of the catheter or by inflation of an eccentric balloon (Barash et al 1981). Pressures of up to 250 mmHg have been recorded inside PAC balloons and so positioning of the balloon near a small artery branch may result in intimal tears which may predispose to wall rupture. Deranged coagulation may increase the likelihood of pulmonary artery damage (Pape et al 1979). In Shah's study (1984), three of the four patients who suffered this complication had been anticoagulated. The degenerative changes in the arterial wall caused by pulmonary hypertension renders the wall less compliant and hence, rather than distend the vessel, the balloon may fracture the intimal lining. Hypothermia during cardiopulmonary bypass is a risk because the flexibility of the catheter is reduced with cooling and this combined with surgical manipulation of the intra-thoracic contents, may precipitate spearing of the vessel wall.

Avoidance of pulmonary artery rupture includes anticipation and recognition of forward migration of the catheter, for example avoiding loops of catheter in the right ventricle, and keeping the catheter tip in the larger branches of the pulmonary artery. Treatment involves isolation of the lung with a double lumen endotracheal tube and application of high levels of PEEP (10–20 cmH$_2$O) prior to emergency thoracotomy and wedge resection (McDaniel et al 1981).

Damage may not cause rupture immediately but in rare instances, may initiate false aneurysm development; Dieden et al (1987) reported a series of nine patients collected over ten years. Most false aneurysms present quickly, (80% in 24 h and 90% by three days) with haemoptysis, pulmonary nodules and dense parenchymal consolidation. The mortality was reported as 24% but, if diagnosed early, such aneurysms can be treated with percutaneous embolization (Davis et al 1987).

Thrombosis

Thrombus may be classified as sleeve or mural clot. Sleeve clot originates at the point of internal injury where the catheter enters the vein and then propagates along the catheter while mural clot may occur anywhere the catheter is in contact with the vein's intimal wall. Generally, sleeve clot appears to be more common than mural clot as Brismar et al (1981) found sleeve clot on 42% of catheters but only 8% were associated with mural clot. Thrombus formation is more common with PAC (33%) than central venous catheters (29%) (Rowley et al 1984).

Sleeve thrombus appears to form quickly; Hoar et al (1981) reported that on direct inspection, obvious thrombus had already formed on PAC 1 to 2 h after placement. Lange et al (1984) prospectively studied 36 patients who died with a PAC in place and noted that there was significant thrombus formation after only two days and that the incidence and extent of thrombus formation significantly increased after 36 h.

Embolism

Minor pulmonary emboli may go unrecognized and may be difficult to diagnose in the complex chest radiograph of a critically ill patient. Boyd et al (1983) reported a 0.2% incidence of pulmonary infarction after PAC placement while two other prospective studies (Elliott et al 1979, Sise et al 1983) made no mention of this complication. However Foote et al (1974) using more invasive measures such as lung scans and postmortem examination reported an incidence of 15% in the 88 patients studied.

Central venous catheters

In most cases, central venous catheters are free from the pulmonary artery complications of PAC. However, damage to the pulmonary artery is indeed possible during central venous cannulation and is occasionally reported (Hirsh & Robinson 1984). The major problems of right-sided catheters are pneumothorax, air embolism, secondary malposition, thrombosis and embolism.

Pneumothorax

The incidence of pneumothorax has been reported as up to 5% (Felicano et al 1979, Puri et al 1980): however, more recently, an incidence of less than 2% has been quoted frequently (Dejong et al 1985, Vazquez & Brodski 1985). As well as the site chosen for catheterization, the operator's expertise and familiarity with the technique used is important. Close supervision by senior staff contributed to a low rate of pneumothoraces (1.25%) in one study (Puri et al 1980).

Air embolism

Air embolism may be the most lethal complication of central venous cannulation. The fatal dose of air in fit healthy adults is between $1-2\,ml\,kg^{-1}/s$; however as little as 20 ml may be required to kill a critically ill patient (Peters & Armstrong 1978). The rate of air injection or aspiration is very important and depends upon the diameter and length of the catheter: for example, 100 ml/s of air may be easily aspirated through a 14-gauge cannula and it takes five times as long to aspirate the same volume of air through a 25 cm cannula compared with a 5 cm one. The most commonly cited reason for air embolism is disconnection or fracture of the hub (75% of cases) (Kashuk & Penn 1984) but it may also occur from faulty insertion technique. Minor air emboli, which cause minimal clinical effects, may occur commonly and may go unnoticed if their presence is not actively sought by such means as ultrasound or echocardiography (Gottodiener et al 1988). On the other hand, Kashuk & Penn described 34 cases of serious air embolism. Seventeen patients perished and half of the survivors were left with neurological deficits.

Secondary malposition

Even if correctly placed initially, secondary migration may occur. Vazquez & Brodski (1985) reported that secondary malposition, which usually occurred in the first 12 to 24 h, occurred in 6% of catheter placements. Such malposition usually involved the subclavian venous catheters migrating towards the head or neck and complaints of discomfort during infusion should alert the physician to possible secondary malposition. However, the authors noted that repositioning of the catheter could usually be achieved by reducing the rate of infusion, discontinuing any hypertonic infusions or repositioning the catheter over a guide wire.

It is probably not justified to routinely check the position of a catheter with a chest radiograph on a daily basis unless indicated for other reasons, especially as the position may be checked by other non-invasive means such as ultrasound. However, routine chest X-ray may give early warning of future problems by, for example, the 'pinch-off sign' which is caused by the pincer action of the clavicle and first rib. Aitken & Minton (1984) reported four patients with the pinch-off sign on routine chest X-ray who went on to develop postural-related difficulty with injection, catheter leak and catheter transection with distal embolization. These authors concluded that the pinch-off sign warranted the removal of the catheter and repositioning at a different site.

Thrombosis

As with PAC, the incidence of thrombosis associated with central venous catheters varies depending on how invasively it is sought, the duration of catheterization and catheter material. If the catheters are examined at postmortem, nearly all catheters show antimortem thrombus formation (Hoshal et al 1971), while if venography is used rates of between 50 to 60% are reported (Bozzetti et al 1983, Conners et al 1985).

Thrombus formation predisposes to catheter-related infection (see below) and vein occlusion. Ducatman et al (1985) reported finding mural thrombi in 45 of 141 patients who had central venous catheters in place at death and who underwent postmortem examinations; they identified organisms in mural clots of five cases. Vanherweghem et al (1986) reported that venous occlusion occurred in 19% of chronic renal failure sufferers after temporary subclavian cannulation for haemodialysis. Such thrombosis may compromise a subsequent arteriovenous shunt or exclude part of the vascular bed for future access.

Various steps have been taken to reduce catheter-related thrombus. Low dose warfarin (2 mg daily) may be used satisfactorily (Bern et al 1986) and this dose should not alter the prothrombin index. Its efficacy may be assessed by the Von Kaulla time, a more usual measure of antithrombin III activity. The addition of heparin to the infusate (e.g. 1 unit per ml) is not effective since thrombus formation occurs on the outer wall of the catheter and the vein's intimal surface, and because this dose is insufficient for satisfactory systemic heparinization. No catheter-related thrombus was found in either those patients who were fully anticoagulated prior to cardiac surgery (Perkins et al 1984) or patients who died with deranged clotting function (Conners et al 1985).

Embolism

The overall incidence of embolism during central venous catheterization is unknown. Mural thrombi adhere to the endothelium and so rarely produce important emboli (Ducatman et al 1985). However, case reports of fatal pulmonary embolism (Kaye & Smith 1988, Bagwell & Marchildon 1989) underline the importance of this complication. Significant pulmonary embolism is more likely during catheter manipulation. Brismar et al (1981) demonstrated that a sleeve clot peeled off the catheter when it was removed and that in several cases parts of a thrombus were carried away in the blood flow. In 3 of 57 patients studied by these authors, lung scintillography confirmed the clinical diagnosis of pulmonary embolism.

Nutrition catheters

The use of parenteral nutrition is increasing; in a group of patients studied by Wolfe et al (1986) the average number of catheters per patient increased from 1.2 to 1.9 over a four-year period. Similarly, Takasugi & O'Connell (1988) reported that in their 4.5-year study, over 50% of catheters were inserted in the last year and a half. Therefore, the prevalence of complications will increase even if the complication rate remains static.

Generally the complication rate of properly maintained nutrition catheters is very low. One recent report gives details of 76 nutrition catheters which remained in place for an average of 16 months; complications were reported on 32 occasions (Stokes et al 1988). Similarly, Wolfe reported 509 complications in 31 112 patient-days, an overall rate of 1.6%. Despite this low complication rate, death due to complications associated with nutrition catheters can occur. Wolfe's study involved 1647 patients and he reported that the nutrition catheter was a primary cause or major contributing factor to the death of four patients (causes of death being tension pneumothorax, subclavian artery laceration, candida sepsis and hyperglycaemic hyperosmolar coma).

The major complications associated specifically with nutrition catheters are outlined below.

Sepsis: The incidence of catheter-related sepsis in nutritional catheters varies between 2.8% (Padberg et al 1981) and 14% (Pettigrew et al 1985), although reports of single episodes without reference to patient-days or differences between colonization, contamination and infection (see below) need careful interpretation. Infection may be reduced by regularly dressing the exit site which dramatically reduces the number of positive cultures taken from the external part of the catheter (Jarrard et al 1980). Careful dressing routines and other aspects of line care have been described more recently (Pennington 1989). Furthermore, it has been shown that catheter-related sepsis rates are lowest when catheter care is entrusted to designated nutrition nurses (Faubion et al 1986).

Breaks in catheter management protocol or the use of the catheter for other purposes increase infective complications. Linares et al (1985) found that the catheter hub was colonized in 70% of patients with catheter-related sepsis. Pemberton et al (1986) found a six-fold increase in catheter sepsis in triple lumen lines when these were used for parenteral nutrition and suggested that this may have been caused by the frequent manipulation of the other ports. This is supported by Wolfe et al (1986) who reported an increase in infection rate from around 3% to over 10% on the introduction of multilumen catheters.

The overall incidence of sepsis is not reduced by subcutaneous tunnelling as it is now appreciated that the major source of catheter infection is due to breaks or junctions in the line. Morgan et al (1987) concluded that although tunnelling did not reduce infection, it prolonged the catheter lifespan. Tunnelling may also have advantages in that it anchors the line and allows the line exit to be conveniently sited for the patient.

Mechanical blockage: Catheters may become blocked by a thrombus, fatty deposits or calcium salts, although the occlusion is generally not sudden, being manifest by ever increasing pressure to maintain a satisfactory infusion rate (Mughal 1989). Catheters blocked by a fibrin sheath may be saved by using a urokinase lock (Glynn et al 1980). Although Glynn used 5000 units of urokinase as a bolus, more recent studies in children have suggested that a continuous infusion of urokinase at 2000 units kg^{-1}/h for 24 h effectively relieves catheter obstruction which had been unresponsive to two previous boluses of urokinase (Bagnell et al 1989). Lines suspected of being blocked and infected may be treated initially by flushing the line with a potent antibiotic such as vancomycin or netilmicin. However, forceful flushing may rupture a completely blocked catheter and therefore in these circumstances the only safe solution is to remove it (Mughal 1989). In the case of lipid containing nutrition fluids, lipid sludging may gradually reduce the flow rate until complete occlusion occurs (Main & Pennington 1984). Flushing the line with 70% ethanol may dissolve the lipid sludge (Pennington & Pithie 1987). If the catheter has not responded to fibrino-lytic therapy, flushing the catheter with 0.1 M hydrochloric acid may dissolve any calcium salts (Mendoza et al 1986).

Major vein thrombosis: While catheter-associated thrombus is common, caval obstruction due to a thrombus is relatively rare. However, once caval obstruction has developed it carries a high mortality; in one study (Stokes et al 1988), superior vena caval thrombosis occurred in six patients, three of whom perished. Inferior vena cava obstruction may be less frequent (Mulvihill & Fonkalsrud 1984) and may also be less serious when it occurs (Fonkalsrud et al 1982).

Mughal (1989) has pointed out that if the catheter is still patent and uninfected but major vein thrombosis is suspected, removal may not be appropriate as this does not necessarily result in resolution of the thrombus and also it prevents local fibrinolytic therapy. Early treatment of partial thrombotic occlusion with systemic anticoagulation may be successful and prevent further propagation of the clot. However, once the vein has become occluded, treatment becomes more difficult; successful recanalization after local thrombolytic therapy has been reported (Theriault & Buzdar 1990) whereas in other instances surgical thrombectomy has been required (de Marie et al 1989, Chamsi-Pasha & Irving 1987). The long term outcome of caval occlusion, either by recanalization or collateral circulation development, is unknown as there have been no longitudinal studies.

INFECTION

Central venous line infection may be classified as follows (Matthay 1983):

(a) Contamination. This occurs when a positive catheter tip culture is presumed to have resulted from pathogen contamination during placement or removal of the line, or during a bacteraemia.

(b) Colonization. Positive catheter tip culture yields the same pathogen as isolated from another primary source in the body such as the respiratory tract.

(c) Catheter-related sepsis. This occurs when the same pathogen is cultured from the blood and catheter tip without prior isolation from another site and the sepsis resolves upon removal of the line.

The usual pathogens are coagulase negative *Staphylococci* and yeasts, but other pathogens such as *Pseudomonas* and *Escherichia* (Clayton et al 1985) may be isolated depending upon the site of venous access and the patients' underlying pathology. Infection may not be confined to the catheter alone. Rowley (1984) noted that 53 of 142 patients who died within one month of PAC placement had some form of right-sided endocardial lesions, e.g. sterile thrombus or subendocardial haemorrhage. Four of these 53 patients had infected vegetations on the pulmonary valve.

The incidence of catheter infection depends upon:

Techniques used to isolate the pathogens: Contamination and colonization are more frequent than catheter-related sepsis and reports vary from between 6% (Myers et al 1985) to 27% (Elliott et al 1979). The highest rates of positive catheter tip culture are reported when the most sensitive techniques are used. For example, Passerini et al (1987) used sonification culture and electron microscopy to demonstrate that 15 out of 20 PAC which had been removed from critically ill patients were infected. Sonification culture involves removing the bacterial glycocalyx from the outer surface of the catheter and disrupting this biofilm using ultrasound prior to scanning with the electron microscope. Cooper & Hopkins (1985) using direct gram-staining of the catheter tip reported this as an extremely sensitive, fast, inexpensive and reliable technique with which they found a contamination rate of 12.4%. A widely used technique for determining catheter tip infection and for distinguishing between contamination and colonization was developed by Maki et al (1977). This technique overcomes the problem that when using an ordinary broth culture bottle, one bacterium contaminating the catheter tip will yield a positive result. The semiquantitative technique involves rolling a 5 cm catheter segment across a blood agar plate, and if after incubation, more than 15 individual colonies are identified, the catheter can be assumed to be colonized. These authors compared this new technique with ordinary broth culture in 250 intravenous catheters and demonstrated its increased specificity. Ninety percent of catheters had low density colonization (< 15 colonies) on semiquantitative culture although just under 20% grew some organisms on broth or plate culture. None of these catheters led to septicaemia; however in 25 catheters which yielded more than 15 colonies by the semiquantitative technique, catheter-related sepsis originated from four.

All the above techniques for detecting infection examine the catheter once it has been removed and so it is inevitable that some 'clean' catheters will be needlessly removed. To avoid such wastage, Mosca et al (1987) have described a sensitive technique for distinguishing between infected and non-infected catheters while they are still in place. Samples of blood are drawn simultaneously through the catheter and a peripheral vein and if the colony count in the catheter blood is five times that in the peripheral blood, catheter infection is extremely likely.

Duration of catheterization: Tully et al (1981) removed all the lines in their study within 72 h and reported infection rates of less than 2%. Michael et al (1981) studied 190 patients and noted that there was a positive relationship between the duration of catheter placement and positive tip cultures if the catheters were left in place for longer than five days. Finally, Kaye et al (1983) reported that if the catheters were in place for less than two days, the catheter tips were only infected in 2.5% of cases, but that if the catheters were in place for more than three days, the observed rates of infection rose to over 20%. Rates of infection appear to increase markedly after a critical period of between two and five days.

RARER COMPLICATIONS

Many other diverse and rarer complications have been reported after central venous catheterization. While no classification of these more rare complications is completely satisfactory, they may be broadly grouped into those categories outlined below (these examples illustrate the variety of complications but are not exhaustive).

Early complications

Early complications are usually due to damage to surrounding structures. During internal jugular vein cannulation, massive haemoptysis and blood aspiration has been reported (Friedman et al 1989). This particular patient required respiratory support on an intensive therapy unit for seven days. Two cases of tracheal puncture during internal jugular vein catheterization were diagnosed by sudden deflation of the endotracheal cuff (Konichezky et al 1983). Early complications after subclavian catheterization include surgical emphysema developing in the absence of a pneumothorax (Chan & Smedley 1989). Unrecognized subclavian artery cannulation and subsequent resuscitation of the patient with 3l of crystalloid infused intra-arterially has been reported (Dedhia & Schiebel 1987).

Late complications

Late complications arising after prolonged catheterization may be divided into local or distant. Examples of local complications include osteomyelitis of the clavicle (Klein et al 1987), extravasation resulting in widespread tissue necrosis (Gemlo et al 1988), erosion of the pericardium (Haeften et al 1988) and a right atrial mass which required surgical removal (Dick et al 1989). An arteriovenous fistula between the right subclavian artery and right brachiocephalic vein has been described (Gramulin et al 1986). This presented 18 months later with progressive congestive heart failure. Arterial damage during attempted internal jugular vein catheterization resulted in formation of a giant false aneurysm of the subclavian artery which presented three weeks later with the patient complaining of dyspnoea and hoarseness (Huddy et al 1989). Another iatrogenic arteriovenous fistula caused brachial plexus compression (Tebib et al 1987) while a mediastinal haematoma has caused temporary phrenic nerve neuropraxia (Seaberg & Generalovich 1989).

Examples of distant complications include a brain abscess which caused right-sided weakness, blurred vision and eventually required surgical drainage. The responsible organism was traced to an infected central line (Perez et al 1988). Also, septic pulmonary emboli from an infected central venous catheter were mistaken for metastatic nodules on the chest X-ray of a young girl undergoing chemotherapy for rhabdomyosarcoma (Stine et al 1989).

Mechanical problems

Mechanical failures at insertion include extravascular knotting of the guide wire (Wang & Einarsson 1987) and disintegration of the guide wire so that part was retained in the patient (Schou 1988). Catheter shearing and fracturing occurs in about 0.1% of all insertions (Lybecker et al 1989). The reported causes of catheter embolization include cutting of the catheter by withdrawal through the needle, improper fixation and severing after repeated intravenous kinking. In the past, surgical exploration for removal was required (Feliciano et al 1979) but with the increased sophistication of interventional radiology, intravascular catheter fragments may be retrieved transvenously (Fischer & Ward 1983). Fisher & Ferreyro (1978) reported that 71% of patients with retained catheter fragment emboli suffered serious complications or died as a result. Embolism may also occur with internal catheters; two cases have been reported. In one case, there was slippage of the retaining 'O' ring and in the other, spontaneous fracture of the catheter occurred (Carr 1989).

Problems with the functioning of the catheter, e.g. blocked cannula lumen, thermistor malfunction and balloon rupture do occur (up to 25% of cases in one study (Sise et al 1981)). There are early case reports of catheter knotting leading to difficulty in withdrawal (Lipp et al 1971) but Shah (1984) failed to detect knotting in his large study even in the presence of another intra-cardiac line which was commonly a temporary pacing wire. Shah also reported PAC obstructing the venous vent during cardio-pulmonary bypass and one catheter was sewn into the atrial wall during closure.

FUTURE DEVELOPMENTS

Catalysts and chemical stabilizers which are used in the manufacture of central venous catheters are now recognized as thrombogenic and a reduction in these constituents may improve catheter performance. As experience with totally implanted catheter systems grows, their advantages will become clearer. Indeed the most recent studies concerning totally implanted systems would suggest that they are now surpassing external catheters for long term use (Guenier et al 1989, Kappers-Klunne et al 1989, Pomp et al 1989). Extension of the specialist team system for the care of prolonged central venous access and the closer surveillance of all catheters for impending complications may help reduce morbidity and mortality.

SUMMARY

Important life threatening complications are associated with the use of all types of central venous catheters. The more serious and frequent complications are encountered with PAC and include arrhythmias, pulmonary artery damage, thrombosis and embolism. The insertion of central venous lines may also be complicated by pneumothorax and air embolism while long term nutrition catheters are commonly complicated by sepsis, thrombosis or mechanical occlusion. Unless special measures are taken in the care of the catheter, the incidence of catheter-related infection will increase with the duration of catheterization. Needless complications may be avoided by careful attention to technique and referral for all aspects of line management to experienced dedicated personnel.

REFERENCES

Aitken D R, Minton J P 1984 The "Pinch-off Sign": A warning of impending problems with permanent subclavian catheters. Am J Surg 148: 633–636
Armstrong R F, Bullen C, Cohen S L, Singer M, Webb A R 1990 Critical care algorithms. Pulmonary artery and central venous catheter monitoring. Clin Intensive Care 1: 93–95

Arrighi D A, Farnell M B, Mucha P, Istrup D M, Anderson D L 1989 Prospective, randomized trial of rapid venous access for patients in hypovolaemic shock. Ann Emerg Med 18: 927–930

Bagnall H A, Gomperts E, Atkinson J B 1989 Continuous infusion of low-dose urokinase in the treatment of central venous catheter thrombosis in infants and children. Pediatrics 83: 963–966

Bagwell C E, Marchildon M B 1989 Mural thrombus in children: Potentially lethal complication of central venous hyperalimentation. Crit Care Med 17: 295–296

Barash P G, Nordi D, Hammond G et al 1981 Catheter-induced pulmonary artery perforation. J Thorac Cardiovasc Surg 82: 5–12

Belani K G, Buckley J J, Gordon R, Casteneda W 1980 Percutaneous cervical central venous line placement: A comparison of the internal and external jugular vein routes. Anesth Analg 59: 40–44

Bennegrad K, Curelan I, Gustaisson B, Linder L E, Zachrisson B F 1982 Material thrombogenicity in central venous catheterization. Acta Anaesthesiol Scand 26: 112–120

Bern M M, Bothe A, Bristrain B, Champayne C D, Keane M S, Blackloan G L 1986 Prophylaxis against central vein thrombosis with low dose warfarin. Surgery 99: 216–220

Bleichroder F 1912 Intra-arterielle Therapie. Bern Klinischen Wochenschrift 1503–1505

Borow M, Crowley J G 1985 Evaluation of central venous catheter thrombogenicity. Acta Anaesthesiol Scand (Suppl.) 81: 59–64

Boyd K D, Thomas S J, Gold J, Boyd A D 1983 A prospective study of complications of pulmonary artery catheterization in 500 consecutive patients. Chest 84: 245–249

Bozzetti F, Scarpa D, Terno G et al 1983 Subclavian venous thrombosis due to indwelling catheter: a prospective study of 52 patients. JPEN 7: 560–562

Brandt R L, Foley W J, Fink G H, Regan W J 1970 Mechanism of perforation of the heart with production of hydropericardia by a venous catheter and its prevention. Am J Surg 119: 311–316

Brismar B, Hardstedt C, Jacobson S 1981 Diagnosis of thrombosis by catheter phlebography after prolonged venous catheterization. Ann Surg 194: 779–783

Carr M E 1989 Catheter embolization from implanted venous access devices: case reports. Angiology 40: 319–323

Cervera M, Dolz M, Herraez J V, Belda R 1989 Evaluation of the elastic behaviour of central venous PVC, polyurethane and silicone catheters. Phys Med Biol 34: 177–183

Chamsi-Pasha H, Irving M H 1987 Right atrial thrombus: a complication of total parenteral nutrition in an adult. Br Med J 195: 308

Chan T Y K, Smedley F H 1989 Surgical emphysema in a patient with an intercostal hernia following insertion of a subclavian central line. Intensive Ther Clin Monit 1: 114–115

Clayton D G, Shanahan E C, Ordman A J, Simpson J C 1985 Contamination of internal jugular cannulae. Anaesthesia 40: 523–528

Conners A F, Castile R J, Farhaf N Z, Tomaashefski N 1985 Complications of right heart catheterization. Chest 88: 567–572

Cooper G L, Hopkins C C 1985 Rapid diagnosis of intravascular catheter associated infection by direct gram staining of catheter segments. N Engl J Med 312: 1142–1147

Cote D D, Torchia M G 1982 Nitroglycerin adsorption to polyvinylchloride seriously interferes with its clinical use. Anesth Analg 61: 541–543

Curelaru I, Gustavsson B, Hansson A H, Linder L E, Stenqvist O, Wojciechowski J 1983 Material thrombogenicity in central venous catheterisation II. A comparison between plain elastomer, and plain polyethylene, long, antebrachial catheters. Acta Anaesthesiol Scand 27: 158–164

Curtas S, Bonaventura M, Meguid M M 1989 Cannulation of inferior vena cava for long term central venous access. Surg Gynecol Obstet 168: 121–124

Damen J 1985 Ventricular arrhythmias during insertion and removal of pulmonary artery catheters. Chest 88: 190–193

Davis S D, Neithamer C D, Schreiber T S, Sos T A 1987 False pulmonary artery aneurysm induced by Swan-Ganz catheters; diagnosis and embolotherapy. Radiology 164: 741–742

Davis S J, Thompson S J, Edney J A 1984 Insertion of Hickman catheters. Comparison of cut-down and percutaneous techniques. Am Surg 15: 673–676

Dedhia H V, Schiebel F 1987 What is wrong with this chest Roentgenogram? Chest 92: 921–922

De Jong P C M, Von Meyenfeldt M R, Rouflart M, Wesdorp R I C, Soeters P B 1985

Complications of central venous catheterization of subclavian vein: the influence of a parenteral nutrition team. Acta Anaesthesiol Scand (Suppl.) 81: 48–52

de Marie S, Hagenouw-Taal J, Schultze Kool L J, Meerdink G, Huysmans H A 1989 Suppurative thrombophlebitis of the superior vena cava. Scand J Infect Dis 21: 107–111

Dick A E, Gross C M, Rubin J W 1989 Echocardiographic detection of an infected superior vena caval thrombus presenting as a right atrial mass. Chest 96: 212–214

Dieden J D, Frilous L A, Renner J W 1987 Pulmonary artery false aneurysms secondary to Swan-Ganz pulmonary artery catheters. Am J Roentgenol 149: 901–906

Donetz A P, Harvey R A, Greco R S 1984 Stability of antibiotics bound to polytetrafluoroethylene with cationic surfactants. J Clin Microbiol 19: 1–3

Ducatman B S, McMichan J C, Edwards W D 1985 Catheter-induced lesions of the right side of the heart. JAMA 253: 791–795

Eichold B H, Berryman C R 1985 Contralateral hydrothorax; an unusual complication of central venous catheter placement. Anesthesiology 62: 673–674

Elliott C G, Zimmerman G A, Clemmer T P 1979 Complications of pulmonary artery catheterization in care of critical ill patients. Chest 76: 647–652

Ellis L M, Vogel S B, Copeland E M 1989 Central venous catheter vascular erosions. Ann Surg 209: 475–478

Emerman C L, Bellon E M, Lukens T W, May T E, Effron D 1990 A prospective study of femoral versus subclavian vein catheterization during cardiac arrest. Ann Emer Med 19: 26–30

Faubion W C, Wesley J R, Khalidi N, Silva J 1986 Total parenteral nutrition catheter sepsis: impact of a team approach. JPEN 10: 642–645

Feliciano D V, Mattox K L, Graham J M, Beall A C, Jordon G L 1979 Major complications of percutaneous subclavian vein catheters. Am J Surg 138: 869–874

Fischer H B, Ward G 1983 Catheter tip embolism—a continuing iatrogenic complication of central venous catheterisation. Intensive Care Med 3: 127–129

Fisher R G, Ferreyro R 1978 Evaluation of techniques for nonsurgical removal of intravascular foreign bodies. Am J Roentgenol 130: 541–548

Fonkalsrud E W, Ament M E, Berquist W E, Burke M 1982 Occlusion of the vena cava in infants receiving central venous hyperalimentation. Surg Gynecol Obstet 154: 189–192

Foote G A, Schabel S I, Hodges M 1974 Pulmonary complications of the flow-directed balloon tipped catheter. N Engl J Med 290: 927–937

Friedman Y, Rackow E C, Weil M H 1989 Massive hemoptysis during catheterization of the internal jugular vein. Chest 95: 1143

Gemlo B T, Rayner A A, Swanson R J, Young J A, Homann J F, Hohn D C 1988 Extravasation. A serious complication of the split sheath introducer technique for venous access. Arch Surg 123: 490–492

Ghani G A, Berry A J 1983 Right hydrothorax after left external jugular vein catheterization. Anesthesiology 58: 93–94

Glynn M F X, Langer B, Jeejeebhoy K N 1980 Therapy for thrombotic occlusion of long term intravenous alimentation catheters. JPEN 4: 387–390

Gore J M, Goldberg R J, Spodick D H, Alpert J S, Dalen J E 1987 A community wide assessment of the use of pulmonary artery catheters in patients with acute myocardial infarction. Chest 92: 721–727

Gottodiener J S, Papademetriou V, Notargiacomo A, Park W Y, Cutler J 1988 Incidence and effects of systemic venous air embolism. Arch Intern Med 148: 795–800

Gramulin Z, Brucher J C, Forster A, Simonet F, Rouge J C 1986 Multiple complications after internal jugular vein catheterisation. Anaesthesia 41: 408–412

Guenier C, Ferreira J, Pector J C 1989 Prolonged venous access in cancer patients. Eur J Surg Oncol 15: 553–555

Gustavsson B, Linder L, Hultman E, Curelaru I 1985 'Half-Way' venous catheters. I. Theoretical premises and aims. Acta Anaesthesiol Scand (Suppl.) 81: 30–31

Gyves J, Ensiminger W, Neidehuber J et al 1982 A totally implanted system for intravenous chemotherapy in patients with cancer. Am J Med 72: 841–845

Hannan A T, Brown M, Bigman O 1984 Pulmonary artery catheter induced hemorrhage. Chest 85: 128–131

Hauser G J, Pollack M M, Sivit C J, Taylor G A, Bulas D I, Guion C J 1989 Routine chest radiographs in pediatric intensive care: A prospective study. Pediatrics 83: 465–470

Hilton E, Haslett T M, Borenstein M T, Tucci V, Isenberg H D, Singer C 1988 Central catheter infections: Single- versus triple-lumen catheters. Am J Med 84: 667–672

Hirsch N P, Robinson P N, 1984 Pulmonary artery puncture following subclavian venous cannulation. Anaesthesia 39: 727–728

Hoar P F, Witren R M, Mangano D T, Avery J G, Szarnichi R J, Hill J D 1981 Heparin bonding reduces thrombogenicity of pulmonary artery catheters. N Engl J Med 305: 993–995

Hoffman M A, Langer J C, Pearl R H, Filler R M 1989 Electrocardiographic guided placement of central venous catheters. Br J Surg 76: 1032–1033

Hoshal V L 1985 The consequences of a cavalier approach to central venous catheterisation. Acta Anaesthesiol Scand (Suppl) 81: 11–13

Hoshal V, Ause R, Hoskins P 1971 Fibrin sleeve formation on indwelling subclavian central venous catheters. Arch Surg 102: 353–357

Huddy S P J, McEwan A, Sabbat J, Parker D J 1989 Giant false aneurysm of the subclavian artery. Anaesthesia 44: 588–589

Iberti T J, Benjamin E, Guppi L, Raskin J M 1985 Ventricular arrhythmias during pulmonary artery catheterization in the intensive care unit. Am J Med 78: 451–454

Jarrard M M, Olson C M, Freeman J B 1980 Daily dressing change effects on skin flora beneath subclavian catheter dressings during total parenteral nutrition. JPEN 4: 391–392

Kappers-Klunne M C, Degener J E, Stijnen T, Abels J 1989 Complications from long term indwelling central venous catheters in hematological patients with special reference to infection. Cancer 64: 1747–1752

Kashuk J L, Penn I 1984 Air embolism after central venous catheterization. Surg Gynecol Obstet 159: 249–252

Kaye C G, Smith D R 1988 Complications of central venous cannulation. Br Med J 297: 572–573

Kaye W E, Wheaton M, Potter-Bynoe G 1983 Radial and pulmonary artery catheter related sepsis. Crit Care Med 11: 249

Klein B, Mittelman M, Katz R, Djaldetti M 1987 Oesteomyelitis of the clavicle as complication of infected subclavian line. Am J Med 83: 1006

Konichezky G E, Saguib S, Soroker D 1983 Tracheal puncture — a complication of internal jugular vein cannulation. Anaesthesia 38: 572–574

Lange H W, Galliani C A, Edwards J E 1984 Local complications associated with indwelling Swan-Ganz catheters; autopsy study of 36 cases. Am J Cardiol 52: 1108–1111

Laster J L, Nichols W K, Silver D 1989 Thrombocytopenia associated with heparin-coated catheters in patients with heparin-associated antiplatelet antibodies. Arch Intern Med 149: 2285–2287

Lavie C, Gersh B 1988 Pacing in left bundle branch block during Swan-Ganz catheterization. Arch Intern Med 148: 981–984

Lee W, Leduc L, Cotton D B 1989 Ultrasonographic guidance for central venous access during pregnancy. Am J Obstet Gynecol 161: 1012–1013

Linares J, Sitges-Sera A, Garau J, Percz J L, Martin R 1985 Pathogenesis of catheter sepsis: A prospective study with quantitative and semi-quantitative cultures of catheter hub segments. J Clin Microbiol 21: 357–360

Lipp H, O'Donoghue K, Resnekov L 1971 Intracardiac knotting of a flow-directed balloon catheter. JAMA 284: 220

Lybecker H, Anderson C, Hansen M K 1989 Transvenous retrieval of intracardiac catheter fragments. Acta Anaesthesiol Scand 33: 565–567

McDaniel D P, Stone J G, Faltas A N et al 1981 Catheter induced pulmonary artery haemorrhage. J Thorac Cardiovasc Surg 82: 1–4

Main J, Pennington C R 1984 Catheter blockage with lipid during long term parenteral nutrition. Br Med J 289: 743

Maki D G, Weise C E, Sarafin H C O 1977 A semiquantitative culture method for identifying intravenous catheter related infection. N Engl J Med 296: 1305–1309

Matthay M A 1983 Invasive hemodynamic monitoring in critically ill patients. Clin Chest Med 4: 233–249

Masud T, Tapson J S 1989 Mediastinal haematoma caused by subclavian catheterization for haemodialysis. Int J Artif Organs 12: 708–710

Mendoza G J B, Soto A, Brown E G, Dolgin S F, Steinfeld L, Sweet A I 1986 Intracardiac thrombi complicating central total parenteral nutrition: resolution without surgery or thrombolysis. J Pediatr Surg 108: 610–613

Micheal L, Marsh M, McMichan M 1981 Infection of pulmonary artery catheters in critically ill patients. JAMA 245: 1032–1036

Morgan K T, McEntee G, Jones B, Hone R, Duignan N, O'Malley E 1987 To tunnel or not to tunnel catheters for parenteral nutrition? Ann R Coll Surg Engl 69: 235–236

Morris D, Mulville D, Lew W Y W 1987 Risk of developing complete heart block during bedside pulmonary artery catheterization in patients with left bundle branch block. Arch Intern Med 147: 2005–2010

Mosca R, Curtas S, Forbes B, Meeguid M M 1987 The benefits of isolator cultures in the management of suspected catheter sepsis. Surgery 102: 718–723

Mughal M M 1989 Complications of intravenous feeding catheters. Br J Surg 76: 15–21

Mulvihill S J, Fonkalsrud E W 1984 Complications of superior versus inferior vena cava occlusion in infants receiving total parenteral nutrition. J Pediatr Surg 19: 752–757

Myers M L, Austin T W, Sibbald W J 1985 Pulmonary artery catheter infections. Ann Surg 201: 237–241

Nickalls R W D 1987 A new percutaneous infraclavicular approach to the axillary vein. Anaesthesia 42: 151–154

Padberg F T, Ruggiero J, Blackburn B R 1981 Central venous catheterization for parenteral nutrition. Ann Surg 193: 264–270

Pape L A, Haffajee C I, Makis J E et al 1979 Fatal pulmonary hemorrhage after use of the flow directed balloon-tipped catheter. Ann Intern Med 90: 344–347

Passerini L, Jackson F L, Casterton J W 1987 Biofilms on right heart flow-directed catheters. Chest 92: 440–446

Patel C, Laboy V, Venus B, Mathru M, Weir D 1986 Acute complications of pulmonary artery catheter insertion in critical ill patients. Crit Care Med 14: 195–197

Pemberton L B, Lyman B, Lander V, Covinsky J 1986 Sepsis from triple- vs single-lumen catheters during total parenteral nutrition in surgical or critically ill patients. Arch Surg 121: 591–594

Pennington C R 1989 Central venous catheters. Scott Med J 34: 419–420

Pennington C R, Pithie A D 1987 Ethanol lock in the management of catheter occlusion. JPEN 11: 507–508

Perez R E, Smith M, McClendon J, Kim J, Eugenio N 1988 Pseudallescheria boydii brain abscess. Am J Med 84: 359–362

Perkins N A K, Cail W S, Bedford R F, Clinger J H, Baschi A J 1984 Internal jugular vein function after Swan-Ganz catheterization. Anesthesiology 61: 456–459

Peters J L, Armstrong R 1978 Air embolism occurring as a complication of central venous catheterization. Ann Surg 187: 375–378

Pettigrew R A, Lang S D, Haydock D A, Parry B R, Bremner D A, Hill G L 1985 Catheter related infection in patients on intravenous nutrition: A prospective study of quantitative catheter cultures and guide wire changes for suspected sepsis. Br J Surg 72: 52–55

Pomp A, Caldwell M D, Albina J E 1989 Subcutaneous infusion ports for administration of parenteral nutrition at home. Surg Gynecol Obstet 169: 329–333

Puri V K, Carlson R W, Bander J J, Weil M H 1980 Complications of vascular catheterization in the critically ill. Crit Care Med 8: 495–499

Robin E D 1987 Death by pulmonary artery flow-directed catheter. Chest 92: 727–731

Rosen M, Latto I G, Ng W S 1981 Handbook of central venous catheterisation. W B Saunders, London

Ross M N, Haase G M, Poole M A, Burrington J D, Odom L F 1988 Comparison of totally implanted reservoirs with external catheters as venous access devices in pediatric oncology patients. Surg Gynecol Obstet 167: 141–144

Rowley K M, Clubb S, Smith G J W, Labin H S 1984 Right sided infective endocarditis as a consequence of flow-directed pulmonary artery catheters. N Engl J Med 311: 1152–1156

Schartz A J, Jobes D R, Greenhow D E, Stephensen L W, Ellison N 1979 Carotid artery puncture with internal jugular cannulation. Anesthesiology 51: S160

Schou H 1988 The double 'J' spring guide wire and its hazards. Partially retained double J-wire: a complication during central venous catheterization. Acta Anaesthesiol Scand 32: 158–160

Seaberg D C, Generalovich T 1989 Hemorrhagic compression of the phrenic nerve after streptokinase therapy. Am J Emerg Med 7: 185–186

Segura B M, Alia A C, Torres R J M, Gil E J, Silges-Sera A 1987 In vitro bacteriological study of a new hub model for intravascular catheters and infusion equipment. Clin Nutr (Suppl.) 104: 99

Selby J B, Tegtmeyer C J, Amodeo C, Bittner L, Atuk N O 1989 Insertion of subclavian hemodialysis catheters in difficult cases. Am J Roentgenol 152: 641–643

Shah K B, Rao T L K, Laughin S, El-Etr A A 1984 A review of pulmonary artery catheterization in 6,245 patients. Anesthesiology 61: 271–275

Shoemaker WC, Appel P L, Bland R, Hopkins J A, Chang P 1982 Clinical trial of an algorithm for outcome prediction in acute circulatory failure. Crit Care Med 10: 390–397

Sise M J, Hollingsworth P, Brimm J E, Peters R M, Virgilio R, Shackford S R 1981 Complications of the flow-directed pulmonary artery catheter. Crit Care Med 9: 315–318

Sprung C L, Pozen R G, Rozanski J J, Punero J R, Eisler B R, Castellanes A 1980 Advanced ventricular arrhythmias during bedside pulmonary artery catheterization. Am J Med 72: 203–208

Sprung C L, Marcial E H, Garcia A A, Sequeira R F, Pozen R G 1983 Prophylactic use of lignocaine to prevent advanced ventricular arrhythmias during pulmonary artery catheterization. Am J Med 75: 906–910

Stenqvist O, Curelaru I, Linder L E, Gustavsson B 1983 Stiffness of central venous catheters. Acta Anaesthesiol Scand 27: 153–157

Stine K C, Friedman H S, Kurtzburg J et al 1989 Pulmonary septic emboli mimicking metastatic rhabdomyosarcoma. J Pediatr Surg 24: 491–493

Stokes M A, Almond D J, Pettit A H et al 1988 Home parenteral nutrition: a review of 100 patient years of treatment in 76 consecutive cases. Br J Surg 75: 481–483

Takasugi J K, O'Connell T X 1988 Prevention of complications in permanent central venous catheters. Surg Gynecol Obstet 167: 6–11

Taylor B L, Yellowlees I 1990 Central venous cannulation using the infraclavicular axillary vein. Anesthesiology 72: 55–58

Taylor T 1989 Pitfalls in invasive vascular procedures. Medical Protection Society (Protection Matters) 23: 12–16

Tebib J G, Bascoulergue J, Dumontet C et al 1987 Brachial plexus compression by iatrogenic arteriovenous fistula. Clin Rheumatol 6: 593–596

Theriault R L, Buzdar A I J 1990 Acute superior vena caval thrombosis after central venous catheter removal: successful treatment with thrombolytic therapy. Med Pediatr Oncol 18: 77–80

Thomson I R, Dalton B C, Lapsas D G, Lowenstein E 1979 Right bundle branch block and complete heart block caused by the Swan-Ganz catheter. Anesthesiology 51: 359–362

Trooskin S Z, Donetz A P, Harvey R A, Greco R S 1985 Prevention of catheter sepsis by antibiotic bonding. Surgery 97: 547–551

Tully J L, Friedland G H, Baldwini L M, Goldman D A 1981 Complications of intravenous therapy with steel needles and teflon catheters. Am J Med 70: 702–706

van Haeften T W, Pampus E C M, Boot H, Strack R J M, Thils L G 1988 Cardiac tamponade from misplaced central venous line in pericardiophrenic vein. Arch Intern Med 148: 1649–1650

Vanherweghem J L, Yassine T, Vandenbosch G, Delcour C, Struyven J, Kinnaert P 1986 Subclavian vein thrombosis: A frequent complication of subclavian vein cannulation for hemodialysis. Clin Nephrol 26: 235–238

Vazquez R M, Brodski E G 1985 Primary and secondary malposition of silicone central venous catheters. Acta Anaesthesiol Scand (Suppl.) 81: 22–25

Wang L P, Einarsson E A 1987 A complication of subclavian vein catheterisation. Extravascular knotting of a guide wire. Acta Anaesthesiol Scand 31: 187–188

Wolfe B M, Ryder M A, Nishikawa R A, Halstead C H, Schmidt B F 1986 Complications of parenteral nutrition. Am J Surg 152: 93–98

14. Update

L. Kaufman

LOCAL ANAESTHESIA

The molecular mechanisms of local anaesthesia are reviewed by Butterworth & Strichartz (1990), outlining the detailed mechanisms of nerve conduction, the structure of Na^+ channel, the binding sites for local anaesthetic agents and how these affect the Na^+ channel. Blockade of Na^+ channels is important for peripheral nerve block, but the action of local anaesthetic agents when used for epidural and spinal anaesthesia is more complex, involving synaptic transmission in the cord by affecting post-synaptic receptors as well as pre-synaptic calcium channels.

Laser–Doppler techniques have been used to trace the absorption of drugs through the skin, and the transient erythema sometimes observed with topical applications is due to an action of the drug on the skin and not a side effect (Woolfson et al 1989).

Cocaine

Cocaine is still used in anaesthesia to produce topical anaesthesia causing constriction of the nasal mucosa; however it is not without side effects. Lange et al (1989) noted that it not only causes constriction of the nasal mucosa but also of the coronary arteries, decreasing coronary blood flow. Cocaine prevents the re-uptake of noradrenaline and it is believed that this mode of action is an alpha-adrenergic effect (see also Isner & Chokshi 1989).

Addiction to drugs in the United States is a major problem, and it has been estimated that in 1986 more than three million people were heroin addicts and that about 15% of the US population had tried cocaine. Between the ages of 25–30 years the percentage rose to 40%, with many of the addicts increasing the dose to raise the level of euphoria (Gawin & Ellinwood 1988).

There is an increase in sudden death in cocaine addicts due to coronary artery obstruction resulting from hyperplasia of the intima, while contraction bands in the media result in cardiomyopathy. Tolerance to tachycardia and the hypertensive action of cocaine are not seen, despite the fact that cocaine prevents the uptake of noradrenaline at the sympathetic nerve terminal (Kumor et al 1988). The diagnosis of cocaine intoxication may be similar to that of phaeochromocytoma (Karch & Billingham 1988).

Other side effects of cocaine intoxication include acute rhabdomyolysis, resulting either from intense vasoconstriction or possibly due to a direct effect on muscle metabolism. Acute renal failure may occur with hypotension, hyperpyrexia and raised serum creatine kinase. This condition may progress to severe liver failure with disseminated intravascular coagulation (Roth et al 1988).

Attempts have been made to reduce the pleasant sensations of cocaine with dopaminergic blocking agents; however, pretreatment with haloperidol has only a limited effect even when given prior to cocaine (Sherer et al 1989).

Lignocaine

Topical lignocaine used during fibreoptic bronchoscopy does not affect the growth of bacteria from bronchoalveolar lavage. It had been feared that the high concentrations of lignocaine which are known to inhibit bacteria and fungi could affect the culture of organisms from the lavage, but the concentrations of lignocaine achieved are inadequate to inhibit bacteria growth (Strange et al 1988).

Topical anaesthesia with 200 mg of lignocaine sprayed on the wound prior to skin closure of hernia operation, resulted in significant lower pain scores and reduced the requirement for analgesia on the first post-operative day. Plasma levels of substance P were unaltered but beta-endorphin levels were significantly increased in the control group (Sinclair et al 1988).

Preparations of local anaesthetic creams are now available which readily penetrate the skin, and the formulation of lignocaine and prilocaine applied under occlusive dressing produces effective analgesia of the skin. This may represent a distinct advantage in that painful injections, venous cannulation, lumbar puncture and even split skin grafts can readily be performed without discomfort (Hanks & White 1988). They even diminish the peripheral flare associated with local histamine release (Harper et al 1989).

Intravenous lignocaine has been advocated by Rimback et al (1990) to reduce the period of post-operative ileus following abdominal surgery. Infusion of lignocaine 3 mg/min prior to induction of anaesthesia and continued for 24 h after surgery appeared to be effective following cholecystectomy. The mechanism of action being suggested is inhibition of sympathetic activity. Lignocaine reduces de-ethylation in the liver allowing steady state levels to be reached rapidly (Saville et al 1989).

There is a possibility that absorption of lignocaine may occur during transurethral prostatectomy if there is damage to the urethral mucosa.

Eardley et al (1989) found that 400 mg of lignocaine gel applied endo-urethrally before the transurethral prostatectomy did not result in toxic reactions. Cardiac arrhythmias occur if the blood level is 2–5 mg/ml and coma results when this reaches 10 mg/ml. Dawling et al (1989) described two cases of deliberate self-poisoning with lignocaine, one by oral ingestion and the other by intravenous injection. In animals, lignocaine resulted in respiratory depression, bradycardia and hypotension without arrythmias, while excess of bupivacaine caused ventricular tachycardia/fibrillation (Nancarrow et al 1989). This may explain the mortality from bupivacaine when administered for Bier's block.

A disturbing survey on the safe use of lignocaine has been reported by Scrimshire (1989), who found that many of the junior doctors of all grades and specialities were ignorant of the safe dose of lignocaine, with or without adrenaline. They were unaware that the strength of the solution used could influence toxicity and that 1% solutions were equivalent to 10 mg/ml. Not surprisingly anaesthetists were better informed!

Bupivacaine

Interpleural anaesthetics have been advocated to reduce post-operative pain following upper abdominal surgery. The interpleural bupivacaine is rapidly absorbed and peak plasma levels can be reduced by the addition of adrenaline (Gin et al 1990). Other detailed studies have been performed by Mogg et al (1990), noting the arterio-venous difference of 20% during the first hour after the administration of the drug. The mean elimination half-life was longer than previously reported.

Winning et al (1988) have studied the effect of inhalation of bupivacaine aerosol on ventilation and breathlessness and found that perception of breathlessness was not affected by anaesthetizing the airways. However, in a similar study in patients following laryngectomy, airway anaesthesia enhanced CO_2 sensitivity and breathlessness (Hamilton et al 1987).

The effects of local anaesthetics on umbilical blood vessels have been overlooked and Monuszko et al (1989) have demonstrated that bupivacaine caused contraction of the umbilical blood vessels. 2-Chloroprocaine relaxed the smooth muscle of blood vessels while the effect of lignocaine was unpredictable.

Procainamide

Procainamide, a longer acting agent than procaine, is widely used in the treatment of cardiac arrhythmias. It may also affect neuromuscular transmission and has in fact resulted in respiratory failure due to dia-phragmatic paralysis (Javaheri et al 1989).

Bier's block

Bier reported on the use of intravenous procaine almost 90 years ago and the safety of the technique relied on the use of procaine, an ester which is rapidly destroyed by cholinesterase. The use of amides such as lignocaine led to reports of sudden cardiac arrest, especially with bupivacaine. However, Hannington-Kiff (1990) drew attention to regional restrictions of the technique, which involve the use of distal and proximal tourniquets. Bier also advocated the use of a distal tourniquet so that any 'unfixed' procaine could be released before coming in contact with the general circulation. An additional trick was to wash out the intertourniquet area with saline, or to release the proximal tourniquet for a short period for the arterial circulation to dilute the procaine in the vein. Hannington-Kiff (1990) also suggested that the veins in the intercuff area should be aspirated and flushed out with saline, again to eliminate the local anaesthetic, in this case bupivacaine which he advocated as the local anaesthetic of choice.

REFERENCES

Butterworth J F IV, Strichartz G R 1990 Molecular mechanisms of local anaesthesia: a review. Anesthesiology 72: 711–734

Dawling S, Flanagan R J, Widdop B 1989 Fatal lignocaine poisoning: report of two cases and review of the literature. Hum Toxicol 8: 389–392

Eardley I, Ramsay J W A, Broome G D, Whitfield H, Murray A, Wilkinson D J 1989 Plasma lignocaine levels during transurethral prostatectomy. Ann R Coll Surg Engl 71: 278–280

Gawin F H, Ellinwood E H Jr 1988 Cocaine and other stimulants—Actions, abuse and treatment. N Engl J Med 318: 1173–1182

Gin T, Chan K, Kan A F, Gregory M A, Wong Y C, Oh T E 1990 Effect of adrenaline on venous plasma concentrations of bupivacaine after interpleural administration. Br J Anaesth 64: 662–666

Hamilton R D, Winning A J, Perry A, Guz A 1987 Aerosol anesthesia increases hypercapnic ventilation and breathlessness in laryngectomized humans. J Appl Physiol 63: 2286–2292

Hanks G W, White I 1988 Local anaesthetic creams—preparations effective on skin should increase use. Br Med J 297: 1215

Hannington-Kiff J G 1990 Bier's block revisited: intercuff block. J R Soc Med 83: 155–158

Harper E I, Beck J S, Spence V A 1989 Effect of topically applied local anaesthesia on histamine flare in man measured by laser Doppler velocimetry. Agents Actions 28: 192–197

Isner J M, Chokshi S K 1989 Cocaine and vasospasm. N Engl J Med 321: 1604–1606

Javaheri S, Logemann T N, Corser B C, Guerra L F, Means E 1989 Diaphragmatic paralysis. Am J Med 86: 623–624

Karch S B, Billingham M E 1988 The pathology and etiology of cocaine-induced heart disease. Arch Pathol Lab Med 112: 225–230

Kumor K, Sherer M, Thompson L, Cone E, Mahaffey J, Jaffe J H 1988 Lack of cardiovascular tolerance during intravenous cocaine infusions in human volunteers. Life Sci 42: 2063–2071

Lange R A, Cigarroa R G, Yancy C W Jr et al 1989 Cocaine-induced coronary-artery vasoconstriction. N Engl J Med 321: 1557–1562

Mogg G A, Triggs E J, Ismail Z, Higbie J, Frost M 1990 Pharmacokinetics of interpleural bupivacaine in patients undergoing cholecystectomy. Br J Anaesth 64: 657–661

Monuszko E, Halevy S, Freese K, Liu-Barnett M, Altura B 1989 Vasoactive actions of local anaesthetics on human isolated umbilical veins and arteries. Br J Pharmacol 97: 319–328

Nancarrow C, Rutten A J, Runciman W B et al 1989 Myocardial and cerebral drug concentrations and the mechanisms of death after fatal intravenous doses of lidocaine, bupivacaine, and ropivacaine in the sheep. Anesth Analg 69: 276–283

Rimback G, Cassuto J, Tollesson P-O 1990 Treatment of postoperative paralytic ileus by intravenous lidocaine infusion. Anesth Analg 70: 414–419

Roth D, Alarcon F J, Fernandez J A, Preston R A, Bourgoignie J J 1988 Acute rhabdomyolysis associated with cocaine intoxication. N Engl J Med 319: 673–677

Saville B A, Gray M R, Tam Y K 1989 Evidence for lidocaine-induced enzyme inactivation. J Pharm Sci 78: 1003–1008

Scrimshire J A 1989 Safe use of lignocaine. Br Med J 298: 1494

Sherer M A, Kumor K M, Jaffe J H 1989 Effects of intravenous cocaine are partially attenuated by haloperidol. Psychiatry Res 27: 117–125

Sinclair R, Cassuto J, Hogstrom S et al 1988 Topical anesthesia with lidocaine aerosol in the control of postoperative pain. Anesthesiology 68: 895–901

Strange C, Barbarash R A, Heffner J E 1988 Lidocaine concentrations in bronchoscopic specimens. Chest 93: 547–549

Winning A J, Hamilton R D, Guz A 1988 Ventilation and breathlessness of maximal exercise in patients with interstitial lung disease after local anaesthetic aerosol inhalation. Clin Sci 74: 275–281

Woolfson A D, McCafferty D F, McGowan K E, Boston V 1989 Non-invasive monitoring of percutaneous local anaesthesia using laser-Doppler velocimetry. Int J Pharm 51: 183–187

NALOXONE

Naloxone has proved to be a useful drug in the identification of opioid receptors and the mode of action of inhalational agents such as nitrous oxide. Experiments with naloxone ($-$) indicate that nitrous oxide analgesia is due to the release of endogenous opioids, although it has a direct effect on opioid receptors (Moody et al 1989). Naloxone has a much higher affinity for the same enzyme binding site as morphine and inhibits the glucuronidation of morphine. This has clinical importance for patients who suffer an overdose of morphine, for although their blood levels may be falling, clearance may be delayed by the use of naloxone which interferes with morphine metabolism (Wahlstrom et al 1989). Naloxone has also been used to demonstrate that prolonged administration of morphine results in reduction in spinal endogenous opioid activity due to tolerance (Bell 1989).

A recent study with naloxone failed to demonstrate that increased endogenous opioids suppressed the respiratory response to CO_2 in patients with chronic obstructive lung disease (Simon et al 1989). In response to submaximal exercise, naloxone increased plasma adrenaline but not blood pressure, heart rate, plasma noradrenaline, plasma renin activity or plasma aldosterone (Bramnert 1988, also see Bouloux et al 1989). High doses of naloxone are required to antagonize buprenorphine which appears to be firmly bound to opioid receptors (Gal 1989). It also suppresses the rise in plasma prolactin following the administration of buprenorphine (Mendelson et al 1989).

Naloxone has other complex actions on the endocrine system. In rats pretreated with morphine, naloxone leads to a massive release of oxytocin (Bicknell et al 1988). In ewes not pretreated with drugs, naloxone has no effect on arginine vasopressin (AVP) or oxytocin (OT), but leads to an increased and prolonged rise in plasma cortisol levels (Thornton & Parrott 1989).

Naloxone has a beneficial effect in the management of septic shock, reducing the amount of inotrope (dopamine)/vasopressor (phenylephrine) required to maintain blood pressure. Roberts et al (1988) recommended a bolus dose of naloxone (30 µg/kg) followed by an infusion of 30 µg kg^{-1}/h.

REFERENCES

Bell J A 1989 Naloxone-induced facilitation of C-fiber reflexes is reduced by chronic morphine. Eur J Pharmacol 168: 101–105
Bicknell R J, Leng G, Lincoln D W, Russell J A 1988 Naloxone excites oxytocin neurones in the supraoptic nucleus of lactating rats after chronic morphine treatment. J Physiol 396: 297–317
Bouloux P M G, Newbould E, Causon R et al 1989 Differential effect of high-dose naloxone on the plasma adrenaline response to the cold-pressor test. Clin Sci 76: 625–630
Bramnert M 1988 The effect of naloxone on blood pressure, heart rate, plasma catecholamines, renin activity and aldosterone following exercise in healthy males. Regul Pept 22: 295–301
Gal T J 1989 Naloxone reversal of buprenorphine-induced respiratory depression. Clin Pharmacol Ther 45: 66–71
Mendelson J H, Mello N K, Teoh S K, Lloyd-Jones J G, Clifford J M 1989 Naloxone suppresses buprenorphine stimulation of plasma prolactin. J Clin Psychopharmacol 9: 105–109
Moody E J, Mattson M, Newman A H, Rice K C, Sholnick P 1989 Stereospecific reversal of nitrous oxide analgesia by naloxone. Life Sci 44: 703–709
Roberts D E, Dobson K E, Hall K W, Light R B 1988 Effects of prolonged naloxone infusion in septic shock. Lancet 2: 699–702
Simon P M, Pope A, Lahive K et al 1989 Naloxone does not alter response to hypercapnia or resistive loading in chronic obstructive pulmonary disease. Am Rev Respir Dis 139: 134–138
Thornton S N, Parrott R F 1989 Naloxone affects the release of cortisol, but not of vasopressin or oxytocin, in dehydrated sheep. Acta Endocrinol 120: 50–54
Wahlstrom A, Persson K, Rane A 1989 Metabolic interaction between morphine and naloxone in human liver. A common pathway of glucuronidation? Drug Metab Dispos 17: 218–220

APPARATUS

Pulse oximeter

The merits and limitations of pulse oximeter have been outlined in *Anaesthesia Review 7* (Kaufman 1990, pp. 227–228). Although pulse oximetry is now considered to be an integral part of essential monitoring, there may be a marked reduction in arterial oxygen saturation before the alarm is activated. This is of particular importance during the disconnection of equipment in a paralyzed patient who has been ventilated (Verhoeff & Sykes 1990) or following oesophageal intubation. Detection of oesophageal intubation is more readily detected by a CO_2 analyzer than a pulse oximeter, and a small portable CO_2 detector is now available (Denman et al 1990). Readings of the pulse oximeter are only accurate at the point of measurement, and there may be delays in detecting hypoxaemia due to a delayed response time of the sensor. Breathing a hypoxic mixture may result in brain damage, even before the finger sensor of the pulse oximeter would generate an alarm signal (see Leading article, Lancet 1990). However, there have been anecdotal episodes where the pulse oximeter has detected intubation of a bronchus: hypoxaemia associated with pleural effusion which developed prior to operation in a patient with Crohn's disease and whose X-ray on admission was normal; primary polycythemia in a patient undergoing minor surgery and on whom a blood count had not been performed. Vasoconstriction due to inadequate perfusion from fluid loss may also lead to a low oxygen saturation reading, responding not to an increase in oxygen in inspired gases but to increasing perfusion with adequate fluid replacement.

In acute bronchiolitis in infants, the $Paco_2$ and pulse oximetry were considered to be the best methods of assessing the initial state of the infant; pulse oximeter was of value in predicting the need for high inspired oxygen (Mulholland et al 1990).

Riley (1989) has expressed concern about the cost of monitoring equipment, and the widespread introduction of pulse oximetry may affect the hospital budget and other high technology equipment. Medical insurance agencies in the United States appear to be on the verge of dictating the type of monitoring that is necessary to minimize the risk of malpractice. The acceptance of minimal monitoring standards (Harvard Standards) has led to a reduction in mishaps during the course of anaesthesia, many of which were due to under-ventilation and could have been anticipated by capnography and oximetry (Eichhorn 1989).

Endotracheal intubation

Tracheal stenosis is a known complication of prolonged intubation. However, Braidy et al (1989) reported laryngeal oedema with granulation tissue at the site of the endotracheal cuff over the posterior aspect of the larynx. The patient developed respiratory distress two months after intubation and on bronchoscopy, a polypoid mass was seen on the anterior aspect of the trachea. The patient responded to inhalation of steroids and beclomethasone. In addition, oral prednisone was commenced and there was improvement in the expiratory and inspiratory flow rates.

Central venous catheterization
(see chapter 13)

Various techniques have been devised for central venous catheterization. Hoffman et al (1989) have devised a catheter, filled with conducting solution, as the exploring electrode and the position of the catheter tip is verified by observing the changes in the P wave on ECG. Erosion of the vessel wall by the catheter may be difficult to detect and Ellis et al (1989) reported ten cases. The diagnosis was made only after approximately 16 h following the onset of symptoms of shortness of breath and chest pain, the catheter being in situ for approximately 60 h. The catheter may migrate to the right atrium or embed in the lateral wall of the vena cava. Despite free aspiration of blood, insertion of the catheter in the left internal jugular vein is said to be more hazardous in that the catheter on insertion may appear to advance down the lumen of the vessel, but in fact only distends the vessel itself.

Dead space

MacFie (1990) has indicated the possibility that drugs given intravenously or by epidural catheter may be ineffectual due to failure to reach the destination on account of dead space. This is particularly true of drugs administered in a volume of 1 ml, although diluting the drugs in larger volumes may lead to errors.

Blood pressure measurement

Turjanmaa (1989) reported on the limitations of non-invasive blood pressure measurement compared with intra-arterial recording, with the subjects in various positions during bicycle ergometer tests and during recovery from exercise. Auscultation techniques with aneroid barometers showed considerable variation from direct arterial readings.

Vaporizers

A limitation of high frequency jet ventilation is the danger of awareness during endoscopy as the technique cannot be used with the vaporizers in current use. Mazloomdoost et al (1989) designed a vaporizer in which the gas is passed over a thin layer of fluid at high velocity, resulting in small droplets which are immediately dispersed and evaporate. The vaporizer had been tried with enflurane in animals, and the inspired concentration could easily be controlled by altering the infusions of the liquid enflurane.

Noise

Hodge & Thompson (1990) have investigated the noise levels in the operating theatre, and found that equipment was often above 75–85 dB which would interfere with the performance and concentration of the surgeons (recommended level should not exceed 30 dB). Equipment such as suckers, alarms on anaesthetic machines and 'intercoms' are the worst offenders. Excessive noise may hamper communication in the operating theatre. Hodge & Thompson (1990) have designated a new term—'noise pollution'! Excessive noise should be avoided especially in patients undergoing surgery under local or regional techniques. It should also be avoided in the recovery and intensive care unit.

Needles and ampoules

It has become apparent that more care and attention needs to be undertaken by staff administering injections or drawing blood for fear of transmission of infections such as hepatitis B or human immunodeficiency virus (HIV). Recapping of needles is a frequent source of injury and is inconsistent with the recommendations from many hospitals (Thurn et al 1989).

Contamination of ampoules may occur when they are opened, especially from the transparent metal etched type. It is recommended that solutions should be aspirated from the ampoule with a filter needle (Sabon et al 1989).

REFERENCES

Braidy J, Breton G, Clement L 1989 Effect of corticosteroids on post-intubation tracheal stenosis. Thorax 44: 753–755
Denman W T, Hayes M, Higgins D, Wilkinson D J 1990 The Fenem CO_2 detector device. An apparatus to prevent unnoticed oesophageal intubation. Anaesthesia 45: 465–467
Eichhorn J H 1989 Prevention of intraoperative anesthesia accidents and related severe injury through safety monitoring. Anesthesiology 70: 572–577
Ellis L M, Vogel S B, Copeland E M III 1989 Central venous catheter vascular erosions — Diagnosis and clinical course. Ann Surg 209: 475–478
Hodge B, Thompson J F 1990 Noise pollution in the operating theatre. Lancet 335: 891–894
Hoffman M A, Langer J C, Pearl R H, Filler R M 1989 Electrocardiographic guided placement of central venous catheters. Br J Surg 76: 1032–1033
Kaufman L (ed) 1990 Update. In: Anaesthesia review 7. Churchill Livingstone, Edinburgh, pp 227–228
Leading article 1990 The trust in pulse oximeters. Lancet 335: 1130–1131
MacFie A G 1990 Equipment deadspace and drug administration. Anaesthesia 45: 145–147
Mazloomdoost M, Klain M, Nemoto E M, Lin M R, Lee-Foon W 1989 Vaporizer for volatile anesthetics during high-frequency jet ventilation. Anesthesiology 71: 150–153
Mulholland E K, Olinsky A, Shann F A 1990 Clinical findings and severity of acute bronchiolitis. Lancet 335: 1259–1261
Riley R 1989 The high price of "sleep": can Australia afford high-technology anaesthesia? Med J Aust 150: 454–457
Sabon R L Jr, Cheng E Y, Stommel K A, Hennen C R 1989 Glass particle contamination: influence of aspiration methods and ampule types. Anesthesiology 70: 859–862
Thurn J, Willenbring K, Crossley K 1989 Needlestick injuries and needle disposal in Minnesota physicians' offices. Am J Med 86: 575–579
Turjanmaa V 1989 Determination of blood pressure level and changes in physiological situations: comparison of the standard cuff method with direct intra-arterial recording. Clin Physiol 9: 373–387
Verhoeff F, Sykes M K 1990 Delayed detection of hypoxic events by pulse oximeters: computer stimulation. Anaesthesia 45: 103–109

GENERAL ANAESTHETIC AGENTS

The mode of action of anaesthesia

Although much information is known about the mechanisms of anaesthesia, no single theory can satisfactorily explain its mode of action. The main consensus from all the studies is the correlation between potency and lipid solubility. Anaesthesia appears to act on the lipid layers of the cell membrane producing reversible changes, but this view has been challenged by Franks & Lieb (1987) who have presented evidence that general anaesthesia may act directly on proteins. Increasing molecular weight appears to increase the anaesthetic potency (Targ et al 1989).

Although it interferes with action potentials, there is little effect on the resting membrane potential. Many anaesthetic agents, excluding halothane however, increase resting intracellular ionized calcium (Daniell & Harris 1988). Landers et al (1989) have discussed the place of calmodulin as a calcium receptor. Although calcium binding to calmodulin is essential for neurotransmitter release at nerve cells, skeletal and cardiac smooth muscle, there is little information on its possible action in the brain where the concentrations are high. High pressure reverses anaesthesia (Albrecht & Miletich 1988). An interesting observation by Newbold (1989) is that large doses of vitamin B12b (hydroxocobalamin) is an antidote to tranquillizers and alcohol.

Bailey (1989) has shown that a five-compartment model comprising lung, vessel-rich tissue, muscle, non-visceral fat and marrow-visceral fat agreed with findings of experiments on the elimination of anaesthetic agents which are not metabolized to any extent. Although theoretical and experimental values are agreed, there may be difficulty in accepting the concept of a marrow-visceral fat compartment.

Effects of general anaesthesia

The effects of general anaesthesia on various body systems are outlined in standard textbooks. Thus the following comments are based only on recent literature.

Blood flow

Measurement of blood flow in the skin can be estimated using heat thermal clearance, and Saumet et al (1988) have shown that anaesthesia affects mainly cutaneous blood flow with very little effect on subcutaneous tissues. Halothane depresses lymphatic contractility (McHale & Thornbury 1989) (see Ch. 7, Sweating and Thermoregulation in Anaesthesia).

General anaesthetic agents depress the responsiveness of cerebral arterioles to increased CO_2 (Levasseur & Kontos 1989).

Renin

Droperidol increases the level of tissue renin rapidly suggesting that it activates inactive tissue renin (Barrett et al 1988), a feature not seen with ether anaesthesia.

Lung function

Anaesthesia results in significant intrapulmonary shunting if the functional residual capacity is reduced below the awake closing capacity. It is directly proportional to the body mass index (weight/height^2), and shunting appears to be due to the reduction in dependent regional lung volume (Dueck et al 1988). Anaesthesia may alter the influence of the autonomic nervous system on pulmonary circulation (Nyhan et al 1989).

Malignant hyperthermia

Inhalational anaesthesia is known to act as a triggering agent for malignant hyperthermia; however, using the response to in vitro contracture tests may help to identify patients who may safely be given volatile anaesthetic drugs. The interpretation of results should be accepted with caution (Allen et al 1990). Isoflurane has joined the list of triggering agents as McGuire & Easy (1990) reported two cases of malignant hyperthermia following its use.

Anaesthesia and age

This has recently been reviewed by Ward & Hutton (1990) who drew attention to the fact that elderly patients often suffered from multiple pathology and are under treatment with a variety of drugs. Age affects all the body systems; changes in the nervous system involves a decrease in the rate of synthesis of neurotransmitters, and the likelihood of Parkinsonism. Decreased respiratory function may be affected in a fall in Pa_{O_2}, while in the cardiovascular system there are changes in myocardial function, occurrence of vascular atherosclerosis and impaired autonomic response. Renal function declines, with a decrease in resting renal blood flow, glomerular filtration rate and tubular reabsorption. Liver blood flow decreases affecting the clearance of drugs. The reduction of body water in muscle mass may lead to changes in the distribution of drugs in the various body compartments, leading to unpredictable effects.

In general, the doses of the anaesthetic agents should be reduced. Hyoscine should be avoided while etomidate appears to offer reasonable cardiovascular stability, but the dose of propofol should be reduced. Atracurium appears to be the relaxant of choice and as for inhalational agents, the MAC decreases with age. Anti-emetics may precipitate Parkinsonism. The duration and extent of regional blockade may be influenced by automical considerations. The half-life of lignocaine is prolonged but clearance is unaffected. Improved monitoring in the peri- and post-operative period have also improved the care of the elderly undergoing surgery.

Anaesthetic agents and the critically ill

Many of the intravenous agents are no longer suitable for sedation for patients in intensive care units, especially etomidate as a result of its effects on adrenocorticol function. Le Normand et al (1988) revived interest in the use of methohexitone which produced little cardiovascular disturbance; there was a decrease in oxygen consumption as the oxygen demand was reduced. However, infusion techniques with methohexitone led to a prolonged period of unconsciousness. Isoflurane (0.1–0.6% in an air–oxygen mixture) was found to be superior to midazolam (0.01–0.02 mg kg^{-1}/h), producing satisfactory sedation in patients who were being ventilated while recovery was also more rapid (Kong et al 1989). Isoflurane has been successfully used to provide sedation in patients undergoing mechanical ventilation, but there has been the possibility that these might lead to increased concentrations of plasma fluoride. Kong et al (1990) were unable to confirm that the increase in fluoride would lead to renal dysfunction.

Propofol was also found to be superior to midazolam, in that weaning from mechanical ventilation was much quicker than with midazolam as was recovery of consciousness (Aitkenhead et al 1989).

Intravenous agents

Propofol

The pharmacodynamic and pharmacokinetic properties of propofol have been reviewed in detail by Langley & Heel (1988). The advantages are rapid induction, rapid recovery and decreased incidence of nausea and vomiting. Although it has no analgesic properties, it is devoid of the anti-analgesia associated with thiopentone. Pain may be produced if it is injected especially into small veins, but this may be alleviated by pretreatment with intravenous lignocaine (Johnson et al 1990) or by administering propofol at a temperature of 4°C (McCrirrick & Hunter 1990).

The pharmacokinetics of propofol during continuous infusion have been studied by Cockshott et al (1990), showing that mean blood concentrations can be predicted based on a three-compartment open model. Morgan et al (1990) also studied the pharmacokinetics of propofol, indicating that there is a large volume of distribution and a long elimination half-life which is of little significance. The half-life of the distribution phase determines the later rise of plasma concentrations, and care should be taken in calculating the regimes for intravenous infusions.

Campbell et al (1988) have reassessed the elimination of propofol, criticizing the previous studies because of the limited post-operative sampling time (8–12 h). It had been suggested that propofol was entirely metabolized but as the clearance was greater than the accepted value of hepatic blood flow, an extrahepatic site for metabolism was postulated. Campbell et al (1988) have demonstrated that although metabolism is a major component in the fate of the drug, the fall in plasma levels during the first 2 h is due to redistribution to peripheral compartments as occurs with thiopentone. Clearance is decreased in the elderly while women had increased clearance rates and volumes of distribution. The elimination half-life during major abdominal surgery was prolonged (Shafer et al 1988).

Kanto & Gepts (1989) have reviewed the pharmacokinetics of propofol, showing that the blood concentration curve corresponds to a three-compartment model. The first phase shows that the drug has a half-life of 2–3 min, the second phase of 34–36 min demonstrates metabolic clearance, and the long third exponential half-life of 184–480 min represents the elimination of the drug from poorly perfused tissues. Seventy percent of the drug is eliminated in the first two phases due to hepatic and extrahepatic metabolism. Although propofol is highly bound to plasma proteins, it does not appear to affect distribution and metabolism.

Propofol prevents a rise in intraocular pressure following the administration of suxamethonium, and it also appears to be a suitable agent for neurosurgical procedures when a rise in intracranial pressure is to be avoided.

Bradycardia has also been reported in the elderly and the dose should be reduced as the cardiac output is depressed. Unlike etomidate, propofol has little effect on adrenocortical function and it does not suppress the increase in plasma cortisol following surgical stimulation (Bray & Loveland, unpublished data).

There have been suggestions that there is a possible interaction between fentanyl and propofol, but Dixon et al (1990) were unable to confirm this. Artificial ventilation may decrease cardiac output and hepatic blood flow, resulting in a reduced clearance of propofol.

Inhalational agents

Trichloroethylene

Although trichloroethylene is less commonly used at the present time, Cavanagh & Buxton (1989) have rekindled interest on the mechanism of side effects of the breakdown product, dichloroethylene, which appears to be responsible for damage, in particular to the fifth cranial nerve. A possible explanation is that this is due to reactivation of the latent virus responsible for herpes simplex and it is not a neurotoxic effect. The herpes virus may affect motor nerves even leading to diaphragmatic paralysis. Unilateral 12th nerve palsy has been noted following halothane anaesthesia (personal series), and the cause of this was only discovered three days later when a row of vesicles was detected on the paralyzed side of the tongue.

Halothane
(see chapter 9)

Although halothane may be hepatotoxic to animals, it is extremely difficult to reproduce the pattern of liver damage known as 'halothane hepatitis'. The reason for the development of severe hepatitis is still unknown.

Studies in progress indicate that the metabolism of halothane is complex, occurring in extrahepatic sites including the mucosa of nose, tongue, cheek, soft palate, pharynx, larynx, oesophagus and tracheobronchial tract. Halothane apparently diffuses over the wall of the large intestine and the caecum. Although cytochrome P-450 is necessary for metabolism, metabolites appear to be formed by intestinal micro-organisms (Ghantous et al 1988). Neuberger (1988) has attempted to elucidate some of the problems associated with halothane hepatitis. Following induction with halothane, there are elevated levels of glutathione-S-transferase. Halothane is metabolized by at least two enzyme systems and it is the reductive route which is associated with direct liver damage. Oxidative metabolism of halothane by cytochrome P-450 to TFA halide metabolites are covalently bound (Hubbard et al 1988). Halothane depresses granulocytes during prolonged anaesthesia and this may be of importance in patients who are on immunosuppressant drugs (Lieners et al 1989). The mechanism of halothane hepatitis appears to be idiosyncratic, and is not dose-dependent but specific antibodies appear to occur in all patients exposed to halothane (Kenna et al 1987). Halothane-induced neoantigens have been identified as trifluoroacetyl-carrier proteins, and the purified form may be of value in identifying patients who are liable to develop halothane hepatitis (Pohl et al 1989).

Halothane alters the shape of the action potential, both in normal patients and in muscle from patients with malignant hyperthermia. These changes are much greater in the diseased muscle, occur at lower concentrations and may be partially prevented by preincubation with dantrolene (Iaizzo et al 1989).

The cardiovascular effects of halothane, enflurane and isoflurane have been studied on the isolated heart, and Sahlman et al (1988) has demonstrated that halothane exerted the most profound depressant effect on myocardium by increasing coronary vascular tone. Isoflurane on the other hand resulted in improved coronary blood flow. Propagation of action potentials in cardiac tissue depends on the low resistant pathway of the gap junction, and the conductance of the junctions are depressed by halothane (and ethrane) without affecting the excitability of the cardiac cells (Burt & Spray 1989).

Warfarin is extensively bound to albumin, and halothane or its metabolite trifluoroacetic acid increases free warfarin levels in the plasma. This is noted an hour after the end of anaesthesia but there is a large increase 24 h later. The increased levels may be due to the displacement of warfarin or inhibition of metabolism (Calvo et al 1989).

New techniques have been introduced for the measurement of blood levels of anaesthetic agents including halothane, enflurane and isoflurane. This involves the use of gas chromatography and Yamada et al (1988) have described a technique in which blood can be analyzed without changing the columns between samples.

Isoflurane

Isoflurane is a coronary vessel dilator affecting the distal arterioles. There is evidence to indicate that isoflurane can cause redistribution of the myocardial blood flow, resulting in myocardial ischaemia in patients with coronary artery disease. Priebe (1989) has reviewed the deleterious effects of isoflurane on the coronary circulation, commenting that the incidence of peri-operative ischaemia does not depend on the anaesthetic agents. The ischaemia may be related to the underlying state of the coronary arteries and the pre-operative management. Priebe (1989) concluded that isoflurane is potentially dangerous but this stricture applies to all other anaesthetic agents.

Anaesthetic agents depress the response of arterial baroreceptors but recovery is more rapid following isoflurane than with enflurane, and this is considered to be a beneficial effect (Takeshima & Dohi 1989).

REFERENCES

Aitkenhead A R, Pepperman M L, Willatts S M et al 1989 Comparison of propofol and midazolam for sedation in critically ill patients. Lancet II: 704–708
Albrecht R F, Miletich D J 1988 Speculations on the molecular nature of anesthesia. Gen Pharmacol 19: 339–346
Allen G C, Rosenberg H, Fletcher J E 1990 Safety of general anaesthesia in patients previously tested negative for malignant hyperthermia susceptibility. Anesthesiology 72: 619–622
Bailey J M 1989 The pharmacokinetics of volatile anesthetic agent elimination: a theoretical study. J Pharmacokinet Biopharm 17: 109–123
Barrett J D, Eggena P, Krall J F 1988 Independent change of plasma and tissue renin in response to anesthetics. Clin Exp Hypertens A10: 757–765
Burt J M, Spray D C 1989 Volatile anesthetics block intercellular communication between neonatal rat myocardial cells. Circu Res 65: 829–837
Calvo R, Aguilera L, Suarez E, Rodriguez-Sasiain J M 1989 Displacement of warfarin from human serum proteins by halothane anaesthesia. Acta Anaesthesiol Scand 33: 575–577
Campbell G A, Morgan D J, Kumar K, Crankshaw D P 1988 Extended blood collection period required to define distribution and elimination kinetics of propofol. Br J Clin Pharmacol 26: 187–190
Cavanagh J B, Buxton P H 1989 Trichloroethylene cranial neuropathy: is it really a toxic neuropathy or does it activate latent herpes virus? J Neurol Neurosurg Psychiatry 52: 297–303
Cockshott D, Douglas E J, Prys-Roberts C, Turtle M, Coates D P 1990 The pharmacokinetics of propofol during and after intravenous infusion in man. Eur J Anaesthesiol 7: 265–275
Daniell L C, Harris R A 1988 Neuronal intracellular calcium concentrations are altered by anesthetics: relationship to membrane fluidization. J Pharmacol Exp Ther 245: 1–7
Dixon J, Roberts F L, Tackley R M, Lewis G T R, Connell H, Prys-Roberts C 1990 Study of the possible interaction between fentanyl and propofol using a computer-controlled infusion of propofol. Br J Anaesth 64: 142–147
Dueck R, Prutow R J, Davies N J H, Clausen J L, Davidson T M 1988 The lung volume at which shunting occurs with inhalation anesthesia. Anesthesiology 69: 854–861

Franks N P, Lieb W R 1987 What is the molecular nature of general anaesthetic target sites? TIPS 8: 169–171

Ghantous H, Lofberg B, Tjalve H, Danielsson B R G, Dencker L 1988 Extrahepatic sites of metabolism of halothane in the rat. Pharmacol Toxicol 62: 135–141

Hubbard A K, Roth T P, Gandolfi A J, Brown B R Jr, Webster N R, Nunn J F 1988 Halothane hepatitis patients generate an antibody response toward a covalently bound metabolite of halothane. Anesthesiology 68: 791–796

Iaizzo P A, Lehmann-Horn F, Taylor S R, Gallant E M 1989 Malignant hyperthermia: Effects of halothane on the surface membrane. Muscle Nerve 12: 178–183

Johnson R A, Harper N J N, Chadwick S, Vohra A 1990 Pain on injection of propofol— methods of alleviation. Anaesthesia 45: 439–442

Kanto J, Gepts E 1989 Pharmacokinetic implications for the clinical use of propofol. Clin Pharmacokinet 17: 308–326

Kenna J G, Neuberger J, Williams R 1987 Specific antibodies to halothane induced liver antigens in halothane associated hepatitis. Br J Anaesth 59: 1286–1290

Kong K L, Willatts S M, Prys-Roberts C 1989 Isoflurane compared with midazolam for sedation in the intensive care unit. Br Med J 298: 1277–1280

Kong K L, Tyler J E, Willatts S M, Prys-Roberts C 1990 Isoflurane sedation for patients undergoing mechanical ventilation: metabolism to inorganic fluoride and renal effects. Br J Anaesth 64: 159–162

Landers D F, Becker G L, Wong K C 1989 Calcium, calmodulin, and anesthesiology. Anesth Analg 69: 100–112

Langley M S, Heel R C 1988 Propofol—a review of its pharmacodynamic and pharmacokinetic properties and use as an intravenous anaesthetic. Drugs 35: 334–372

Le Normand Y, de Villepoix C, Pinaud M et al 1988 Pharmacokinetics and haemodynamic effects of prolonged methohexitone infusion. Br J Clin Pharmacol 26: 589–594

Levasseur J E, Kontos H A 1989 Effects of anesthesia on cerebral arteriolar responses to hypercapnia. Am J Physiol 257: H85–H88

Lieners C, Redl H, Schlag G, Hammerschmidt D E 1989 Inhibition by halothane, but not by isoflurane, of oxidative response to opsonized zymosan in whole blood. Inflammation 13: 621–630

McCrirrick A, Hunter S 1990 Pain on injection of propofol: the effect of injectate temperature. Anaesthesia 45: 443–444

McGuire N, Easy W R 1990 Malignant hyperthermia during isoflurane anaesthesia. Anaesthesia 45: 124–127

McHale N G, Thornbury K D 1989 The effect of anesthetics on lymphatic contractility. Microvasc Res 37: 70–76

Morgan D J, Campbell G A, Crankshaw D P 1990 Pharmacokinetics of propofol when given by intravenous infusion. Br J Clin Pharmacol 30: 144–148

Neuberger J 1988 Halothane hepatitis. ISI Atlas of Science. Pharmacology 2: 309–313

Newbold H L 1989 Vitamin B-12b as an antidote for over-sedation. Med Hypotheses 30: 1–3

Nyhan D P, Goll H M, Chen B B, Fehr D M, Clougherty P W, Murray P A 1989 Pentobarbital anesthesia alters pulmonary vascular response to neural antagonists. Am J Physiol 256: H1384–H1392

Pohl L R, Kenna J G, Satoh H, Christ D, Martin J L 1989 Neoantigens associated with halothane hepatitis. Drug Metab Rev 20: 203–217

Priebe H-J 1989 Isoflurane and coronary hemodynamics. Anesthesiology 71: 960–976

Sahlman L, Henriksson B A, Martner J, Ricksten S E 1988 Effects of halothane, enflurane, and isoflurane on coronary vascular tone, myocardial performance, and oxygen consumption during controlled changes in aortic and left atrial pressure. Anesthesiology 69: 1–10

Saumet J L, Leftheriotis G, Dubost J, Kalfon F, Banssillon V, Freidel M 1988 Cutaneous and subcutaneous blood flow during general anaesthesia. Eur J Appl Physiol 57: 601–605

Shafer A, Doze V A, Shafer S L, White P F 1988 Pharmacokinetics and pharmacodynamics of propofol infusions during general anesthesia. Anesthesiology 69: 348–356

Takeshima R, Dohi S 1989 Comparison of arterial baroreflex function in humans anaesthetized with enflurane or isoflurane. Anesth Analg 69: 284–290

Targ A G, Yasuda N, Eger E I II et al 1989 Halogenation and anesthetic potency. Anesth Analg 68: 599–602

Ward R M, Hutton P 1990 Factors modifying the use of anaesthetic drugs in the elderly. Br Med Bull 46: 156–168
Yamada T, Hirai Y, Sakano S et al 1988 Direct determination of the blood concentration of halogenated anesthetic agents by gas chromatography. Acta Med Okayama 42: 183–192

Nitrous oxide

The analgesic properties of nitrous oxide may be due to the release of endogenous opioids as it leads to a significant elevation of serum prolactin and a decrease in cortisol levels, which also occur following the administration of opioids (Gillman et al 1988). Thirty percent nitrous oxide–oxygen provides adequate relief of ischaemic chest pain associated with myocardial infarction. However, the relief of pain following myocardial infarction was accompanied by a fall in serum endorphin levels. No adverse effects were reported, although inhalation of nitrous oxide may lead to psychological impairment. Estrin et al (1988) noted that the amplitude of the P-330 waves were reduced and there was an increase in P-latency. There is also suppression of the motor evoked potentials which may be of value for intra-operative monitoring during neurosurgery (Zentner et al 1989).

Nitrous oxide is known to inhibit methionine synthase leading to neurological and haematopoietic disorders. Brennt & Smith (1989) have shown that other agents such as methylmercury may have similar actions. This suggests that in dental departments there may be chronic mercury vapour exposure which may be hazardous if there is also chronic exposure to nitrous oxide.

Attempts to administer nitrous oxide as a sole anaesthetic agent in a hyperbaric condition has proved to be unsatisfactory. Side effects included tachypnoea, tachycardia, increase in blood pressure, clonus and opisthotonus (Russell et al 1990).

REFERENCES

Brennt C E, Smith J R 1989 The inhibitory effects of nitrous oxide and methylmercury in vivo on methionine synthase (EC 2.1.1.13) activity in the brain, liver, ovary and spinal cord of the rat. Gen Pharmacol 20: 427–431
Estrin W J, Moore P, Letz R, Wasch H H 1988 The P-300 event-related potential in experimental nitrous oxide exposure. Clin Pharmacol Ther 43: 86–90
Gillman M A, Katzeff I, Vermaak W J H, Becker P J, Susani E 1988 Hormonal responses to analgesic nitrous oxide in man. Horm Metab Res 20: 751–754
Russell G B, Snider M T, Richard R B, Loomis J L 1990 Hyperbaric nitrous oxide as a sole anesthetic agent in humans. Anesth Analg 70: 289–295
Zentner J, Kiss I, Ebner A 1989 Influence of anesthetics—nitrous oxide in particular—on electromyographic response evoked by transcranial electrical stimulation of the cortex. Neurosurgery 24: 253–256

BENZODIAZEPINES

Benzodiazepines have in the past been considered safe because of the view that they cause minimal cardiorespiratory depression. These drugs should still be administered cautiously especially in patients with chronic obstructive respiratory disorders, and should not be administered by the operator anaesthetist. The recent CEPOD report (Confidential Enquiry into Perioperative Deaths 1987) revealed that their use in providing sedation while minor surgery was being performed under local analgesia, led to an unacceptable mortality rate. Different benzodiazepines, even though they have equivalent anxiolytic properties, vary in action on sedation, performance and amnesia (Greenblatt et al 1988). They probably act by increasing the affinity of GABA for GABA receptors, acting as receptor agonists (see Oreland 1987). EEG changes were maximal 1 min following diazepam infusion and 5–10 min following midazolam, but there were significant changes for 5 h following the former drug and only for 2 h following the latter drug (Greenblatt et al 1989). Peripheral benzodiazepine binding sites in platelets are increased following stress, despite normal levels of cortisol, growth hormone and prolactin (Karp et al 1989). There are also peripheral benzodiazepine receptors in tumours and central receptors in astrocytomas and glioblastomas (Ferrarese et al 1989).

The pharmacokinetics of the newer benzodiazepines have been reviewed by Garzone & Kroboth (1989) who outlined the detailed actions of alprazolam, triazolam, midazolam and loprazolam.

Clobazam and clonazepam

Clobazam and clonazepam have been widely used in the treatment of epilepsy with the former causing less sedation and psychomotor side-effects. Both drugs have little effect on the respiratory response to CO_2 (Wildin et al 1990).

Oxazepam

The kinetics of oxazepam are unaffected by propranolol or labetalol, but the simple reaction time test was increased when oxazepam was combined with beta-adrenoceptor blocking agents (Sonne et al 1990).

Lorazepam

Lorazepam is rapidly absorbed following oral administration, with a peak concentration at 0.5–2 h. The volume of distribution is large and it is 80% protein bound. The elimination half-life of lorazepam varied between 4–15 h, possibly due to the activity of metabolites (Garzone & Kroboth 1989).

It might have been expected that metabolism will be depressed in patients suffering from burns, but with lorazepam glucuronidation was unaffected and in fact there was an increased clearance (Martyn & Greenblatt 1988).

Diazepam

Sedative doses of diazepam (and midazolam) produce a maximal reduction in blood pressure and an increase in Pa_{CO_2}, and this correlates with the plasma concentrations of the drugs. However, with repeated doses of diazepam, acute tolerance developed (Sunzel et al 1988). Gilmartin et al (1988) confirmed the respiratory depressant effect of diazepam and this was due to an action on chemoreceptors and not as might be thought by impairing muscle function. They also found, in contrast, that chlormethiazole while also producing drowsiness, had little effect on the respiratory response to CO_2 or on maximum static pressures.

There is a possibility that diazepam may increase the plasma concentrations of local anaesthetic agents. Giaufre et al (1988) found that children who received caudal blockade with 1 ml/kg of a mixture of 50% lignocaine (1%) and 50% bupivacaine (0.25%) had a higher plasma level of bupivacaine but not lignocaine, compared with those who did not have diazepam for premedication. Although it is possible that diazepam may affect the distribution of bupivacaine or plasma binding, it is most likely that diazepam in fact inhibits the metabolism of local anaesthetics such as bupivacaine.

Nuotto & Saarialho-Kere (1988) studied the interactions of indomethacin and diazepam in healthy volunteers and found that diazepam (10–15 mg) caused drowsiness, mental slowness, clumsiness and impaired performance. These effects were not augmented in the presence of indomethacin but the combined use of the drugs led to increased dizziness.

A dose of 10 mg of oral diazepam had no effect on baseline levels of cortisol but significantly reduced the increase in cortisol due to exposure to painful electrical stimulus. There is no effect on growth hormone, beta-endorphin or ACTH and thus diazepam may have a significant effect on suppressing the endocrine response to surgery (Roy-Byrne et al 1988).

Intravenous sedation with diazepam (or midazolam) is used with increasing frequency for investigations and for endoscopy. It has been noted that, particularly during endoscopy for upper gastrointestinal investigations, there is a marked depression of respiration and a profound fall in oxygen saturation. Bell et al (1988a) have recommended the use of oximetry and supplementary oxygen during this technique which is often performed by the operator—'sedator'. Hypoxia has also been noted during endoscopic cholangio-pancreatography (Griffin et al 1990), peritoneoscopy (Brady et al 1989) and colonoscopy (Berg, unpublished data). These possible respiratory hazards have prompted Shelley et al

(1989) to issue a series of guidelines to improve safety during endoscopy involving more detailed pre-operative assessment, emergency equipment in endoscopy units, training of personnel, the use of oxygen and monitoring, and facilities for recovery, especially in day case patients.

Midazolam

The water-soluble agent midazolam which has a short half-life, reaches peak plasma concentrations at 20–60 min. It can be given rectally as absorption is also rapid by this route (Clausen et al 1988). The volume of distribution is large and it is 80% protein bound. The metabolism of midazolam is by hydroxylation followed by glucuronidation (Garzone & Kroboth 1989).

Midazolam may be used to provide sedation for endoscopy in intensive care situations or during plastic surgical procedures. Compared with ketamine, sedation was more profound and was associated with less pain on injection (White et al 1988).

During endoscopic procedures, respiratory depressant effects have been widely reported when oxygen saturation fell rapidly, especially in elderly patients (Loveland, personal studies). Milligan et al (1988) advocated the use of alfentanil as the means of reducing the dose of midazolam for sedation during upper gastrointestinal endoscopy. Alfentanil led to improved operating conditions and rapid recovery, although there was a higher incidence of recall during the procedure which apparently did not detract from the acceptability of the technique.

Continuous infusions of midazolam have been used to provide sedation in intensive care units when patients are being ventilated. Oldenhof et al (1988) however found that half of their patients were still drowsy 10 h after the infusion had been discontinued, despite the fact that the elimination half-life is said to be approximately 2 h. It has been suggested that this is due to the metabolite alpha-hydroxymidazolam glucuronide; this has a short half-life and it is not known if it has any influence on the level of consciousness. It has been suggested that the metabolism of the drug is slow, but Wills et al (1990) felt that prolonged drowsiness was due to an increase in volume of distribution, especially in patients with a low plasma albumin (25 g/l) (Vree et al 1989).

Ho et al (1990) compared the effect of intravenous midazolam or inhalation of isoflurane in dental patients, and found that there was a significant impairment of memory following midazolam.

Shelly et al (1989) have demonstrated that following liver transplantation, there is still a potential for midazolam to be metabolized suggesting that the metabolic activity of the newly transplanted liver is unimpaired. There may be some extrahepatic metabolism but caution in the use of benzodiazepines is urged by Park et al (1989), in patients who have had liver transplantation or are suffering from severe liver disease.

Alprazolam and triazolam

These drugs are rapidly absorbed, reaching peak concentrations 1 h after administration; in fact following sublingual administration the peak levels are higher and occur quicker than after oral administration. The volume of distribution is approximately 1 l and both are extensively protein bound. Alprazolam is extensively metabolized and has an elimination half-life of 9.5–12 h. Its duration of action is prolonged by liver damage but not renal disease. On the other hand, triazolam has an elimination half-life of 1.8–5.9 h and its metabolites do not accumulate. Liver dysfunction but not renal disease prolongs the action of triazolam (Garzone & Kroboth 1989).

Benzodiazepine antagonists

The search for other anxiolytics led to the discovery of a specific benzodiazepine receptor antagonist, flumazenil (Haefely & Hunkeler 1988). It acts by competitive antagonism at the specific receptor site and antagonizes all the central benzodiazepine effects. The minimum effective dose appears to be 0.2 mg intravenously followed by further low doses of 0.1 mg at 1 min intervals (Amrein et al 1988). Despite the fact that it has a high therapeutic index, the Lancet (Leading article, 1988) sought to discredit this new antagonist by warning of the possible dangers of re-sedation when the antagonism wore off, and the fact that it might encourage the use of larger doses of benzodiazepines because of knowledge that antagonists were available. This editorial provoked spirited comments of unfair bias (Bardhan & Hinchliffe 1988, Bell et al 1988b, McCloy & Pearson 1988, Daneshmend & Logan 1988). Mattila et al (1989) found that the reversal of diazepam in the course of spinal anaesthesia had little effect on post-operative orientation, comprehension and anterograde amnesia. Although flumazenil does not appear to cause major haemodynamic responses, increased levels of plasma catecholamines have been reported (Marty & Joyon 1988). White et al (1989) following the reversal of midazolam by flumazenil noted that acute anxiety did not develop, nor was there any increased levels of plasma adrenaline, noradrenaline, vasopressin or beta-endorphin.

Surprisingly, flumazenil improved patients with hepatic encephalopathy from acute or chronic liver failure, although patients with brain oedema did not respond. The mechanisms of this improvement is still obscure but it may displace 'endogenous benzodiazepine-like substance from the $GABA_A$-benzodiazepine receptor' (Grimm et al 1988). The involvement of GABA and benzodiazepine receptor complex in the causation of hepatic encephalopathy has been reviewed by Basile & Gammal (1988), who confirmed the usefulness of benzodiazepine receptor antagonists (see Jones et al 1990).

The use of flumazenil may reveal information about the mode of action of anaesthetic agents. It did not reduce the anaesthetic potency of halothane, and only partially antagonized the potentiating action of diazepam when given with halothane; complete antagonism was achieved when the dose of flumazenil was increased markedly. However, flumazenil does improve the emergence from halothane anaesthesia. There is a possibility therefore that flumazenil does affect the actions of halothane in the same range of concentrations that produce anaesthesia (Geller et al 1989).

REFERENCES

Amrein R, Hetzel W, Hartmann D T L F, Hoffmann-La Roche & Co Ltd 1988 Clinical pharmacology of flumazenil. Eur J Anaesthesiol (suppl 2): 65–80
Bardhan K D, Hinchliffe R F C 1988 Letters to the editor: Midazolam antagonism. Lancet 2: 388
Basile A S, Gammal S H 1988 Evidence for the involvement of the benzodiazepine receptor complex in hepatic encephalopathy—Implications for treatment with benzodiazepine receptor antagonists. Clin Neuropharmacol 11: 401–422
Bell G D, Morden A, Coady T, Lee J, Logan R F A 1988a A comparison of diazepam and midazolam as endoscopy premedication assessing changes in ventilation and oxygen saturation. Br J Clin Pharmacol 26: 595–600
Bell G D, Morden A, Carter A, Coady T 1988b Letters to the editor: Midazolam antagonism. Lancet 2: 388
Brady C E III, Harkleroad L E, Pierson W P 1989 Alterations in oxygen saturation and ventilation after intravenous sedation for peritoneoscopy. Arch Intern Med 149: 1029–1032
Clausen T G, Wolff J, Hansen P B et al 1988 Pharmacokinetics of midazolam and alpha-hydroxy-midazolam following rectal and intravenous administration. Br J Clin Pharmacol 25: 457–463
Confidential Enquiry into Perioperative Death 1987 Association of Surgeons of Great Britain and Ireland and Association of Anaesthetists of Great Britain and Ireland
Daneshmend T K, Logan R F A 1988 Letters to the editor: Midazolam antagonism. Lancet 2: 389
Ferrarese C, Appollonio I, Frigo M, Gaini S M, Piolti R, Frattola L 1989 Benzodiazepine receptors and diazepam-binding inhibitor in human cerebral tumors. Ann Neurol 26: 564–568
Garzone P D, Kroboth P D 1989 Pharmacokinetics of new benzodiazepines. Clin Pharmacokinet 16: 337–364
Geller E, Schiff B, Halpern P, Speiser Z, Cohen S 1989 A benzodiazepine receptor antagonist improves emergence of mice from halothane anaesthesia. Neuropharmacology 28: 271–274
Giaufre E, Bruguerolle B, Morisson-Lacombe G, Rousset-Rouviere B 1988 The influence of diazepam on the plasma concentrations of bupivacaine and lignocaine after caudal injection of a mixture of the local anaesthetics in children. Br J Clin Pharmacol 26: 116–118
Gilmartin J J, Corris P A, Stone T N, Veale D, Gibson G J 1988 Effects of diazepam and chlormethiazole on ventilatory control in normal subjects. Br J Clin Pharmacol 25: 766–770
Greenblatt D J, Harmatz J S, Dorsey C, Shader R I 1988 Comparative single-dose kinetics and dynamics of lorazepam alprazolam, prazepam and placebo. Clin Pharmacol Ther 44: 326–334
Greenblatt D J, Ehrenberg B L, Gunderman J et al 1989 Pharmacokinetic and electroencephalographic study of intravenous diazepam, midazolam and placebo. Clin Pharmacol Ther 45: 356–365
Griffin S M, Chung S C S, Leung J W C, Li A K C 1990 Effect of intranasal oxygen on hypoxia and tachycardia during endoscopic cholangiopancreatography. Br Med J 300: 83–84
Grimm G, Katzenschlager R, Schneeweiss B 1988 Improvement of hepatic encephalopathy treated with flumazenil. Lancet 2: 1392–1394
Haefely W, Hunkeler W 1988 The story of flumazenil. Eur J Anaesthesiol (suppl 2): 3–14

Ho E T F, Parbrook G D, Still D M, Parbrook E O 1990 Memory function after I.V. midazolam or inhalation of isoflurane for sedation during dental surgery. Br J Anaesth 64: 337–340

Jones E A, Basile A S, Mullen K, Gammal S H 1990 Flumazenil: potential implications for hepatic encephalopathy. Pharmacol Ther 45: 331–343

Karp L, Weizman A, Tyano S, Gavish M 1989 Examination stress, platelet peripheral benzodiazepine binding sites, and plasma hormone levels. Life Sci 44: 1077–1082

Leading article 1988 Midazolam—is antagonism justified? Lancet 2: 140–142

McCloy R F, Pearson R C 1988 Letters to the editor: Midazolam antagonism. Lancet 2: 389

Marty J, Joyon D 1988 Haemodynamic responses following reversal of benzodiazepine-induced anaesthesia or sedation with flumazenil. Eur J Anaesthesiol (suppl 2): 167–171

Martyn J, Greenblatt D J 1988 Lorazepam conjugation is unimpaired in burn trauma. Clin Pharmacol Ther 43: 250–255

Mattila M J, Levanen J J, Makela M-L, Helske M 1989 Limited antagonism by flumazenil of diazepam-induced sedation in patients operated on under spinal anesthesia. Curr Ther Res 46: 717–723

Milligan K, Howe J P, McLoughlin J, Holmes W, Dundee J W 1988 Midazolam sedation for outpatient fibreoptic endoscopy: evaluation of alfentanil supplementation. Ann R Coll Surg Engl 70: 304–306

Nuotto E, Saarialho-Kere U 1988 Actions and interactions of indomethacin and diazepam on performance in healthy volunteers. Pharmacol Toxicol 62: 293–297

Oldenhof H, de Jong M, Steenhock A, Janknegt R 1988 Clinical pharmacokinetics of midazolam in intensive care patients, a wide interpatient variability? Clin Pharmacol Ther 43: 263–269

Oreland L 1987 The benzodiazepines: a pharmacological overview. Acta Anaesthesiol Scand 32 (suppl 88): 13–16

Park G R, Manara A R, Dawling S 1989 Extra-hepatic metabolism of midazolam. Br J Clin Pharmacol 27: 634–637

Roy-Byrne P P, Risch S C, Uhde T W 1988 Neuroendocrine effects of diazepam in normal subjects following brief painful stress. J Clin Psychopharmacol 8: 331–335

Shelley M P, Wilson P, Norman J 1989 Editorial: Sedation for fibreoptic bronchoscopy. Thorax 44: 769–775

Shelly M P, Dixon J S, Park G R 1989 The pharmacokinetics of midazolam following orthotopic liver transplantation. Br J Clin Pharmacol 27: 629–633

Sonne J, Dossing M, Loft K, Olesen K L et al 1990 Single dose pharmacokinetics and pharmacodynamics of oral oxazepam during concomitant administration of propranolol and labetalol. Br J Clin Pharmacol 29: 33–37

Sunzel M, Paalzow L, Berggren L, Eriksson I 1988 Respiratory and cardiovascular effects in relation to plasma levels of midazolam and diazepam. Br J Clin Pharmacol 25: 561–569

Vree T B, Shimoda M, Driessen J J et al 1989 Decreased plasma albumin concentration results in increased volume of distribution and decreased elimination of midazolam in intensive care patients. Clin Pharmacol Ther 46: 537–544

White P F, Vasconez L O, Mathes S A, Way W L, Wender L A 1988 Comparison of midazolam and diazepam for sedation during plastic surgery. Plast Reconstr Surg 81: 703–710

White P F, Shafer A, Boyle W A III, Doze V A, Duncan S 1989 Benzodiazepine antagonism does not provoke a stress response. Anesthesiology 70: 636–639

Wildin J D, Pleuvry B J, Mawer G E, Onon T, Millington L 1990 Respiratory and sedative effects of clobazam and clonazepam in volunteers. Br J Clin Pharmacol 29: 169–177

Wills R J, Khoo K-C, Soni P P, Patel I H 1990 Increased volume of distribution prolongs midazolam half-life. Br J Clin Pharmacol 29: 269–272

OPHTHALMOLOGY

Surgery and anticoagulants

Potential problems arise when elderly patients who are on anticoagulants such as warfarin present for cataract extraction and possible lens replacement. Discontinuing the anticoagulants may result in cerebral thrombosis or embolism but on the other hand, there is a possibility that the surgical procedure may be ruined by excessive bleeding. Robinson & Nylander (1989) maintained that cataract surgery can be successfully undertaken without discontinuing the warfarin, provided that prothrombin levels are within the range recommended by the British Society of Haematology. In a series of ten patients, four operations were performed under local anaesthesia and no cases of retrobulbar haemorrhage were reported. However, three patients developed hyphaema but this did not appear to affect the outcome of surgery. In a similar study, Gainey et al (1989) found that the incidence of haemorrhagic complications was greater in patients on warfarin than those in the control group, but there was no significant difference between those patients who were still on warfarin and those whose therapy had been discontinued.

Obstetrics

It had been believed that patients who have surgery for retinal detachment might have a pre-disposition to further retinal detachment during spontaneous vaginal delivery. Although responses to the questionnaire suggested that a history of retinal detachment was an indication for instrumental delivery, Inglesby et al (1990) reported that there was no clinical evidence or theoretical reason to support this view, and that previous operation for retinal detachment was not a contraindication to spontaneous vaginal delivery.

Beta-adrenoceptor blocking agents and the eye

Timolol, a non-cardioselective beta-blocker, is applied topically to reduce intraocular pressure by inhibiting the formation of aqueous humour. Gaul et al (1989) noted that non-cardioselective drugs were more potent than those with beta-1 actions. Timolol is rapidly absorbed via the nasal mucosa and conjunctiva resulting in cardiovascular, respiratory and central side effects. Pretreatment with ephedrine reduces absorption while pilocarpine increases peak concentrations in the plasma (Urtti & Kyyronen 1989). Soderstrom et al (1989) have advocated the combined use of timolol and pilocarpine.

Intraocular pressure

It is surprising that there have been few studies on the measurement of plasma levels of drugs following ocular instillation. A recent study by Lahdes et al (1988) showed that instillation of 40 μl 1% atropine into the eye resulted in a peak plasma concentration of 860 ± 420 pg/ml within 8 min, which is as rapid as intramuscular injection. There was no effect on pulse or blood pressure although this had previously been reported as well as other side effects, including hyperpyrexia, mental confusion, skin flushing and decreased motility of the gut. The topical instillation of an angiotensin converting enzyme (ACE) inhibitor lowered the intraocular pressure without producing systemic side effects (Watkins et al 1988) while timolol and carteolol, a recently introduced topical beta-blocker, also reduced intraocular pressure without significantly altering the resting heart rate or blood pressure (Brazier & Smith 1988). However, topical ocular instillation of beta-blockers has been reported to cause bradycardia and bronchoconstriction in asthmatic patients (Le Jeunne et al 1989).

Intubation often leads to hypertensive response and Mostafa et al (1990) have demonstrated that lignocaine given by aerosol prior to anaesthesia, not only prevented the rise in intraocular pressure but also demonstrated that after intubation, the pressure was also less than the control group.

Endocrine response

It has been assumed that metabolic response to surgery is of importance following major abdominal surgery, but Barker et al (1990) have demonstrated that during cataract extraction, there was a rise in circulating cortisol and glucose in patients receiving general anaesthesia whereas this response was absent in patients who had the operation performed under local analgesia with retrobulbar and facial blocks.

REFERENCES

Barker J P, Robinson P N, Vafidis G C, Hart F R, Sapsed-Byrne S, Hall G M 1990 Local analgesia prevents the cortisol and glycaemic responses to cataract surgery. Br J Anaesth 64: 442–445
Brazier D J, Smith S E 1988 Ocular and cardiovascular response to topical carteolol 2% and timolol 0.5% in healthy volunteers. Br J Ophthalmol 72: 101–103
Gainey S P, Robertson D M, Fay W, Ilstrup D 1989 Ocular surgery on patients receiving long-term warfarin therapy. Am J Ophthalmol 108: 142–146
Gaul G R, Will N J, Brubaker R F 1989 Comparison of a noncardioselective β-adrenoceptor blocker and a cardioselective blocker in reducing aqueous flow in humans. Arch Ophthalmol 107: 1308–1311
Inglesby D V, Little B C, Chignell A H 1990 Surgery for detachment of the retina should not affect a normal delivery. Br Med J 300: 980
Lahdes K, Kaila T, Huupponen R, Salminen L, Iisalo E 1988 Systemic absorption of topically applied ocular atropine. Clin Pharmacol Ther 44: 310–314
Le Jeunne C L, Hugues F C, Fufier J L, Munera Y, Bringer L 1989 Bronchial and cardiovascular effects of ocular topical beta-antagonists in asthmatic subjects: comparison of timolol, carteolol, and metipranolol. J Clin Pharmacol 29: 97–101
Mostafa S M, Wiles J R, Dowd T, Bates R, Bricker S 1990 Effects of nebulized lignocaine on the intraocular pressure responses to tracheal intubation. Br J Anaesth 64: 515–517
Robinson G A, Nylander A 1989 Warfarin and cataract extraction. Br J Ophthalmol 73: 702–703
Soderstrom M B, Wallin O, Granstrom P-A, Thorburn W 1989 Timolol-pilocarpine combined vs timolol and pilocarpine given separately. Am J Ophthalmol 107: 465–470
Urtti A, Kyyronen K 1989 Ophthalmic epinephrine, phenylephrine, and pilocarpine affect the systemic absorption of ocularly applied timolol. J Ocular Pharmacol 5: 127–132

Watkins R W, Baum T, Tedesco R P, Pula K, Barnett A 1988 Systemic effects resulting from topical ocular administration of SCH 33861, a novel ACE inhibitor ocular hypotensive agent. J Ocular Pharmacol 4: 93–100

Index